Half a Century of
Medical Research

Volume Two

Contents of Volume Two

Illustrations in Volume Two

Introductory Note

Volume One of this work, published earlier (under the date 1973), had the subtitle *Origins and Policy of the Medical Research Council (UK)* and dealt with constitutional and administrative aspects. It contained an author's preface (including acknowledgements) and an introduction by Sir Harold Himsworth, both of which apply to the work as a whole; otherwise each volume is largely self-contained.

The present volume is concerned with the development of the Council's scientific programme, considered as a contribution to the international endeavour for the advancement of knowledge in the biomedical field. To help any readers coming to it direct, a brief explanation of the origins, status and functions of the Medical Research Council may be useful here.

The Medical Research Council is the official agency charged by HM Government in the United Kingdom with the promotion of research aimed at the advancement of knowledge in the biomedical field. It also advises the Government, or Government departments, in matters involving the most recent information or requiring special investigation. Its members are appointed in a manner that ensures its status as an independent scientific body.

The Council was established in 1920 under a provision of the Ministry of Health Act 1919 and was incorporated by Royal Charter. It was the direct successor of the Medical Research Committee, appointed in 1913 to implement a provision of the National Insurance Act 1911 whereby a penny per annum per head of the insured population was allocated, from parliamentary funds, to purposes of research. Until 1965 the Council was responsible to a ministerial Committee of the Privy Council; thereafter, by virtue of the Science and Technology Act 1965, the functions of that body were absorbed by the Secretary of State for Education and Science. In 1966 the Council was granted a new Charter.

From the earliest days of the predecessor Medical Research Committee, three main ways of promoting research have been employed. Firstly, the Council maintains a central institute—the National Institute for Medical Research, now at Mill Hill in the

northwestern suburbs of London—with a permanent staff for work
in the laboratory branches of medical science. This has recently been
paralleled by a Clinical Research Centre within a district general
hospital in the same area.

Secondly, in addition to the National Institute and Clinical
Research Centre the Council maintains a staff that is mostly grouped
in research units and similar establishments, which are as a rule
attached to universities, hospitals or research institutes not under the
Council's own control. A few of these units are overseas.

Thirdly, the Council makes grants in support of work by persons
not in its own employ, on either a short- or a long-term basis, for
investigations proposed by the recipients. Grants may be for personal
remuneration, for assistance or for expenses; there are also various
awards for training and for travel. Also, in special circumstances,
there are block grants as subsidies to institutions, and when appropriate the grant aid may be on a long-term basis.

Papers giving the results of research promoted in these ways are
contributed by the workers to scientific journals in the usual manner.
Only a small fraction of the output has been published by the Council
in its own series of special reports.

Lists of senior scientific staff are given in the appendices of this
volume. A list of senior members of the headquarters staff forms
an appendix to Volume One. The successive Secretaries of the
Council—all distinguished medical scientists—have been Sir Walter
Fletcher (1914–33), Sir Edward Mellanby (1933–49), Sir Harold
Himsworth (1949–68) and Sir John Gray (from 1968); and under the
first three of these the present writer was chief of the supporting
administrative staff (1919–57).

As stated in the preface in Volume One, the period covered by
this history is the first half-century, or slightly more, of the existence
of the Council as such—that is, from 1920, plus the seven years of the
predecessor Committee from 1913. The primary concern in the present volume is with the beginnings of major developments in the
Council's scientific programme. The account does not purport to be
comprehensive, and in the choice of examples much important work
—especially in the category of grant-aided projects—necessarily goes
unmentioned.

Postscript The acknowledgements made in the preface to Volume
One cover the whole work; but special thanks are due to Julia Smith
on this occasion for undertaking the bulk of the indexing.

L. T.

Medical Research Council Headquarters Office
20 Park Crescent
London W1N 4AL

Corrections to Volume One

page 6, para. 1, line 15
"Chapter 12" should read "Volume Two"

page 25, para. 2 (*Early proceedings of the Committee*) line 4
"Addision" should read "Addison"

plate 2a (facing p. 65)
"KCMB" should read "KCMG"

page 84, para. 1, line 4
"as it" should read "which"

page 95, line 1, and p. 113, line 2
before "Laboratories" insert "Research"

plate 3 (facing page 96)
The photograph purporting to be of Sir Edward Mellanby is actually, by a most regrettable error, one of his brother Professor John Mellanby, MD, FRS, also a distinguished physiologist (and a member of the Medical Research Council, 1936–39). A correct photograph is included in Volume Two.

page 105, para. 1: *The use of animals in experimental research*—lines 11 and 12 should read:
"animal experimentation). Both in the research work for which it is responsible and in the exercise of its official advisory functions the" (This was the subject of a loose correction slip issued with the book.)

page 116, para. 1, line 6
"Didgeon" should read "Ridgeon"

page 128, para. 1, lines 10 and 11
"chemical elucidation" should read "preparation"
and
"the structure" should read "a highly potent specimen"

page 174, para. 4, line 3
"Her Majesty's" should read "His Majesty's" (*at date*)

page 249, lines 32 and 34
    "Dobel" (twice) should read "Dobell"

page 284, line 1
    "Vicsount" should read "Viscount"

page 284, penultimate lines
    "Learmouth" (twice) should read "Learmonth"

page 285, line 10
    insert "(later Sir John Gaddum)"

page 286, 6th line from bottom
    delete "Mr"

page 295, line 27
    "Victora" should read "Victoria"

page 301, col. 1, line 25
    after "Melville" insert "A."

page 302, line 21
    "Zackary" should read "Zachary"

page 302, col. 1, 13th line from bottom, and page 305, col. 2, line 28
    (entry for Minoprio, G.)
    "Carroll" should read "Caroll"

page 302, col. 2, line 1
    after "Chick" insert "(Dame Harriette C.)"

page 303, col. 2, line 12
    after "Gaddum, J. H." insert "(Sir John G.)"

page 305, col. 1, line 23
    after "Hugh" insert "L."

Part I
The General Field

Part I

The General Field

Chapter 1
Origins of the Programme

Definition of medical research—The original research schemes—The schemes
in retrospect—Comparison with present programme—The historical role of
tuberculosis research—Statistical assessments in tuberculosis—The unorthodox
fringe in treatment of tuberculosis—The place of cancer research—Main fields
of development

Definition of medical research

The scope of the Council's activities has already been discussed under
administrative headings in Volume One; in the present and following chapters the programme is considered with respect to its scientific content. This has been largely a matter of natural development,
as neither the Council nor the predecessor Committee was given any
terms of reference defining the precise nature and scope of its
scientific activities; the constitutional instruments dealt exclusively
with administrative matters. The National Insurance Act 1911 made
provision simply "for the purposes of research"; and that this meant
medical research was an obvious inference from the general nature
of the measure.

At the outset a legal opinion was given that no restriction to
tuberculosis was implied by the inclusion of the provision for research
in a section of the Act dealing with the treatment (sanatorium
benefit) of that disease. The terms of the ruling did, however, suggest
that there might be a limitation to the diseases of insured persons;
but in practice this was interpreted so widely as to constitute no
limitation at all. In any event, no condition relating to national insurance considerations could reasonably have been regarded as
passing to the Council when its constitution was granted in a fresh
context in 1920.

The lawyers' apparent assumption that medical research must
necessarily be directed to diseases as such was, of course, scientifically
naïve; it ignored research aimed at the advancement of natural
knowledge that might eventually, and perhaps only indirectly, help
towards the solution of practical problems of medicine. If any
narrow interpretation of that sort were ever in mind, it was effectively
ruled out by the Medical Research Committee's own definition,
contained in the general scheme of research that was submitted
formally to the Minister in November 1913. This document has
already been more fully quoted in Volume One, but the important
definition must here be given again:

> The object of the research is the extension of medical knowledge with the view
> of increasing our powers of preserving health and preventing or combating

3

disease. But otherwise than that this is to be the guiding aim, the actual field of research is not limited and is to be wide enough to include, so far as may from time to time be found desirable, all researches bearing on health and disease, whether or not such researches have any direct or immediate bearing on any particular disease or class of disease provided that they are judged to be useful in promoting the attainment of the above object.

By the Minister's approval of the whole submission, the Committee's assumption of its own scientific terms of reference could be regarded as endorsed by HM Government. The scientific policy of the Council, whether expressed in these or equivalent words, remains the same to this day.

The subject matter covered by the definition has, however, progressively expanded. In its Report for 1929–30 the Council was already able to say:

> On the one hand, the sphere of medicine has grown by extension; it has increased in comprehensiveness so as to take into its charge more and more widely all the problems of human life that call for better knowledge of the human body and its functions, seen and unseen. On the other hand medicine has been growing intensively, by taking more and more fully into her service the methods and resources of the primary sciences.

Since then, the process has steadily continued.

The original research schemes

The first research schemes submitted to the Minister by the Medical Research Committee were in general terms; and these were followed in July 1914 by a submission reporting progress towards the establishment of the centralised part of the Committee's general programme of research. In October 1914, however, a very detailed statement of research schemes was submitted, and in due course approved. The document opened with a general statement, including a list of scientific staff appointed to the departments of the 'central institute', some comments on the allocation of funds, and a preliminary expression of policy on the manner and conditions of award of research grants. It then proceeded to set out in detail, under subject heads, the 'research schemes' themselves—in effect, although the participation of the central institute is indicated, a programme of external research grants in aid of particular investigations. The subject classification was followed by a restatement of much the same information under geographical heads; the grants were listed in alphabetical order of places within the main divisions —England, Scotland, Ireland, Wales and (a solitary item) Switzerland. This in turn was followed by a financial summary and, finally, by a short account of emergency work undertaken in connection with the war (see Part III).

The list of grants (excluding items of work to be undertaken by the central institute) may be summarised, under main subject heads, as follows:

Subject	No. of grants	Total
Tuberculosis	44	£8 875
Rickets	19	3 425
Hygienic relations of milk	8	2 100
Rheumatic infections	3	600
Diseases of the nervous system	6	1 250
Thyroid secretion	3	200
Chronic (rheumatoid) arthritis	1	250
Dust inhalation and pulmonary disease	4	700
Oral sepsis	1	250
Epidemic infantile diarrhoea	1	150
Status lymphaticus	3	300
Diabetes	2	350
General pathological researches	9	900
	104	£19 350

It is obvious that the several schemes varied widely in their magnitude and importance; the heavy weighting on the first three subjects is significant. A fuller statement of those schemes that were actually brought into being, in spite of the outbreak of war, is given in the Report for 1914–15; this shows two extra headings—anaphylaxis and diseases of the heart.

The original schemes in retrospect

It is of curious interest to note the outcome of these various initial projects, without at this stage considering the many new ones subsequently added. Some of the original subjects are still under active research, but their problems have naturally become very different. Other projects were brought to a successful conclusion, or the problems were solved by research work elsewhere—and one problem, for adventitious reasons, simply ceased to exist. Others again dropped out, proving either to be intractable within the resources of knowledge and methods then available or to have been misconceived according to later ideas.

Tuberculosis Research in this subject still continues to hold a not unimportant place, but the problems have changed. The work done under the auspices of the Council has made a substantial contribution to world knowledge of tuberculosis, and has helped to diminish the relative importance of the disease. Fuller reference to the historical role of tuberculosis research in the Council's programme is made later in the present chapter.

Rickets The problem was completely solved during the next few years and within the Council's programme. It would not have been possible in advance to place this then highly controversial question squarely within the field of nutritional research; but the solution did so. Nutrition, in fact, soon became the major subject in the general programme, and some account of the development of research in it, including that on rickets, is given in a later chapter.

HCMR—B

The hygienic relations of milk A projected monograph, mentioned in the document, was duly published under the aegis of the Committee. Certain special inquiries also mentioned, with others added later, were concluded in due course. Knowledge of the subject is now abundant, and compulsory pasteurisation has solved the practical problem.

Rheumatic infections Research in rheumatic conditions of infectious or other origin has continued to figure in the Council's programme, and the attention therein given to the subject has much increased.

Diseases of the nervous system The particular investigations, three of them relating to the microchemistry of the cerebrospinal fluid, have long since been concluded. The general subject of neurology, however, naturally remains an important area of research.

Thyroid secretion The particular projects came to little, but the whole subject was revolutionised by work, outside the Council's programme, determining the chemical nature of thyroxine (Kendall, 1915; and especially Harington, 1926–27).

Chronic (rheumatoid) arthritis The subject proved to be unassailable by clinical attack, and in 1927 the Research Hospital at Cambridge became the Strangeways Research Laboratory, largely supported by the Council (Volume One). The reorientation of the scientific approach has been described by Dame Honor Fell, Director of the Laboratory from 1927 to 1970, as follows:

> Strangeways abandoned his clinical research on rheumatoid arthritis and turned his attention to cell biology, because he felt that the clinical investigations were blocked by ignorance of the basic facts of cellular physiology. The pure research that he initiated has been expanded in many directions that he could not have foreseen, but it is interesting that at the present time so much of our work still refers to skeletal tissue. Studies now in progress have provided information about the physiology of the cells of cartilage and bone that will almost certainly prove to be relevant to the problems for the investigation of which the Cambridge Research Hospital was originally founded.

Dust inhalation and pulmonary disease This subject has received increasing attention, and in later years a research unit (in relation to coal-mining in South Wales) has been among the resources directed to it by the Council.

Oral sepsis A much wider programme of work on dental disease was later promoted by the Council, although with more emphasis on nutritional factors than on infection.

Epidemic infantile diarrhoea This killing seasonal disease of small children had a peak in Britain in the hot summer of 1911, which was doubtless a reason for its inclusion among the schemes although ordinarily it was difficult to find material for even a brief investigation. Another peak in 1921 caused the Council to prepare for an intensive study in the following year; but then almost no cases occurred. Since that time the disease has practically ceased to exist, probably as a result of the wide replacement of raw cow's milk by heat-treated milk in the feeding of infants.

Status lymphaticus The object of this inquiry had been to determine the reality of a supposed condition of over-development of the thymus gland, often cited at coroners' inquests as a cause of unexplained sudden death. The collective work of a group of pathologists was coordinated by a special committee appointed by the Council jointly with the Pathological Society of Great Britain and Ireland. The Committee reported in 1931 that the data provided "no evidence that so-called 'status thymicolymphaticus' has any existence as a pathological entity" (Report for 1930–31).

Diabetes The single investigation mentioned was not pursued. The whole question of diabetes was radically altered in 1921 by the discovery and first preparation of insulin in Toronto. The introduction of this successful treatment into Britain, and various developments of its methods, became a major responsibility of the Council for several years following.

General pathological researches This is a miscellaneous heading that would have its equivalent today, or at any intervening time, although the particular items of work mentioned in the original schemes were long ago concluded in one way or another.

In general retrospect, the Council said in its Report for 1932–33:

> In the twenty years since the establishment of the original Medical Research Committee, the problems of medical research, although remaining fundamentally the same, have altered in some notable respects. Many diseases have greatly diminished in deadliness. In some cases no cause can be assigned for the change; in others the difference is clearly due to improved social conditions; in a further number the credit may be given to definite measures of preventive medicine, representing the practical application of earlier scientific knowledge. There remains an important group in which the change is the direct result of new knowledge acquired by recent research: to this advance it may be confidently claimed that workers in this country—very many of them aided by the Council—have largely contributed.

Comparison with present programme
It is not practicable to produce a statement of the present research programme in a form closely comparable with the original 'research schemes'. In such summaries as have recently been prepared, any particular item may appear under two or more heads to provide an index to the current programme. Moreover, it would not be possible to cost separate items of work undertaken in the Council's own establishments, which nowadays constitute a large proportion of the total, although there are also very many separate research grants to independent workers.

Some impression of the field covered by the programme more recently may nevertheless be conveyed by the following list of the headings used in the "Index to Main Subjects of Research

Programme" in the Report for 1963–65 (the most recent report in which these broad headings were in the subject index):

Anaesthesia
Anatomy
Bacteriology
Biochemistry
Biological engineering
Biological standardisa-
    tion
Biomechanics
Biophysics
Burns
Cancer
Cardiovascular diseases
Chemotherapy
Climatological medicine
Computer science
Dental research
Dermatology
Endocrinology and hor-
    mone diseases

Gastroenterology
Genetics
Haematology
Immunology
Metabolic disorders
Molecular biology
Mycology
Neurology
Nutrition
Obstetrics and gynae-
    cology
Occupational health and
    industrial medicine
Ophthalmology and
    physiology of vision
Oto-rhino-laryngology
Paediatrics
Parasitology
Pathology

Pharmacology
Physiology
Psychiatry and psycho-
    logy
Public health
Radiobiology
Radiotherapy
Respiratory disorders
Rheumatic conditions
Service medicine
Social medicine
Statistics
Surgery
Toxicology
Tropical medicine
Tuberculosis
Urology
Virology

Historical role of tuberculosis research

A special place must be given to research on tuberculosis, in recognition of the predominant part that it played in the early constitutional history of the Council (Volume One). There was indeed, at the outset, a natural assumption that in the allocation of resources tuberculosis research was entitled to priority, or at least to an important place; the latter it has certainly always had.

At the present date, some may find it surprising that tuberculosis should have played such a leading role in the motivation of state support for medical research. It is easy to forget that, in the opening decades of this century, so-called consumption was still regarded as "captain of all those men of death" (Bunyan). While tuberculosis is of course still an important disease, it no longer stands in the very forefront of medical problems. This recession is doubtless attributable to a combination of measures—on the preventive side better housing, improved nutrition, hygiene of milk, and vaccine prophylaxis; on the curative side earlier diagnosis, sanatorium treatment, antibiotics, chemotherapy, and new surgical procedures. The Council's programme over half a century reflects this progress, in nearly all its aspects, as shown in subsequent chapters.

Statistical assessments in tuberculosis

In planning the original scientific organisation, stress had been laid on the need for a statistical department; and such a department was in fact provided. It was not surprising that one of its first tasks should have been a study of the epidemiology of 'phthisis' (pulmonary tuberculosis) in Great Britain and Ireland; Dr John Brownlee's two reports on this subject, based on the mortality returns of the respective Registrars-General, were published for the Committee in 1918 and 1920. Even earlier, the very first publication of the Committee, in 1915, was a report by a special investigation committee that it had appointed to study the incidence of phthisis in relation to occupation; this report dealt with the boot and shoe industry. It was followed in 1919 by a report on the prevalence and aetiology of tuberculosis in industry, particularly among female munition workers.

The statistical approach was likewise used in assessments of the results of treatment, and in the first instance—appropriately enough —of sanatorium treatment. In the period 1919–24, reports appeared relating to patients at two well known sanatoria in Surrey and among insured persons in Bradford; these were said to "form a trilogy which gives a fairly complete picture of the results that may be expected from sanatorium treatment in this country". A report in 1922 sought to evaluate the results of the then relatively new treatment known as artificial pneumothorax, in which one lung is collapsed to give it rest, and this was followed in 1936 by a statistical analysis of the considerable experience of the method that had by that date been gained by the medical service of the London County Council. In 1924 a clinical report analysed the experience of treating a long series of cases of tuberculosis of the larynx. And, in respect of diagnosis, a report in 1932 assessed the value of tuberculin testing in man. In more recent years, statistical methods have been used in assessing the effects of such new therapeutic agents as streptomycin and isoniazid; and there have also been extensive statistical assessments of the value of BCG vaccine in prophylaxis (Chapter 11).

The unorthodox fringe in treatment of tuberculosis
During the period between the wars, tuberculosis was a favourite field for the exploitation of unorthodox medication, to which it unfortunately lent itself at that time. It was a serious disease, but too unpredictable in its manifestations for the progress of cases to be easily assessed; and there was an admitted lack of recognised therapeutic substances of real efficacy. In some instances, the pressures exerted on behalf of alleged remedies were sufficient to constitute a substantial nuisance.

At one end of the range there were immunological treatments advocated and used by a few qualified medical men, but unsupported by evidence that their more critical colleagues could accept. The proponents had access to the professional forum, and to this they were invariably referred by the Council. At the other end there were the secret preparations put forward, for tuberculosis or as veritable panaceas, by persons of obscure qualifications and commonly domiciled in the less developed countries of Europe and Asia. These had one feature in common, that nothing would be divulged until a large sum of money had been paid; and such overtures could be rejected out of hand.

More troublesome were some forms of treatment in a midway category, promoted by unqualified people and supported by 'evidence' of testimonial quality. The promoters tended to stimulate pressure groups of patients and busybodies, anxious to champion the supposed pioneer against the alleged tyranny of the professional 'closed shop'. There was, for example, a vaccine introduced into Britain by a citizen of a medically advanced foreign country, in which he was evidently a prophet without honour. And there was a powder said to be prepared from the root of a South African plant known to the indigenous tribes, a statement to which a resonant Zulu name bore witness.

Latterly, the growing success of scientific medicine in dealing with tuberculosis has restricted the scope for unorthodox methods and for sheer quackery. Their commercial exploitation has also been inhibited by the ban, placed by statute since 1941, on the advertisement of preparations claimed to cure this and certain other diseases.

The place of cancer research

Like the dog in the Sherlock Holmes story which did nothing in the night, the remarkable thing about cancer is that it does not figure at all in the original research schemes. Not only so, but the omission does not seem to have been publicly questioned, or publicly explained until this was done in the Report for 1921–22. The reason for it was in fact quite simple, although apparently for several years recorded only in oral tradition.

When the Medical Research Committee came into being, cancer was the one field of medical research for which there was already, by the standards of those days, ample financial provision. This was the result of voluntary contributions from the public, in a cause that has always made a strong appeal to the charitable. The Imperial Cancer Research Fund, established in 1902, was the principal body engaged in raising funds, and these it applied chiefly to the maintenance of a scientific staff and laboratories in London. There were also departments for cancer research attached to various hospitals, notably the one at the Royal Cancer (later Royal Marsden) Hospital, in London, that became the Institute of Cancer Research. The subject was also richly endowed in the United States of America and in countries in continental Europe. It was indeed remarked that if money could solve the cancer problem it would have been solved long before.

The Committee was thus content, for the time being, to leave cancer research to its existing promoters. To have done otherwise, without any ideas for new lines of work, would merely have led to duplication of effort; and meanwhile many other important branches of medical research were starving for funds and could immediately benefit from the Committee's help. Close relations have always been maintained with the Imperial Cancer Research Fund and other institutions specially concerned with the subject; and a part of the Council's land at Mill Hill was leased to the Fund in 1923 as a site for new laboratories.

When the Council succeeded the Committee in 1920 it had its first opportunity of entering the field of cancer research with a line of work that was not already being supported in the United Kingdom. This resulted from the acquisition of a quantity of radium that had been collected during the war by the Ministry of Munitions. The use of this material in the treatment of malignant conditions was the beginning of what eventually developed into a wide programme of work in radiotherapy and radiobiology (Chapters 4, 6).

The Council's next important incursion into the cancer field did not originate from any deliberate policy decision, but from the spontaneous interest of members of the scientific staff. This was when, in 1925, W. E. Gye and J. E. Barnard of the National Institute for Medical Research took up the question of the possible role of a filter-passing virus in the aetiology of some malignant conditions (Chapter 7). In succeeding years various items of cancer research received grant-aid, but it was not until much later that the Council gave support to any major project other than that concerned with the effects of irradiation.

In 1923 another fund-raising body was set up as the British Empire Cancer Campaign (now Cancer Research Campaign). Its programme differed from that of the Imperial Cancer Research Fund in not including (until very much later) any research centre controlled by the Campaign itself but in consisting entirely of the allocation of grants. (The complementary nature of the functions of the two bodies was expressed in a joint letter in *The Times* of 10 April 1967, replying to a criticism of the multiplicity of appeals.) The initiative came from a group of eminent medical practitioners and others, with support from the British Red Cross Society. The opening moves were somewhat inept; the Council was not consulted at any early stage, nor were such clearly interested parties as the Imperial Cancer Research Fund and the Middlesex Hospital (with its important cancer research department) fully informed. A strong desire for independence was clearly evinced, existing organisations being apparently suspected of wishing to impose some form of control. The Council, for its part, had no acquisitive ambitions and no reason to do other than welcome another body likely to bring fresh resources to medical research—always provided that the scientific approach was soundly based.

The promoters of the Campaign, as it happened, were shortly forced into a more cooperative attitude by their desire for royal patronage. The latter was of course not obtainable except on the advice of ministers, particularly the Minister of Health, and before this was given the Council was naturally consulted through official channels. The upshot of protracted and often acrimonious negotiations was that the Campaign agreed to be guided by a Scientific Advisory Committee of which half the members would be nominated jointly by the Royal Society and the Council. Despite its initial reluctance to accept this formula, the Campaign soon appreciated that the externally nominated members of the Committee were well qualified to be helpful and that they were truly serving as individual counsellors and not as representatives, being neither briefed nor expected to report back. Cooperation between the Council and the Campaign was quickly established; and among other things it was arranged that the Council's Radiology Committee should advise both organisations in its special field. Amicable relations have subsisted from that time; the Council and the Campaign have regularly consulted, and they have on many occasions supported the same projects by making complementary grants. In 1969 a joint committee was set up for the award of grants.

From 1951 the Council assumed the major responsibility for maintaining the Institute of Cancer Research: Royal Cancer Hospital, as described in Volume One; the British Empire Cancer Campaign has been the next largest supporter. So, for the first time, the Council's programme included support of an establishment devoted to cancer research in all its aspects.

In 1965 the Council became responsible for the United Kingdom's financial contribution to a new international project, the International Agency for Research on Cancer, with its headquarters at Lyons.

Main fields of development

In the succeeding chapters the development of the programme is considered under strategic heads corresponding with broad divisions of medical research. The general field is divisible under the heads of curative medicine, preventive medicine and basic science.

Certain special fields are, so to speak, extracted in Part II from the main fields of research since they represent a different approach, relating to the particular circumstances in which the problems—be they clinical, preventive or basic—tend to arise. Industrial and social medicine, here grouped together, deal with mankind in relation to the structure of modern society, including the conditions of occupation. Tropical medicine, obviously, is concerned with conditions in hot climates and usually in a much less controlled environment. The production, evaluation and biological standardisation of medicinal substances and the Public Health Laboratory Service are also discussed. War medicine and services research are also dealt with separately, in Part III.

This classification of fields of work is not necessarily valid except for the purposes of the present history. Some such logical framework was clearly requisite for a coherent account in the following chapters, but it is no more than a rationalisation. It is certainly far from representing any 'master plan' that was consciously in mind at the actual inception of the programme; indeed, although the scheme seems to fit the research that has in fact developed, this chapter shows that the original approach was much more empirical.

Chapter 2
Curative Medicine: Clinical Science

The circumstances of clinical research—The availability of clinical research
workers—The idea of a research hospital—The Council's Department of Clinical
Research—The role of teaching units and departments—A reassessment—
Deployment of further research units—Training awards in clinical science—
Research in general practice—The influence of Thomas Lewis—Research in
the National Health Service—The Clinical Research Board—Research in
surgery—Research into mental disorders—Responsibility in investigations on
human subjects—Clinical Research Centre

The circumstances of clinical research

Clinical research, the direct study of disease in the human subject,
is a discipline of primary importance in any comprehensive programme of research in medicine; it has always been recognised as
such by the Council, as by its predecessor Committee. Its promotion,
however, faces obstacles of a special kind. There is the practical
difficulty that it is necessary to have control of hospital beds, with all
attendant facilities for the scientific investigation of cases. There is
the ethical consideration that the interests of the individual patient
must always come first whenever these happen to conflict with the
claims of a general research objective; and whoever is in medical
charge must be at the same time a skilful physician or surgeon and
a research worker with a broad scientific outlook.

There was at first a shortage of research-minded and scientifically
trained clinicians; the whole emphasis of clinical training had been
placed on the peculiar manifestations and needs of the individual
case, and this had tended to militate against an outlook directed
towards the study of any disease as a generalised entity. Moreover,
clinicians on the then honorary staffs of hospitals had to earn their
living in private consulting practice; those who held paid teaching
appointments usually did so on a part-time basis. The general
practitioner, in addition to other handicaps, was no less subject to
the exacting demands of his primary avocation.

The history of the Council's promotion of clinical research is thus
one of constant endeavour to overcome the special difficulties mentioned above. This was at first an uphill fight, but in its Report for
1952–53 the Council felt able to record a substantial improvement
in the general circumstances of the subject:

During the present century progress in medical research has been more rapid
than at any other time in history. Beyond question this is due to the increasing
application of the scientific method to the study of biological phenomena. Yet
in the various branches of medical research the rate of progress has differed
widely. Generally speaking, the advance has been early and rapid in those
branches centred in the laboratory; slower and more delayed in those directly

13

concerned with sick persons. In the last two or three decades, however, scientific progress in the clinical field has been gathering momentum; it is now generally extending beyond the stage of observation and description of syndromes, so fruitfully practised by the great clinicians of the nineteenth century, into a stage characterised by planned investigations of illness. The direct investigation of disease is today becoming increasingly feasible, and it may be expected to yield as rich a harvest in the future as investigations of the normal have yielded in the past. No longer need the clinical investigator be entirely dependent for his data on the chance occurrence of natural events or on discoveries suitable for clinical application being made in other fields of medical research.

The availability of clinical research workers

The crux was not so much the provision of the physical facilities for clinical research as the availability of suitably qualified research workers. In its Report for 1919–20 the Council stated its belief that clinical science could advance only if those in charge of patients came trained in the methods of controlled observation and with knowledge of the ancillary laboratory arts—and came young enough, and free from outside preoccupations other than those of relevant higher teaching. Again, in its Report for 1928–29, the Council contrasted the task of the practising physician with that of the clinical research worker; the latter, although primarily solicitous of his patients' welfare, must concentrate his thoughts upon getting new knowledge bearing on the general subject which was his chosen study.

The problem therefore resolved itself into: (*a*) the creation of career opportunities; (*b*) special training of candidates for the posts; (*c*) finding or establishing a suitable environment for their life's work; and (*d*) the provision therein of all the necessary facilities for doing research.

The idea of a research hospital

When the Medical Research Committee first entered the field, the tempting solution was the provision of a special research hospital with a whole-time staff, following the example of the Rockefeller Institute in New York. And already it possessed—for the future National Institute for Medical Research—a hospital building of which part could be used again for wards. Also, at the point when there appeared to be the alternative possibility of taking over the Lister Institute of Preventive Medicine as the Committee's central establishment, Lord Iveagh had offered to provide a hospital of 50 beds on an adjacent site (Volume One).

There were, however, various objections to adopting any such plan. One was the high cost, involving provision for clinical research out of proportion to that for the other research which the Committee had in view. Another was the risk that a hospital specially designated for research might acquire an undeserved reputation for being too little concerned with the welfare of the patients. The hospital, moreover, would necessarily have been a relatively small one, lacking the overall resources and multiplicity of stimulating contacts found in, particularly, a teaching hospital. So the Report for 1918–19 records that the idea of establishing a research hospital had been definitely abandoned; the same object, it was believed, could be achieved—and with advantages—by attaching a Department of Clinical Research to University College Hospital, London. Not only has the Council never thought it advisable to have its own hospital, but when its staff have had medical care of patients they have normally exercised that care as honorary members of the staff of the hospital in which they work.

There have been a very few exceptions to the rule just stated, for the most part limited to providing some share of the cost; an example was the payment to St Mary's Hospital for the maintenance of 25 beds under the care of Sir Almroth Wright (Volume One). The only instance in which the Council has itself maintained a hospital is at its Laboratories in The Gambia, where the circumstances are exceptional (Chapter 10).

The Council's Department of Clinical Research

The development of the Council's system of research units has already been discussed in Volume One (see also Appendix C); the clinical units among them are here considered from a different angle. The decision against having a special research hospital had its corollary in the attachment of the Council's first clinical research department to an existing institution—University College Hospital, London, where Sir Thomas Lewis was already a member of the honorary staff. There was at first no thought of setting up similar departments elsewhere; as with the National Institute for Medical Research for the laboratory sciences, the conception was that of a single central establishment which would be supplemented peripherally by grants to clinical research workers holding part-time teaching appointments in medical schools. There was, however, originally an intention to strengthen the central establishment by creating a second senior research post alongside that held by Lewis; Dr T. R. Elliott was in fact appointed in this capacity in 1919, but almost at once resigned to become Director of the new professorial Medical Unit at the same hospital.

The title 'Department of Clinical Research' (at one stage extended by the words 'and Experimental Medicine') expresses a relationship with both the Council and the Hospital's Medical School. It originated in relation to the Council, the department being until 1930 known in the Hospital as the Cardiographic Department. A change in the status of Sir Thomas Lewis took place in 1932 when the Rockefeller Foundation endowed the post and the Council was for a time left to do little more than add superannuation provision; later on, with rising salary levels, the Council contributed the major share.

The influence of the Department on the advancement of clinical science in the United Kingdom, and indeed internationally, has been immense. It has been exerted partly by the output of original work, partly by force of example, and partly by the men whom it has produced. Among the latter are: Dr A. N. (later Sir Alan) Drury, who turned to experimental pathology at Cambridge and was later Director of the Lister Institute; Dr R. T. Grant, who became Director of a cognate Council unit at Guy's Hospital; Dr G. W. (later Sir George) Pickering, who was appointed Professor of Medicine at St Mary's Hospital, London, and later Regius Professor at Oxford; Dr E. J. (later Sir Edward) Wayne, who became successively Professor of Pharmacology at Sheffield and Professor of the Practice of Medicine at Glasgow; Dr E. E. (later Sir Edward) Pochin, who succeeded as Director of the Department itself; and Dr J. R. Squire, who directed another of the Council's units, became Professor of Experimental Pathology at Birmingham, and at the date of his untimely death was Director-designate of the Council's new Clinical Research Centre. Of Lewis himself more is said later.

The role of teaching units and departments
Having provided its own central establishment for clinical research, the Medical Research Committee turned its attention to aiding the subject elsewhere. There were at that time no full-time professors of clinical subjects, and so no organised academic departments; the universities and medical schools were not sufficiently active either in encouraging clinical research or in training men for it. Thought was accordingly directed towards the improvement of clinical teaching, as stated in the Report for 1919–20:

> It was with this in view that the Medical Research Committee gave whatever cooperation was in their power to the prospective formation in medical and surgical hospital wards of what, for want of a better, or even a good, name, are being called 'units'. Early in 1917 they had addressed to the Minister for Education at his request a statement in which they expressed the opinion that the general cause of medical research was being gravely retarded by the traditional mode of study in hospital wards, for want of a system in which research work could proceed under the conditions necessary for scientific progress and linked closely at the same time with higher teaching based upon it and exchanging fertilisation with it. It was pointed out that the absence of such a system at the chief centres of medical treatment and medical education impeded advance not only by sterilising the immediate opportunities for research but not less by yielding no proper supply of trained men fitted to make use of opportunities elsewhere.

The Council itself adopted the policy of supplementing the part-time salaries of selected temporary assistants to the whole-time professorial directors of teaching units in certain London hospitals; promising men were thus enabled to devote themselves for a time wholly to teaching and research. Thus at University College Hospital, where Professor T. R. Elliott headed the Medical Unit, a grant for work on liver conditions was made to Dr J. W. (later Sir John) McNee, who afterwards became Professor of Medicine in the University of Glasgow. Both at St Bartholomew's Hospital and at the London Hospital, grants were made to assistants—Dr F. R. (later Sir Francis) Fraser, and Dr A. W. M. (later Sir Arthur) Ellis —who before long succeeded their respective chiefs. Also in the Medical Unit at the London Hospital, Dr George Riddoch received a personal grant for research in neurology. The Council was also able to help indirectly by influencing the allocation of private benefactions to the provision of laboratories for the clinical teaching units at two of the hospitals.

The situation outside London was slower in developing. The university departments in clinical subjects had part-time teaching staffs who were largely engaged in practice. A movement towards the establishment of whole-time chairs was nevertheless gaining ground; and in its Report for 1931–32 the Council was glad to note that the University of Aberdeen had been able to improve the conditions attaching to its Regius Chairs of Medicine and Surgery so as to be in a position to invite applications from a wide field of candidates who had shown ability to advance their subject by personal research. Both appointments were given to men who had received grants from the Council; Dr L. S. P. (later Sir Stanley) Davidson was appointed Professor of Medicine in 1930, and Mr J. R. (later Sir James) Learmonth came back from the Mayo Clinic in America to become Professor of Surgery in 1932; both of them later went on to corresponding chairs at Edinburgh. Much of this was due to the influence of Professor J. J. R. Macleod, a Nobel laureate who had himself recently returned from Toronto to the Chair of Physiology at Aberdeen; he had become a member of the Council and was in close accord with its officers.

In its Report for 1932–33 the Council recorded that there was a general increase in the number of whole-time or nearly whole-time professorial and other clinical posts. And its Report for 1933–34 mentioned a series of instances in which, sometimes by aid of benefactions, the opportunities for careers in clinical science had been augmented. Most important of all had been the opening of the British Postgraduate Medical School (now Royal Postgraduate Medical School) at Hammersmith Hospital; this provided a galaxy of departments in clinical and paraclinical subjects, with a distinguished whole-time staff and good facilities for research work. Although the Council was not initially associated in the enterprise, it later came to have many close and fruitful relations with the School.

Again, in its Report for 1935–36 the Council warmly welcomed Lord Nuffield's large gift to the University of Oxford for research and postgraduate teaching in medical science; the then Secretary of the Council was appointed a trustee of the endowment. At Cambridge a department of clinical research had been formed under the direction of the Regius Professor of Physic.

In London, the innovations were filling a vacuum rather than directly replacing any pre-existing department. In the provinces, except at Oxford and Cambridge, and in Scotland the change involved a frontal attack on the entrenched positions of part-time staff, and this could be pressed home only on the occurrence of professorial vacancies. There was, however, an earlier outflanking movement to give charge of hospital beds to whole-time professors of pharmacology, traditionally a laboratory subject, or of pharmacology and therapeutics. For example, Professor (later Sir) Edward Mellanby was in this position at Sheffield from 1920; the chair was indeed created for him and was intended to be in effect one of experimental medicine. Nor was this the earliest instance.

A reassessment

While the reform of clinical teaching was spreading throughout the country, the Council had undertaken a reassessment of the benefits. In 1929, stimulated by new proposals from Sir Thomas Lewis, it appointed a subcommittee to consider future policy. The question was whether the Council should increase its help to the teaching units and departments, or could with greater advantage work towards the establishment of one or two stable positions primarily for research, comparable with that held by Lewis himself. The five professorial heads of medical teaching units in London were consulted; and the conclusion was inescapable that the Council's support of research in these units had helped to produce valuable work but had done little towards recruitment to clinical research in the long term. The men who had done part-time research in these units had later tended to take up private practice or else academic careers in such subjects as physiology or pathology. This could be attributed, at least in part, to the dearth of posts with prospects for careers in whole-time clinical research or teaching.

Accordingly, in its Report for 1928–29 the Council stated its belief that "there can never be a successful and maintained recruitment of young men of ability for clinical research until there are at least a few stable positions in sight, the occupation of which at middle-age will provide reasonable remuneration and adequate power of educating a family". The Council hoped "that some advance towards the solution of this national problem may be made by a clear statement of their intention to do what is in their power to encourage still further the scientific and direct study of disease in man". To this end the Council was seeking to recruit young men of ability prepared to test themselves in this line of work.

Deployment of further research units

The Council was thus committed to building up a staff of whole-time clinical research workers, and this implied the establishment of further research units at different hospitals; the scarcity of suitable leaders made it inevitable that progress would be slow. The first of the new establishments was the Neurological Research Unit set up in 1933 at the National Hospital for Nervous Diseases, Queen Square, London, under the direction of Dr E. A. Carmichael; here the Council acted at the invitation of the Hospital. This was a specialised unit, and Lewis pressed the view that there was still urgent need for one with more general terms of reference. This led to the establishment of the Clinical Research Unit at Guy's Hospital under Dr R. T. Grant. The Surgical Research Unit established at Edinburgh in 1938 was, for fortuitous reasons, short-lived.

The deployment of clinical (and other) research units gathered momentum after the Second World War. It is noteworthy that no new units had such wide titular scope as those at University College Hospital and Guy's Hospital; even these two had programmes that were at first strongly slanted towards a particular specialty, namely cardiovascular conditions. Similarly, the Department of Experimental Medicine, which the Council set up at Cambridge in 1945 under Professor R. A. McCance, was concerned mainly with problems of nutrition and metabolism. All the others had some limitation of subject explicit in their titles, and this had clearly become the trend of policy. Some units were only in part clinical.

Having regard to the information given elsewhere, it will suffice here to classify the subjects with which the wholly or partly clinical units, other than those just mentioned, were concerned:

(a) Broad fields such as industrial medicine, tropical medicine, obstetric medicine.
(b) Particular conditions such as malnutrition, burns, pneumoconiosis, tuberculosis, atheroma, rheumatism, demyelinating diseases.
(c) Specified organs, systems or functions of the body such as eyes, ears, teeth, skin, digestive tract, cardiovascular system, nervous system, temperature regulation.
(d) Certain forms of treatment such as radiotherapy, clinical chemotherapy, applications of clinical endocrinology, blood transfusion, electrical treatment.
(e) Various aspects of mental defect and mental disorder (see later).

Training awards in clinical science
In 1936 the Council turned its attention to assistance in training men for work in the field thus being opened up (Volume One); in brief, the Council in 1936 established six Postgraduate Studentships for training in methods of research in clinical medicine and experimental pathology, and four Research Fellowships in the same fields for more senior men already with some experience in research. These awards came to an end during the Second World War; but in 1950 the Council instituted Clinical Research Fellowships that were in effect temporary research appointments.

Research in general practice
Towards the end of 1914, Dr (later Sir) James Mackenzie presented to the Medical Research Committee a *Memorandum on a Method for*

Research in Clinical Medicine. This, he said, was based on his own experience, as for nearly thirty years he had been investigating disease on the lines that he was now suggesting. While a general practitioner, he had found that disease presented itself to him in a manner totally different from that in hospital practice; and he had had to train himself in methods of investigation very different from those taught in medical schools. He considered that there were two fields of practical medicine in which knowledge at that time was markedly deficient—the early stages of disease and the course pursued in protracted disease; only the general practitioner had the opportunities for improving the bases of diagnosis and prognosis in these respects.

A subcommittee of two, Sir Clifford Allbutt and Mr C. J. Bond, discussed Mackenzie's proposals with him. It reported in general agreement with Mackenzie's views and suggested the names of three general practitioners who might be invited to undertake part-time work on the lines proposed. At the same time it recorded its opinion "that the following negative propositions would secure general agreement: (i) that no random assignment of enquiries to general practitioners or to panel doctors is likely to have any good results; and (ii) that no advance in knowledge is likely to come from the amassing of clinical facts by untrained observers or by observers out of touch with modern knowledge and modern methods".

It was impracticable to proceed with the scheme during the war, but the Report for 1919–20 recorded that part-time grants were being made to two of the practitioners originally suggested by the subcommittee—Dr H. J. Starling of Norwich and Dr E. E. Laslett of Hull. Other grants were also mentioned, and "Research Work in Professional Practice" continued to be a separate subheading in annual reports up to that for 1925–26.

Again, in 1920 Mackenzie sent to the Council a *Memorandum on some Medical Aspects of the National Health Insurance Act.* This was "drawn up with a view to indicate the principal defects in medical knowledge which exist at the present time and which impair the success of the Act, and also to indicate some steps which can be taken to remedy them". (In the seventeenth James Mackenzie Lecture, delivered before the Royal College of General Practitioners on 14 November 1970, Dr E. V. Kuenssberg quoted from this document, with comments.) In 1922 Mackenzie presented to the Council a memorandum on medical records in general practice (quoted in full by Mair, 1962).

Mackenzie moved to Scotland on his retirement from consulting practice in London; at St Andrews his material support and inspiring leadership created for a time an active centre of research in a small community. The Council helped with grants for particular parts of the programme but avoided commitment to any form of general subsidy. After Mackenzie's death in 1925, an attempt was made locally to keep the centre in being, under the title of 'St

Andrews (James Mackenzie) Institute for Clinical Research'—but the mainspring had gone. Soon the Institute became merely a place where four practitioners saw their panel patients and kept their routine records; apart from that, occasional meetings were addressed by visiting lecturers. The Council was invited to take over the Institute, but after careful inquiry by a visiting subcommittee decided that the project was no longer viable.

There were of course pioneers before Mackenzie in making notable additions to knowledge in the course of their practice, but these did not start any wide movement in their own generations. There was little that the Council could do to foster such a movement; the urge had to grow from within, as in time it did.

In more recent years the Council sponsored a fruitful project in collaboration with the Public Health Laboratory Service (originally under its own direction). In 1947 an Epidemiological Research Unit was established at Cirencester, Gloucestershire, in charge of Dr R. E. Hope-Simpson, who was in general practice there and part-time pathologist at the local hospital. He became responsible for a series of epidemiological researches on various infectious diseases, throwing light on serial intervals between epidemics and on incubation periods; among other things, he demonstrated that herpes zoster and varicella (chickenpox) were due to an identical virus.

In 1951 the Council had set up a Working Party on Research in General Practice under the chairmanship of Sir James Spence; and in 1957 this became a full committee, with Professor Sir Robert (later Lord) Platt as chairman and Dr Hope-Simpson as secretary. Meanwhile, the (now Royal) College of General Practitioners had come into being in 1952, and it was soon sponsoring a number of investigations, of which results have since been published. In the Report for 1957–58, in which this field was reviewed, the Council noted that much further work was in progress under various auspices.

The influence of Thomas Lewis

Thomas Lewis (1881–1945) was for nearly thirty years engaged in whole-time clinical research for the Council (and its predecessor Committee), directing its earliest establishment in that field. Throughout, he strenuously advocated the claims of clinical science to be regarded as an important independent discipline, for which full research opportunities should be provided. He was characterised by what Himsworth called an "earnest impatience"; he set a brilliant example by a prodigious output of original work of the highest quality; he was an inspiring albeit demanding leader; he wrote lucidly and spoke convincingly. A man of medium physique and quiet voice, he was single-minded in the extreme—forthright, often brusque, almost resenting any distraction from the work in hand or from the furtherance of his chosen cause. Yet at times he could fully relax, reveal wide interests, and indulge in sports and hobbies; among other things he was a skilful bird-photographer. A full obituary has been provided by two of his earliest assistants in the Council's service (Drury and Grant); and in its Report for 1940–45 the Council paid its own tribute.

Between the two world wars Lewis was active in promulgating his views on the steps necessary for the better promotion of research work in clinical medicine. Among other things, he wrote a letter in 1929 which was circulated to members of Council. In this he maintained that the relative lack of progress was "the direct or indirect outcome of the almost constant association between clinical research work and the opportunist atmosphere of practical or curative medicine". He expressed unease about the stability of the Council's then sole department in the subject, which depended too much on himself. He foretold that the Council would find it necessary "sooner or later to develop a department or departments of clinical and experimental work on a broader and sounder basis than at present exists". He had in mind not merely a proliferation of research units, which in fact became the next step, but eventually "an institute, the atmosphere within which shall not be influenced by the immediate needs of consulting Medicine or Surgery, but shall be derived from the purer sources from which the atmosphere in other institutes (in which the natural sciences are studied) is derived". Within such an institute the workers would be "free from the distractions presented by the petty and mainly diagnostic problems of diverse and obscure cases"; they would thus be enabled to "settle down to a more profound and uninterrupted study of the natural history of selected diseases". He envisaged such an institute as necessarily connected with a general hospital commanding a large selection of clinical material, but not one in which large numbers of students were trained as practitioners.

Lewis went on to say that there were not at the moment enough men in sight to staff such an institute—"young and able men who are aspiring to research in clinical medicine as a life-time career". This was largely because the possibility of such a career was not evident. The Council, he urged, should therefore emphatically announce that its policy was to develop departments of clinical medicine and surgery on the basis of providing life-time careers. This led to the appointment of a subcommittee, mentioned earlier, on whose advice the Council took such action as was immediately practicable.

Again, in 1942, Lewis submitted a memorandum to the Council making proposals for the advancement of clinical research when the end of the war should permit. This document was circulated to the members serving at the time and noted for future consideration; but it was in fact never resuscitated after the war, in the difficult conditions then prevailing. Lewis had believed that the time would be opportune for placing clinical science on a firmer basis in the United Kingdom. At the outbreak of war, according to him, there had been in Britain "the most promising group of young clinical research workers that this country has ever seen".

The question, as Lewis saw it, was whether the Council could make improved arrangements by some form of centralisation. The research workers themselves should possess greater control over the conditions of their work; and it was doubtful whether full facilities could be obtained except in an institution primarily intended for research. He accordingly envisaged "a central unit of clinical science" providing adequate facilities. This could be merely a meeting house with a library and workshops; or it might comprise a small or large complement of hospital beds and laboratories, or perhaps only the latter. There were several possibilities to be considered, and the memorandum did not carry the discussion beyond that point. It concluded as follows: "It is my firm conviction that the power of modern methods to explore the nature of disease in man far transcends anything which is at all generally credited to it."

Tom Lewis did not live to urge his proposals further in time of peace; but although little could be done immediately after the war, there can be no doubt that he would have thoroughly approved of much that has been accomplished since. In retrospect, it was said in the Report for 1951–52 that: "Thomas Lewis was in advance of his age; but it was largely due to him and men of his way of thinking—particularly to the professors in the new university clinical units in the medical schools—that a generation of research workers was won to clinical research and trained in the application of scientific methods to clinical problems."

Research in the National Health Service

The National Health Service Act 1946, and the National Health Service (Scotland) Act 1947, came into force in 1948 (Volume One); and Northern Ireland followed suit. These measures made a drastic change in the conditions of work of the nation's hospitals. The consulting staffs became salaried instead of honorary; and various degrees of part-time employment made it possible to undertake private practice or other outside work—or to engage in research.

There were also explicit powers "to conduct research". Ministers (who in fact already had powers under earlier legislation) could not only conduct research but could assist other persons to do so; and in Scotland this double power was given also to Regional Hospital Boards and Boards of Management forming part of the new organisation. In England and Wales, however, Boards of Governors of teaching hospitals, Regional Hospital Boards and Hospital Management Committees had power only to conduct research. The legal ruling was that these bodies had thus no power to give grants for work conducted solely by other bodies: "The circumstances must be such that it can reasonably be said that the Board or Committee, alone or in conjunction with someone else, has promoted or sponsored the research project and has general control over its character and the carrying out of it."

At first the powers had no financial teeth, and the Treasury would clearly be unwilling to provide public funds for the purpose until assured that satisfactory arrangements for control and coordination had been made. There were, however, substantial endowment funds of private origin in the hands of former voluntary hospitals, and with all the routine necessities now being provided by the Exchequer the income was wholly available for amenities and research. The amount of free income of this kind varied widely between different hospitals and without relation to their respective opportunities for promoting research. In Scotland, where there was a precedent from the educational field, a substantial part of these endowment funds was removed from the control of the separate hospital authorities and pooled under a body created for the purpose, the Scottish Hospital Endowments Research Trust.

In the changed circumstances arising from the Act, the Council received with pleasure an invitation from the Standing Medical Advisory Committee of the Ministry of Health to take part in discussion of new arrangements. A Joint Committee was set up under the chairmanship of Professor Sir Henry Cohen (later Lord Cohen of Birkenhead); and two of the Council's representatives were also members of the Advisory Committee on Medical Research in Scotland, so bringing the Department of Health there into liaison. By 1952 it was thus possible to present a single and unanimous report to the three Ministers concerned—the Lord President of the Council, the Secretary of State for Scotland and the Minister of Health. The Ministers accepted the recommendations in principle, leaving details of implementation for further discussion. The main conclusions were summarised in the Council's Report for 1951–52 as follows:

(1) A central organisation for the promotion of clinical research should be established as part of the Medical Research Council. A Clinical Research Board, for the detailed supervision of centrally organised clinical research, should be appointed by the Council after consultation, and in agreement, with the Health Departments. The Medical Research Council should be the financial authority for centrally organised clinical research and should be the employing authority of the research workers engaged on its projects. The necessary additional funds should be made available to develop clinical research.

(2) Provision should be made for decentralised research at the level of Regional Hospital Boards, Boards of Governors of teaching hospitals and Hospital Management Committees. Within this field there should be the greatest possible freedom from detailed supervision. In England and Wales responsibility for the distribution of Exchequer moneys for research purposes should lie with the Regional Hospital Boards and Boards of Governors; and each Board should set up a research committee after consultation, and in agreement, with the associated University or Medical School, to advise on the spending of the research budget. In Scotland the distribution of Exchequer Funds through Regional Hospital Boards and Boards of Management would continue to be

made by the Department of Health for Scotland on the advice of the Advisory Committee on Medical Research.

(3) Careers in clinical research should be equated with careers in the National Health Service.

The report, *Clinical Research in Relation to the National Health Service*, was published as an official 'white paper' in 1953 and copies were distributed to hospital authorities. Consultations were continued to produce a detailed scheme, and in 1957 it was possible to circulate this to the hospital boards and committees in memoranda from the Ministry of Health and the Department of Health for Scotland. The whole position was reviewed by the Council in its Report for 1955–56.

Centralised research was to be financed and controlled by the Council, with the advice and help of the new Clinical Research Board. Workers appointed by the Council would be members of its staff, and research units maintained by the Council would be part of its organisation. Suitably qualified research workers would also be given honorary appointments by the hospital authorities concerned. Senior members of hospital staffs would still be free to make individual applications to the Council for grants, subject to their authorities approving any arrangements proposed to be made.

Decentralised research financed from Exchequer funds, provided to hospital authorities through National Health Service channels, was to be limited to relatively minor projects in order to avoid duplication of programmes and to ensure that candidates for senior research posts would be judged against a national standard. It was expected that research projects under these arrangements would normally arise mainly from, and be closely related to, medical practice in hospitals. Within these limits the greatest possible freedom was to be allowed, but hospital authorities could seek advice from the Clinical Research Board if they wished to do so.

In circulating its memorandum, the Ministry of Health referred to the importance of the continuation and development of clinical research to the efficiency of the health service; all concerned should therefore be informed of the powers and duties of hospital authorities and of the opportunities for coordination. The Scottish document was equally forthright: "The Secretary of State regards clinical research as an essential and inseparable aspect of the medical services provided in hospitals." The Council, in its Report, expressed the view that in recent years the development of clinical research in university and hospital departments had been so conspicuous that it now formed a sound foundation on which to build.

For financing the development of clinical research under centralised arrangements, the Treasury provided the Council with an additional £50 000 in 1954–55; and it recognised that the requirement was likely to rise to about £250 000 within a few years. The provision of Exchequer funds to the National Health Service for decentralised research was a separate operation and was longer in taking effect.

The Clinical Research Board

It had been agreed with the Health Departments that the Council should be reinforced by a Clinical Research Board in the discharge of its widening responsibility for clinical and paraclinical research. This body was accordingly set up in 1953 "to advise and assist the Council in the promotion of clinical research". The Chairman was to be appointed by the Council; and if he were not a member of Council, he was to be *ex officio* an assessor to it. Five members were to be appointed on the nomination of the Health Departments, and five on the nomination of the Council; the latter would normally include the clinicians serving on the Council for the time being. The nominations were then to be agreed between the parties before the Council made the definitive appointments. The period of office was to be three years, but this was later increased to four years for members of Council in order to run with their service on that body. The Chief Medical Officers of the two Health Departments in Great Britain, and of the Ministry of Health and Local Government for Northern Ireland, were to be official assessors. A senior medical officer on the Council's headquarters staff (Dr F. J. C. Herrald) was to be Secretary of the Board; and the Secretary of the Council would attend meetings. The Chairman of the Board during its first six years was Sir Geoffrey Jefferson, a distinguished surgeon who had formerly served on the Council.

Research in surgery

What has been said in this chapter refers primarily to clinical medicine, as distinct from surgery. In the latter, research is more closely bound up with treatment, although surgeons themselves or physiologists may prepare the way for new operational procedures by experimental work in the laboratory. In its Report for 1936–37 the Council made the following comment:

> It is well known that since the introduction of antisepsis and asepsis the progress of surgery has been both great and rapid. So much so, indeed, that the statement a few years ago by the late Lord Moynihan, that advance in surgical technique was approaching finality, was received with some surprise by the general public. Nevertheless, it is certainly true that substantial innovations in surgical methods have become sufficiently rare to be matters of considerable interest.

In the light of many subsequent developments, it would seem that the instincts of the general public were sound.

The Council's Report for 1936–37 spoke of the Council's active interest in new work on the surgery of the heart that was being undertaken by Mr Laurence O'Shaughnessy at the Lambeth Cardiovascular Clinic of the London County Council. The subject was then in its infancy; unhappily this pioneer was soon to become a casualty of war.

In 1938 the Council established its Surgical Research Unit at Edinburgh, to which reference has already been made. Although the particular project did not continue, there have been others. For instance, as particularly noticed in the Report for 1952–53, Mr E. J. Delorme of the Council's external staff worked on the use of hypothermia in surgery in the Wilkie Surgical Research Laboratory of the University of Edinburgh. This bears relation to a programme of physiological researches on the effects of low temperatures, undertaken at the National Institute for Medical Research. Similarly, there have been surgical applications of experimental results in skin grafting and organ transplantation; the work on the former subject, which earned Professor P. B. (later Sir Peter) Medawar a Nobel Prize, was grant-aided by the Council. The Council sponsored a Research Group on the Experimental and Clinical Problems of Transplantation, under Professor M. F. A. Woodruff, later taken over by the University of Edinburgh; and it has made grants for work on renal transplantation under Professor R. Y. Calne at Addenbrooke's Hospital, Cambridge. Study of the metabolic effects of surgical procedures was for a time the programme of one of the Council's units.

Yet the special nature of clinical research in surgery remains. As was said in a memorandum presented to the Council by one of its members in 1957: "The surgeon's laboratory is still, to a considerable extent, the operating theatre." The Report for 1959–60 contained a review article on "A changing outlook on the surgical treatment of duodenal ulcer."

Research into mental disorders

Disorders of the mind, as well as those of the body, have always been regarded as falling within the Council's sphere. This was formally confirmed in 1920, when responsibility for a small number of research projects was transferred to the Council from the Board of Control, a financial adjustment being made by the Treasury. The grants that the Board had hitherto been making were maintained by the Council for varying periods of years.

In 1921, after consultation with the Board of Control, the Council appointed a Mental Disorders Committee to advise it in this field. This included eminent psychiatrists and neurologists reinforced, on the Council's usual plan, by members drawn from other disciplines. It cannot be said, however, that this body was notably successful in bringing important proposals to the notice of the Council; nor did the latter then have many promising applications on which to seek the Committee's advice. The Committee was reconstituted in 1934.

The subject was indeed scientifically immature. The clinical arts needed in the approach to mental illness were different from those used in dealing with primarily physical conditions; and the terminology used was (in the strict sense) peculiar. Research was handicapped by a lack of definite base-lines and objective criteria; the psychiatrist's concepts existed within his own frames of reference. The deep divisions between rival schools of thought were symptomatic of an inexact science. Above all, there was an absence of men combining knowledge of the subject matter with capacity for research.

In its Report for 1929–30 the Council said: "Medicine, too, has to deal with the interplay of mind and body, a primary duty belonging to the clinical field and in the management of life, which is still very far from adequate fulfilment, whether in medical education or in medical research." But the situation was not one that could be quickly improved; the subject had to develop, and there was not much in the Council's power that would accelerate the process. One approach was by investigations of orthodox type, in the attempt to correlate mental disorders with possible underlying physical abnormalities ascertainable by the methods of pathology, biochemistry or physiology; the earlier projects aided by the Council were mostly of this kind, but there was no certainty that important answers were to be found in this way. The direct approach to mental disorders as such, from a base in psychology, was clearly important; but it was elusively difficult. Mention has been made of one early project, at the level of mental defect, in Volume One.

In recent years the emergence of suitably qualified men, coupled with the opportunities of the National Health Service, has enabled the Council to promote a number of research projects of both types. Units have been established in such fields as occupational psychiatry, clinical psychiatry, neuropsychiatry and the chemical pathology of mental disorders; and other investigations have been grant-aided. In 1970 the Council issued, as a booklet, the report of a committee chaired by Professor D. A. K. (later Sir Douglas) Black, surveying the field of biochemical research in psychiatry and making proposals for further development.

Another approach has been epidemiological—determining the incidence of various conditions, by the classical methods of census and survey, in the search for correlations with possible aetiological factors. Further, much of the work on human genetics that the Council has promoted over the years has special relevance to mental defect.

A division of psychiatric research is included in the new Clinical Research Centre, with wards in the associated hospital (see later).

Responsibility in investigations on human subjects
It is obvious that there are limitations on the kind of investigations that may properly be made on human subjects for the advancement of knowledge; but to define the limits is far from easy. Clinical research workers may thus often be faced with ethical, and sometimes even legal, questions calling for authoritative advice. In 1953,

accordingly, the Council circulated to its staff and others a statement of the considerations which should, in its opinion, govern the conduct of scientific investigations on patients. Subsequently, the range and scope of technically feasible procedures steadily increased; and there was also a need for guidance on the conduct of investigations on healthy persons. The Council, therefore, again reviewed the whole question, in consultation with its legal advisers and the Health Departments, and in its Report for 1962–63 published a comprehensive statement of its opinions in this regard. One feels that Hippocrates (b. 460 B.C.), who himself used the methods of research, could have endorsed this judicious pronouncement. Only a summary can be given here.

During the last fifty years medical knowledge has advanced more rapidly than ever before, and this is without doubt largely due to the marriage of the newer methods of science with the traditional methods of medicine. The use of new procedures must clearly continue, so great are the benefits to be gained, yet their potentialities go far beyond the marginal variations in established practice that were tried in earlier days.

A distinction is drawn between procedures undertaken as part of patient-care to benefit the individual, whether by treatment, prevention or assessment, and those undertaken either on patients or on healthy subjects to contribute to medical knowledge. The former are governed by the ordinary code of professional conduct in medicine, whereas the latter fall within the ambit of investigations on volunteers.

In the use of procedures directly connected with the management of the condition in a particular patient, the latter's willingness to be guided by the judgement of his medical attendant is implicit. If the medical attendant has reasonable grounds for believing that a new procedure will contribute to the benefit of the patient, the position is the same as if the procedure were entirely established practice; the novelty is relevant only in that it entails special care, and to obtain the prior agreement of the patient (or of a parent or guardian in the case of a child) is no more than a considerate and provident requirement of good medical practice. The same ethical and legal considerations apply to the administration of new preventives to persons not at the moment suffering from the relevant disease but potentially at risk.

The trial of new treatments or preventives is often greatly facilitated by comparison with control groups of subjects not receiving these; a more speedy and precise evaluation can thus be obtained than by the gradual accumulation of experience. Such controlled trials, however, are permissible only where there is a genuine doubt within the profession as to which of two procedures is the better; it is then justifiable to give the new treatment or preventive to a proportion of the subjects, on the understanding that the remainder receive what was previously accepted as best. So far as practicable, the purpose of the trial should be frankly explained to the patients, and their cooperation obtained. The Council also consider that controlled clinical trials should always be planned and supervised by a group of investigators and never by an individual alone.

While the preceding considerations cover the majority of clinical investigations, it is often important to use human subjects to determine normal values and their variations, so that abnormal values can be recognised as such. The subjects must sometimes be ill persons, when variations in a morbid condition are in question, but at other times they may be either entirely healthy persons or sufferers from some condition irrelevant to the point under study. The common feature is that the investigation is of no direct benefit to the particular individual, who must therefore volunteer in the full sense of the word. This means that true consent, freely given with proper understanding of what is involved, must be obtained; without it, the possibility or probability that the investigation will be of benefit to humanity would afford no defence.

It is important that clear evidence of the fact and circumstances of consent should be recorded. Particular care is necessary in this respect when the volunteer stands in special relation to the investigator, as a patient to his doctor or a student to his teacher. The situation is also particularly difficult where minors or mentally abnormal persons are involved. There is in any event a heavy responsibility not only on the investigators, but on the heads of departments, on grant-giving bodies such as the Council itself, on specialised societies which mould opinion in particular fields, and on the editors of medical and scientific journals. With regard to the last, published accounts of investigations should make it clear that the appropriate requirements have been fulfilled. The statement concludes:

> The progress of medical knowledge has depended, and will continue to depend, in no small measure upon the confidence which the public has in those who carry out investigations on human subjects, be these healthy or sick. Only in so far as it is known that such investigations are submitted to the highest ethical scrutiny and self-discipline will this confidence be maintained. Mistaken, or misunderstood, investigations could do incalculable harm to medical progress. It is our collective duty as a profession to see that this does not happen and so to continue to deserve the confidence that we now enjoy.

New Clinical Research Centre

In 1957 the Council reverted to the subject of a possible centralised organisation for clinical research, associated with a hospital. The members may have had no clear awareness that their predecessors had earlier, as noted above, given some thought to similar ideas at the instance of Thomas Lewis; but now the time was ripe for an ambitious scheme. On this occasion the initiative came from the Secretary, Sir Harold Himsworth, who had since his appointment been working steadily towards the creation of better facilities for clinical research. Incidentally, as Professor of Medicine at University College Hospital, he had been a younger colleague of Thomas Lewis.

Himsworth's memorandum pointed to the limitations of the system of clinical research units on which the Council had hitherto relied. Some of the difficulties were implicit in the guest–host relationship, which among other things often involved setting unconventional people within an orthodox professional pattern. A mere unit did not itself command large enough resources in the way of equipment, or of collaboration in such related fields as pathology; and there was a degree of impermanence in a small team built round a director who might have no obvious successor. Specialties tended to wither in isolation, and there was need for a research community of adequate size. Such a community should stand in a relation to a hospital similar to that of a medical school; to avoid the complications of a triangular relationship, a teaching hospital should not be chosen.

Clinical members of Council submitted memoranda of their several views. A centralised scheme should not diminish the Council's support of clinical research in university institutions. The new centre should not be attached to the National Institute for Medical Research, which was already big enough for one Director; and Mill Hill was the wrong kind of area for such a hospital as would be required. The idea of a special research hospital should be ruled out, for the same reasons as had operated earlier.

The project thereafter took shape, and in its Report for 1958–59 the Council announced the conclusion, reached in consultation with the Clinical Research Board, "that a centre should be set up, which would comprise an adequate and appropriately comprehensive concentration of relevant clinical and paraclinical disciplines". And also that this centre "would be incorporated within a general hospital which was providing, and would continue to provide, a full range of services to the community".

In 1960, with the tripartite agreement of the Ministry of Health, the North-West Metropolitan Regional Hospital Board and the Council, and with the approval of the Treasury, the decision was taken to go ahead with a particular scheme. So as this history closes, there is in being a major additional facility for research in the clinical field—the Council's Clinical Research Centre, associated with the Regional Board's new Northwick Park Hospital. After some years of intensive planning, constructional work began early in 1966. The combined project began to become operative in 1970, and the building was formally opened by Her Majesty the Queen on 23 October; completion of the present scheme was expected in 1974. The site is a fine one, less than ten miles from the centre of London, and incidentally about five miles from the National Institute for Medical Research.

This is a joint venture by a hospital authority and a research organisation; each is responsible for its own part, but these parts have been planned in the closest integration and are intended to work together in intimate accord. Northwick Park Hospital is a district general hospital of the National Health Service, primarily serving the growing London Boroughs of Brent and Harrow. Patients in the locality have the benefit of the latest advances in medical science and access to the special facilities for diagnosis and treatment available in the research centre. The research workers, for their part, gain by being brought into immediate contact with everyday medical problems.

The hospital provides the normal range of services, including general medicine, surgery, psychiatry, paediatrics and obstetrics. The object of the Research Centre is the intensive study of disease. Patients in need of special investigations or complicated treatment are admitted to the Research Centre either from the wards of the hospital itself, from the local community at the request of their own doctors or from other parts of the country by arrangement. The staff of the centre includes medically qualified and other scientists, the latter drawn from such disciplines as physics, chemistry, biology and mathematics. Many skills can thus be combined in the investigation of the increasingly complicated problems of medicine; and an essential feature of the whole scheme is the opportunity for the free interchange of ideas between medical and other scientific workers.

The general hospital is planned eventually to provide 686 ordinary and 48 additional beds, and the Research Centre to have 180 beds and 5 special care baby cots. The Research Centre's beds, like the others, are maintained by the National Health Service, which also provides nursing, but the patients are in the care of specialists who are in the main members of the Council's staff holding honorary appointments with the Regional Board. The non-medical research and ancillary staff of the centre are likewise in the employ of the Council.

The site is one of 46 acres and thus leaves ample space for future expansion, allowance for which has also been made in the design of the buildings in view of the expected need to accommodate future changes in the practice of medicine. It was implicit in the original concept of the joint enterprise that the general hospital and the Research Centre should not be separate and self-contained, but should be integrated in a single architectural complex. The various specialist departments are therefore accommodated in a series of carefully related buildings linked together; the central block, seven storeys high, houses wards and the main part of the Research Centre. The design embodies may attractive features on the hospital aspect as well as meeting the scientific requirements of the research side. The architects were Llewellyn-Davies, Weeks, Forestier-Walker and Bar.

The Clinical Research Centre is not intended to replace the Council's existing arrangements in this field. It does, however, represent a culmination of the endeavours of many years to make more adequate provision for clinical research in face of all the circumstantial difficulties. It is an outcome, one feels, that would have been welcomed by Lewis as a fulfilment of his ambitions for the future of his subject. It is also a fruit of the endeavours of Himsworth, who as a clinician coming to be Secretary of the Council was naturally greatly concerned with fostering such schemes. The detailed planning of the centre owes a great deal to the late Professor J. R. Squire —one of Lewis's disciples and successively Director and Honorary Director of research units of the Council (Appendix C); he had been Director-designate of the Clinical Research Centre since 1960, but died suddenly in January 1966, at the age of 50, just when the project to which he had contributed so much thought was beginning to take tangible form. In March 1966 Professor G. M. Bull was appointed by the Council in his place. Dr (now Sir) Richard Doll had been nominated as Deputy Director, but on his appointment as Regius Professor of Medicine at Oxford this post was filled by Dr D. A. J. Tyrrell.

The Clinical Research Centre at present comprises divisions concerned with anaesthesia, animals, bioengineering, cell pathology, clinical chemistry, clinical investigation, communicable diseases (including the Common Cold Unit at Salisbury), computing and statistics, cryobiology, hospital infection, immunology, inherited metabolic diseases, radioisotopes, and surgical sciences; and also sections dealing with electron microscopy, haematology and radiology. A Division of Psychiatry was being set up early in 1974, and future plans include work on infant development and dermatology.

Chapter 3
Curative Medicine: Therapeutic Agents (Chemical and Biological)

The clinician's armamentarium—Pharmacology—Anaesthetics—Hormone preparations: insulin—Liver extracts—Sex hormones—Cortisone—A second thryoid hormone—Blood constituents—Chemotherapy: the empirical era—Sulphonamide therapy—Later developments in chemotherapy—Chemotherapy of cancer—Antibiotics: penicillin—Other antibiotics

The clinician's armamentarium

Research in curative medicine both begins and ends with the clinician, who alone can observe the symptoms and course of a disease in man and alone can assess the results of treatment; but he employs today methods of diagnosis and therapy based on scientific work that is not itself clinical, and indeed often not medical in a professional sense. Lord Platt, himself an eminent clinician and closely associated with the Council, has stated reasons for the view that "the phenomenal success of modern medical treatment seems to have depended almost wholly on non-clinical, often non-medical scientists, frequently working in, or in close collaboration with, the pharmaceutical industry". As Sir George Godber, Chief Medical Officer of the (then) Ministry of Health, put it: "Medicine will never again be self-sufficient. It has not only a large group of professions supplementary to medicine but also a great and increasing need for the aid of other scientists from disciplines only occasionally concerned with the care of patients or with health."

In the particular sphere of therapeutic agents, medicine is indebted to a galaxy of biological, chemical and physical branches of science. One need only consider the range of the medicinal substances now available: physiologically active drugs occurring in nature, commonly in plants; gases used as anaesthetics; hormone preparations from animal glands; vitamins found in vegetable and animal foodstuffs; immunological products dependent on the reactions between infective microorganisms and the human or animal body; synthetic chemical compounds with specific effects; and the antibiotics, extracted from moulds and potently bactericidal. And again, on the physical side, there are such agents as radiations of different kinds and various mechanical aids, as well as powerful instruments for refined methods of laboratory diagnosis (Chapter 4).

In each of these fields the Council has always supported research, whether by employing staff with appropriate interests or by making grants in response to applications. In all of them there have been times when initiative on the Council's part has been required, in order to promote some special scheme of work. Selected examples of

34

this kind must for the most part suffice in the following sections relating to agents of different types. Vitamin preparations and immunological products play a greater part in preventive than in curative medicine and are therefore dealt with under that head (Chapters 5, 7).

Collaboration with the pharmaceutical industry in research, the use of the patent law in the medical field, the clinical evaluation of remedies, and the biological standardisation of therapeutic substances not assayable by chemical tests—this last a particularly noteworthy item in the Council's programme—are dealt with separately (Chapters 11, 12).

Pharmacology
The 'galenical' drugs, mostly physiologically active substances extracted from certain plants, represented the materia medica of traditional pharmacology. That science has acquired much wider horizons, but drugs of the older type have continued to provide important subjects for research, undertaken with the aid of modern chemical and biochemical methods. A Department of Biochemistry and Pharmacology, under the direction of Dr H. H. (later Sir Henry) Dale, figured prominently in the original organisation of the National Institute for Medical Research. A few examples of its work may be mentioned.

Ergot, a drug prepared from a fungus parasitic on rye, had for long been used empirically in medicine as a stimulant of the contractile activity of the uterus, during and after labour; and its components were known to include two alkaloids each capable of producing stimulating effects—but, unlike the whole extract, not when administered orally. In 1932 the Council's Therapeutic Trials Committee invited Dr Chassar Moir, then in the Obstetric Unit of University College Hospital, to compare the actions of these two alkaloids on the puerperal uteri of normal patients willing to cooperate; he showed that their actions were indistinguishable. Moir went on from there to demonstrate clinically the presence in ergot of a hitherto unrecognised principle which was effective when given by mouth, and which had a higher oxytocic activity and a lower toxicity than the other alkaloids. At the National Institute Dr H. W. Dudley undertook the chemical pursuit of the principle, guided at every step by Moir's clinical records. As a result, a water-soluble alkaloid was isolated, characterised and named. This combined effort thus added a safe and potent remedy, pure ergometrine, to the obstetrician's armamentarium.

Also at the National Institute, but in the following decade, Dr Harold King made chemical analyses of *Strychnos* material used in pharmacological and clinical work by Dr R. G. R. West at Oxford and at the National Hospital for Nervous Diseases, London. He proceeded to study various alkaloids found in arrow-poisons made from plants by indigenous tribes of South America and known by the general name 'curare' (woorara, woorali). The poison's paralytic action is essentially one of antagonism to the normal actions of acetylcholine in the body. The original introduction of the substance into experimental physiology had been the subject of lurid suspicion and protest (Tennyson, for example, wrote of "the hellish oorali"); but King's isolation and chemical characterisation of one of the alkaloids, tubocurarine, was an important factor in the spectacular improvement in methods of producing a safe and effective surgical anaesthesia, with full muscular relaxation, in abdominal operations.

This success aroused widespread interest regarding chemical substances of similar type, and led to attempts at replacing the naturally occurring alkaloids by synthetic compounds. At the National Institute, shortly after the Second World War, Dr King, Dr W. D. M. Paton and Dr E. J. Zaimis synthesised and studied the series of compounds that have since become known as the methonium drugs. The actions of these were also investigated elsewhere, but Paton and Zaimis were responsible for a particularly extensive pharmacological study. In short, it was eventually shown that some members of the series hindered the transmission of excitation through the nerve ganglia, thus having a remedial effect against high blood pressure, while others had actions that made them potential substitutes for curarine.

In 1958 the Council established a Neuropharmacology Research Unit under the honorary direction of Professor P. B. Bradley in the University of Birmingham. This is concerned with the actions of drugs on the central nervous system, investigating these by the methods of neurophysiology, psychology, and biochemistry. Studies have been made of substances thought to be synaptic transmitters (facilitating the passage of nervous impulses across junctions between nerves and brain), and of representative drugs used in psychiatric treatment; the psychological effects of some of the drugs have been examined experimentally. Attempts are being made to relate biochemical data to the findings of the physiological and behavioural investigations. Other units followed (Appendix C).

Anaesthetics
A special branch of pharmacological study relates to the use of certain gases in the production of anaesthesia. This was actively taken up by the Council in 1924, when it arranged with the Anaesthetics Section of the Royal Society of Medicine for the joint appointment of a special committee to promote research into the value, effects and possible dangers of different anaesthetic methods; the Council also provided grants, and the cooperation of its staff, for the investigations. The Anaesthetics Committee maintained its work for many years, and in 1935 its secretary (later chairman), Dr C. F. Hadfield, published a review of its progress up to that time.

One of the first tasks was an investigation of the purity of supplies of nitrous oxide placed on the market for anaesthetic use. Although the quality of the gas was generally excellent, cases of contamination with very small amounts of deleterious substances were brought to light, and methods for removing these impurities were recommended. Similar attention was given to supplies of anaesthetic ether, and with these little fault was found. Later, the Committee gave advice to the Pharmacopoeia Commission on the standards of purity which should be laid down in the *British Pharmacopoeia* for various anaesthetic gases.

The Committee also arranged for clinical trials of some of the less known gases possessing anaesthetic properties, and likewise of new preparations introduced as the result of chemical research. Physiological investigations were made into such problems as the effects of anaesthesia on metabolism, on respiration, and on kidney function. The dangers of explosions in operating theatres received much attention.

Of the Anaesthetics Committee, the Council said in its Report for 1934–35: "The organisation set up is an example of a standing committee which keeps continuously in view the questions requiring investigation in a particular field, and takes action regarding these when necessary."

The joint committee was not formally discharged until 1956, but for some time before that its function had dwindled to vanishing point. It was followed by two bodies dealing with particular aspects of the subject, of which one was the Committee on Non-Explosive Anaesthetic Agents set up in 1955. This Committee was concerned chiefly with the trial of new fluorine compounds made under the direction of Professor M. Stacey in the University of Birmingham. A special task was to advise the Medical Department of the Royal Navy on non-explosive anaesthetic agents for use in nuclear submarines.

Earlier, in 1949, the Council had appointed a Committee on Analgesia in Midwifery, in response to a request for investigation by a Working Party set up by the Health Departments to consider the acute shortage of midwives and their proper status and functions in relation to the doctor and the health visitor. The problem was the practical one "of finding a safe and effective analgesic agent for midwifery and devising for its administration apparatus that is light, simple and requires a minimum of maintenance". The only method available to unsupervised midwives at this time, 'gas and air', involved inconvenient apparatus and was therefore too seldom used in domiciliary practice. The Committee decided that trilene was the most suitable agent and proceeded to draw up a detailed specification of a suitable inhaler, prescribing the permitted concentrations and defining the range of conditions under which the mechanism must be guaranteed to function consistently. After laboratory tests, three prototypes submitted by manufacturers were approved; and the National Birthday Trust Fund helped to meet the cost of providing a sufficient number of inhalers for a large-scale trial. The

Royal College of Obstetricians and Gynaecologists, the Ministry of Health and the Central Midwives Board joined in the organisation of the trials, together with authorities in Scotland. An account of the work, with the Committee's recommendations, was published in 1954 in the Council's series of memoranda. This body was disbanded in 1959 but soon replaced by a Committee on Nitrous Oxide/Oxygen Analgesia in Midwifery, which reported in 1968.

Hormone preparations: insulin

The so-called 'biologicals', as contrasted with the galenicals, are typified by the hormone preparations. These represent another group of medicinal substances found in nature, but in this instance in the animal body; their use in medicine reflects their role in normal physiology. Early examples of endocrine substances prepared for medical use are the active principles of the hormones secreted by the thyroid gland and by the posterior lobe of the pituitary body.

The Council's first major interest in this field arose from Canadian work leading to the introduction of insulin, a principle extracted from the islet tissue of the pancreas of animals, for replacement therapy in diabetes mellitus. The existence of this hormone had for sometime been hypothetically postulated as indispensable for carbohydrate metabolism; and the name had even been coined (by Schafer, in Britain) ten years before a long series of researches in various countries culminated in a practical result. This was achieved in the University of Toronto in 1921, when by experiments on dogs Dr F. G. (later Sir Frederick) Banting, with his colleague Dr C. H. Best, definitely demonstrated the existence of an active principle in the pancreas that was essential for the proper disposal of sugar within the body, its absence or deficiency causing the distressing and often fatal condition of diabetes. And in the same laboratory Dr J. B. Collip and Professor J. R. R. Macleod had succeeded in extracting this principle from the pancreas of the ox in a form suitable for therapeutic use in alleviating the disease in man. Commercial production followed in Canada and the United States, and clinical trials became possible—and thereafter general clinical use.

At the invitation of the University, the Council sent Dr H. H. Dale and Dr H. W. Dudley to Toronto in the autumn of 1922 to bring back detailed information. There was a need to confirm and evaluate the clinical results reported from Canada, to assist British commercial firms in undertaking manufacture, and to make arrangements for standardising the product (Chapter 12). These measures were all put in hand by the Council as matters of special urgency.

The clinical trials were organised at eight centres where there were laboratory facilities for the preparation of insulin on a small scale for local use. Five of these centres were teaching hospitals in London—where opportunities that would not have been found a few years earlier were provided by the recently instituted units for clinical teaching—and the others were at Sheffield, Edinburgh and

Glasgow respectively. For the London centres, the collection of the raw material from slaughterhouses and its distribution under proper conditions were undertaken by the National Institute for Medical Research. When commercial supplies became available, the clinical investigations were continued with these; and a report embodying the early clinical experience at the special centres was published in the medical press as a guide to the use of insulin by the medical profession.

For commercial production, the Council approached the principal firms of manufacturing chemists thought to have the necessary special facilities and experience; of these, three London firms (two acting together) and three in other parts of Great Britain decided to take up production—although some later dropped out. All received in equal degree the technical advice of the Council's staff and early reports of research work at the National Institute. As a result, British production soon met the whole of the home demand, so that American insulin had no longer to be imported except for special purposes; there was indeed a surplus available for export. During the short period when commercial supplies were inadequate, issue had to be restricted to hospitals and physicians having facilities for their effective use; to advise on such matters, outside the field of research, a departmental committee was set up by the Minister of Health at the Council's request.

In dealing with the commercial aspect, the Council's hand was strengthened by the possession of patent rights in the method of preparing insulin. World-wide patents had been taken out by the University of Toronto, which assigned the United Kingdom rights to the Council. The latter licensed the manufacturing firms under the patent, charging no royalties and imposing no conditions except as regards submission of the product for tests of quality. (The Council did indeed reserve the right to fix a maximum selling price, but there was never occasion to exercise this.) The Council also held a supplementary patent covering an improved method of purification devised by Dudley at the National Institute. At one point, Best came over from Toronto to work for a time with the staff at the National Institute on the mode of action of insulin, and this collaboration had important results.

The benefit of the breakthrough by the Toronto research workers had been made widely available within a remarkably short time. In the Council's Report for 1922–23, which gave a detailed account of the events summarised above, the outcome was acclaimed in these words:

The public have become suddenly aware that a substance named insulin has been introduced to use, or, as is commonly said, 'discovered', and that daily miracles are being achieved by its means. Men declining quickly or slowly through stages of weakness and pain to early death have been brought within a few days back to full working power; sufferers carried to hospital actually dying of diabetes, already helpless and unconscious, have been resuscitated as by some magic and have been brought back almost at once to normal life by help of this remedy. This boon appears as a sudden gift: diabetic men, women, and children in these recent months have been granted alleviation which has been denied to all their suffering predecessors during all recorded time.

At no other time has the Council's administrative office been so closely involved in the drama of a new remedy giving spectacular relief, or been so massively exposed to the pathos of severe illness with its attendant fears and hopes. The Canadian discovery had naturally attracted wide public attention, and the Council's endeavours to bring the benefits to British diabetics were in turn made known. Inquiring, appealing, often heartrending letters arrived by the sackful, so that ordinary correspondence became submerged. The only possible answer was to advise an approach to one of the hospital centres that were for the moment the sole sources of treatment, although not every applicant could be accepted. A few patients came in person to the office, including one emaciated individual led in by his wife and obviously far advanced in his illness; he was referred to a hospital, and some time later he strode briskly into the office to shake one firmly by the hand and express his gratitude to medical research.

For many years the production, testing and clinical use of insulin continued to demand much attention from the Council. Although "in all competent hands, insulin gave dramatic results in the restoration of health and in the prolongation of life during its continued use", the Council's Reports for 1929–30 and 1931–32 expressed dissatisfaction with the picture in the country as a whole. The demand had risen only gradually; this showed that insulin, although by then in abundant supply, had not been reaching many of those who needed it. Further, it seemed that many were receiving insulin but not under proper conditions of biochemical control and dietetic balance. These facts were reflected in the apparent steadiness of the general death-rates recorded for diabetes, which was at the time often cited by the enemies of research as evidence of the alleged uselessness of insulin. Various other factors masked the important result that, in barely eight years, the mortality from diabetes in England and Wales had been reduced by 37 per cent in males (21 per cent in females) under 55, and by 45 per cent in males in the age group 25–45. Thus, in spite of as yet inadequate use of insulin, the death-rates were already showing the prolongation of life among diabetics.

Insulin was also providing a valuable new tool in experimental physiology, and its availability stimulated a series of investigations of intermediate carbohydrate metabolism at the National Institute for Medical Research. Subsequently, Dr F. G. (later Sir Frank) Young of the Institute's staff used a hormone of the anterior lobe of the pituitary gland to produce a condition of diabetes in dogs. Although insulin had proved highly successful in replacement therapy in the naturally occurring disease in human beings, little was yet known of the causes or possible means of preventing diabetes; a new means of studying the condition experimentally was therefore a valuable asset.

In 1958, Dr F. Sanger of the Council's external staff, working in the University of Cambridge on proteins, was awarded the Nobel Prize in Chemistry for his elucidation of the structure of insulin.

Liver extracts

A few years after the introduction of insulin the Council became involved in an analogous development, this time originating in a discovery made in the United States. In 1926, at Boston, Minot and Murphy reported that patients suffering from pernicious anaemia, a disease hitherto regarded as incurable, could be quickly restored to vigorous health by liver substance in their food. The Council remarked in its Report for 1927–28:

> It is of curious but tragic interest in human history that no accident of observation had previously served to bring this relief to sufferers. The discovery was made by directly applying in hospital practice the results of experiments made with dogs which Whipple and Robscheit-Robbins of Rochester, N.Y., had just published. Here again, as in so many other instances, the experimental method had brought a practical advance where observational study through all the years had brought none. Here, too, is a fresh instance of service to mankind for which the dog was found to be specially fitted.

Quickly following this, Cohn and others at Boston found that suitable extracts of liver contain in small volume the factor which has this curative effect; the treatment was thus made available for patients unable to tolerate a large daily consumption of uncooked liver in their diet. By the courtesy of Harvard Medical School, the Council was given early information and was invited to cooperate in trials of this liver extract with a view to introducing the remedy to general use.

Experimental work at the National Institute led to a useful modification of the original American process of extraction. Meanwhile, the Council had invited the cooperation of the appropriate British firms and had arranged for clinical trials of their products by selected physicians at various hospitals in England, Scotland and Ireland. A report of satisfactory results in these trials was published in the medical press early in 1928 and led to general adoption of the treatment in the United Kingdom.

In its Report for 1934–35, the Council related that during the past year Dakin and West had published in America a method for preparing from liver the active haemopoietic agent—a complex chemical substance—in a much purer state than hitherto. Dr Dakin came to England and supervised the use of this method on a manufacturing scale by a British firm, "a member of whose staff had previously discovered an important stage of the chemical procedure". Again the Council invited a few physicians with special experience to make clinical trials of the preparation. The results showed that weekly injections of as little as 0·1–0·2 grams of the purer product could constitute adequate replacement therapy. As the Council's Report said: "to anyone mindful of the almost certain death that followed the development of pernicious anaemia, even so recently as ten years ago, the recovery that follows these minute injections of anti-anaemic principle seems little short of miraculous".

Several of the Council's workers took part in the subsequent investigation, in different countries, of the nature of the intrinsic and extrinsic factors involved; and progress in elucidating this complex question was reviewed in the Report for 1953–54.

Sex hormones

In its Report for 1931–32, the Council reported a significant development:

> During the past year new provision has been made at the Institute for the study of sex hormones, those chemical substances in the body which control the functions of the reproductive system. This highly specialized branch of research has been acquiring growing importance for medicine. It is also one for which the Ronan Building at Hampstead, and the provision at the Farm Laboratories for the breeding of small animals, both wild and domesticated, give unusual facilities. The Council accordingly made an offer to the Royal Society to accommodate at the Institute the work of the Society's Foulerton Student, Dr A. S. Parkes, hitherto done in the Physiological Institute at University College, London. The offer was accepted, and at the beginning of 1932 Dr Parkes, retaining his Foulerton Studentship for the normal term, moved into the laboratories at Hampstead.
>
> This new subdepartment will not only give additional scope to primary investigations in an important field, but it will also make expert advice available to the Department of Biological Standards in the creation of standards for those members of the complex system of sex hormones that come to have practical importance in medicine.

Dr A. S. (later Sir Alan) Parkes was appointed to the Council's staff at the National Institute on the expiration of his studentship; and he remained head of a subdepartment or division (with various titles) until he left in 1961 for a chair at Cambridge.

The Council reviewed progress in this field in its Report for 1937–38:

> Advancement of knowledge of hormonal action has been astonishing in recent years, and few but the experts can hope to keep abreast of the discoveries. Nor is the subject made easier of comprehension by the interaction of these substances one with another. The complications have been made even worse by the overlapping of physiological action of the different hormones, especially in the case of the sex hormones, where it is common to find female-stimulating (gynaecogenic) properties in substances primarily male (androgenic) in action. The clarification of these ambisexual problems in terms of chemistry is engaging the interest of many investigators throughout the world.

In its next Report, for 1938–39, the Council reviewed some of the applications of the work on sex hormones, particularly in the agricultural field, as a result of collaboration between Dr Parkes and Dr J. (later Sir John) Hammond of the Animal Nutrition Institute at Cambridge. Valuable practical possibilities of stimulating and controlling the reproductive powers of sheep emerged from this collaboration. It was considered possible that the methods might ultimately be extended to women, and in this regard the following remark was made:

> The interest of man has too often been engaged in the development of scientific methods for preventing fertility, and only last year the Council reported the production of a new oestrogenic compound which had the property of counteracting the effect of a hormone of the ovary and ending pregnancy. It is satisfactory to observe that research in this field is also producing knowledge of the means of increasing fertility rather than suppressing it, and the work described above suggests that such knowledge is approaching the stage of practical application.

Among substances under investigation was a synthetic oestrogen, diethylstilboestrol, prepared by Professor E. C. (later Sir Charles) Dodds and others. Dodds and Parkes were associated in the experimental investigation of the effects of this on the female reproductive processes. This led to its clinical use in the treatment of menstrual disorders (and later of forms of cancer—notably of the prostate gland in men and of the breast in women).

In the Council's staff organisation, the provision for experimental work on hormones at the National Institute was supplemented by the Clinical Endocrinology Research Unit established at Edinburgh in 1946. Among other things, much work was done there on the control of ovarian function in women. A small Neuroendocrinology Research Unit was established at Oxford in 1962.

Cortisone

Towards the end of 1949 a new field of work in endocrinology was opened up by the American discovery of cortisone (a steroid hormone of the adrenal glands) and ACTH (adrenocorticotrophic hormone of the pituitary gland). These related substances had been shown to be capable of suppressing the pain symptoms of rheumatoid arthritis and to have useful effects in some other diseases. The Council was anxious to have this treatment tested and evaluated, but progress was hampered by the extreme scarcity of the material, extracted from animal glands of small size. Complete synthesis was thought likely to be difficult, and the best hope seemed to be preparation on the basis of some steroid compound occurring more widely in nature. The Council accordingly sent Dr R. K. Callow and other members of its scientific staff to Africa in quest of plant species containing suitable steroids; hecogenin from sisal was found to be a useful starting point for the synthesis, and this discovery was eventually developed commercially.

The situation was eased when the American firm of Merck & Co. presented a kilogram of cortisone jointly to the Council and the

Nuffield Foundation. These bodies together appointed a committee, under the chairmanship of Sir Henry Cohen (later Lord Cohen of Birkenhead) to organise investigation of the use and value of cortisone in the treatment of chronic rheumatic diseases. By invitation, the Council also joined with the National Heart Institute of the US Public Health Service, and with the American Heart Association, in controlled trials of therapy for acute rheumatic fever, with particular reference to the prevention of permanent damage to the heart.

Two years later it was concluded that cortisone had no specific effect in rheumatoid arthritis. It remained one—and a powerful one, not without attendant dangers—of the substances useful for alleviation. Work promoted by the Council at a number of centres in Great Britain subsequently showed that cortisone had some value in a minority of cases of ulcerative colitis, an obscure chronic disease subject to natural remissions.

A second thyroid hormone

In 1952–53, Dr Rosalind Pitt-Rivers of the National Institute and Dr J. Gross (working in the United States with a Canadian fellowship) jointly discovered a second hormone (triiodothyronine) of the thyroid gland, related to thyroxine but more active than it. This opened up a fruitful field of research and has proved to be of importance in the treatment of thyroid deficiency.

Blood constituents

Analysis of the complex series of factors involved in blood clotting, much of which was done by the Council's Blood Coagulation Research Unit at Oxford in association with the Blood Products Laboratory at Elstree, has made it possible to treat haemophilia and Christmas disease by replacement therapy with the specific factors that are deficient in these conditions.

Chemotherapy: the empirical era

The term 'chemotherapy' is usually restricted to the medical use of synthetic compounds having specific actions against particular infective organisms. Although most of them are used in treatment, a few—such as suppressive antimalarials in the tropics—are given prophylactically during periods of exposure. Some are administered by injection, while others can be taken orally. The discovery of an increasing number of useful chemotherapeutic agents has been an outstanding achievement of medical research in the present century.

The British contribution to the subject was at first small, and the endeavour to increase it formed, from an early stage, an important part of the Council's programme. The policy of research promotion in this field developed through a number of phases which may be briefly indicated.

Before the Council's time, in 1905, Thomas and Breinl in Liverpool had shown that an already known organic derivative of arsenic acid, 'atoxyl', was more potent against trypanosome infections of laboratory animals than was arsenic in inorganic form; but this did not lead to any notable development of British research in chemotherapy. It was Ehrlich and his colleagues in Germany who, in 1909, really opened up the field by their introduction of salvarsan, an organically bound compound of arsenic, for the treatment of syphilis. Ehrlich had first built on his own observations of the special affinity of dyes for certain cells and tissues, but this proved to have no practical significance for chemotherapy; he had then built on the discovery of atoxyl.

During the next quarter of a century only a few important successes were achieved. These included the German antimony compounds for helminth and *Leishmania* infections, and the American (tryparsamide), German (germanin and suramin), and—in a veterinary context—British (antrycide) drugs for trypanosome infections. Synthetic compounds were also beginning to replace the naturally occurring cinchona alkaloids (quinine, quinidine, etc.) used against malaria—first the German plasmoquin (pamaquine) and atebrine (mepacrine), and later the British proguanil (paludrine) and pyrimethamine (daraprim). It is noteworthy that all these compounds were effective against protozoal, spirochaetal or helminthic infections, and therefore had their chief application in tropical medicine. A real chemotherapeutic agent against any bacterial infection was not yet in sight. And in this regard it may be recalled that Almroth Wright had promulgated it as a doctrine that artificial chemotherapy would never be effective against ordinary bacteria, which in his view could be dealt with only by immunological techniques.

The Report of the Medical Research Committee for 1918–19 records the provision of a chemical assistant to Professor E. J. MacWeeny, in Dublin, for the preparation of a series of synthetic dyes to be tested for their powers of restraining the growth of the tubercle bacillus. It also mentions support given to the cooperation between a bacteriologist and a chemist—Professor C. H. Browning of Glasgow (earlier of London) and Professor J. B. Cohen of Leeds —in a study of the bactericidal properties of various compounds in relation to their chemical structure; this likewise came to be orientated to tuberculosis. Such work, however, scarcely carried chemotherapy beyond the use of local antiseptics.

The Council's Report for 1923–24 mentions work by King, at the National Institute, in the classical field of chemotherapy. He was then engaged in the production of compounds resembling atoxyl and tryparsamide for use against experimental trypanosomiasis. At the Institute there were good opportunities for collaboration between chemists and biologists; but except in isolated cases, such as the Browning–Cohen linkage, this was not easy to arrange over a wider field. The Council therefore turned to the Department of Scientific and Industrial Research for help in providing collaboration on the chemical side. So in the Report for 1926–27 one reads that a Joint Committee of the Council and the Department was drawing up a scheme, and in the following year that a joint scheme had been adopted by both parties. Under this arrangement, chemists employed or aided by the Department worked on the production of compounds in series of which members showed promise, while the Council provided biologists in like manner for the experimental trials. The two sets of workers had a clearing house for information and ideas in the form of a continuing joint committee. But the whole undertaking was purely empirical in its methods, and on a minute scale compared with the screening operations of German industry.

In its Report for 1936–37 the Council stressed the importance of chemotherapy for a country with large responsibilities in tropical territories, contrasted with the backwardness of British science and industry in this field:

The discovery and production of chemical compounds of value in this way, on the other hand, has depended almost entirely on German science and industry, and still so depends. Add to this that the most notable exception (tryparsamide, for sleeping sickness) is of American origin, and that the best example of a natural product for like purposes (quinine, for malaria) is practically a Dutch monopoly, and it will be realised that the special needs of the British Empire in this respect have to be met almost entirely from foreign sources. This is all the more remarkable because several fundamental discoveries in chemotherapy have been made in this country. British chemists and pharmacologists have played a distinguished part in opening up new fields in chemotherapy, and there is every reason to suppose that they will be equally successful in developing such fields as soon as the opportunities for organised research on these problems are provided.

The Report proceeds to define the requirement:

The scientific problem in chemotherapy is itself of a special nature. The aim is to find substances which are lethal for particular parasites, but yet not seriously toxic for the human patient. It is a case of finding substances with which the margin between efficacy and safety is sufficiently great to be exploited for medical purposes. The difficulty in the way of finding such substances is the apparent absence of any rational connection between chemical structure and therapeutic value, among the members of those groups of compounds which show effects of the kind required. This makes the search largely empirical, involving the production and testing of an almost infinite number of different substances. The type of research organisation required is thus very different from that which is usually effective in medical science, although with increased knowledge of a fundamental type this subject may ultimately be developed into one of scientific order.

Thereafter the Council's plan is unfolded:

In the absence of effective cooperation by industry, it was considered that a central research laboratory, with a staff able to give their whole time and thought to chemotherapy, would be an essential factor in a national scheme. It was proposed, none the less, that parts of the work should still be allocated to different academic centres. It was strongly held that one of the chief advantages of a central laboratory would be the opportunity for the close daily association of biological investigators with those engaged in the synthetic production of new compounds. It is not sufficient that chemists who are not experts on the biological side of the problem, and to whom 'trypanocidal' and 'antimalarial' actions are little more than words, should make their own programmes on the basis of merely chemical analogy with substances which have proved effective in one direction or another. Under such conditions the biological work of testing the compounds becomes a dull routine having none of the character of a truly cooperative research.

It was envisaged that a scheme such as this would attempt to follow, with Government support, the general line of action of a great commercial organisation taking up this subject of research. There would, however, be the extremely important difference that a commercial scheme aims solely at practically remunerative success and suppresses the scientifically valuable information incidentally obtained; whereas a publicly supported scheme, whatever the measure of its practical success, would be certain to produce material of much more than immediate value for the theoretical basis of the whole problem. The main question why a particular chemical structure produces a specific chemo-therapeutic effect, which a small departure from that structure weakens or destroys, cannot be approached without mass data such as at present do not exist.

Sulphonamide therapy
While the movement for a more deliberate and sustained integration of chemical and biological experimental work was building up, a crucial development took place in which the contribution from the Council's side was mainly clinical, showing that an underrated product of German chemistry was in fact of the greatest practical importance in medicine.

Visiting the Bayer works at Elberfeld in the early 1930s, Sir Henry Dale was introduced to Dr G. Domagk, who had obtained curative results in streptococcal infections in mice with a red dye compound named 'prontosil'. The discoverer was hesitant in claiming this success, and his colleagues appeared to be sceptically inclined; but in 1935 a publication was made in restrained terms. Early in the same year Dale was told that the Bayer Company was ready to supply prontosil to the Council for clinical testing under the arrangements of its Therapeutics Trials Committee and he induced Dr Leonard Colebrook of the Council's staff, working in the Bernhard Baron Memorial Research Laboratories of Queen Charlotte's Hospital, London, to undertake the task; Colebrook agreed, although as a devout disciple of Almroth Wright he had no expectation of success. About the same time, also, Professor Trefouel and his colleagues at the Pasteur Institute in Paris had found—and told Dale during a visit there—that the experimental results were not due to the dye component, but were equally obtainable when that had been separated off; what was left was a known compound, sulphanilamide, which was subject to no proprietary restrictions. The German hesitation may have been due to prior awareness of this fact; and a subsequent endeavour to attach the name 'prontosil album' to sulphanilamide (the original compound becoming 'red prontosil') may be interpreted as an attempt to retain some measure of commercial control over the rich fruits of Domagk's discovery.

Be that as it may, Colebrook's team soon obtained dramatic results in the treatment of puerperal streptococcal infections, first with the red compound and then with colourless sulphanilamide. During the first few months, it is true, the preliminary experiments with mice gave disappointing results; but by the beginning of 1936 these had improved to a point at which use on patients was justified. Reports of clinical success with prontosil were published by Colebrook, Kenny and colleagues in June and December 1936; and in 1937 the work was continued with sulphanilamide, yielding equally good results.

Colebrook had been well placed to make a trial of this kind, as he already had available a succession of patients with puerperal fever and his team was engaged in assessing the value of various immunological techniques in dealing with this dangerous streptococcal infection. On the strength of the experimental evidence, it was thus possible to treat comparable groups of patients by immunological and chemotherapeutic methods respectively. Very soon after his success became known, sulphanilamide was widely tried in different forms of streptococcal and other infections, and the medical profession found itself with a potent new weapon against septicaemia.

This breakthrough, establishing the first artificial chemotherapeutic agent specifically effective in bacterial infections, had far-reaching consequences. Sulphanilamide was efficacious against only a certain range of bacterial species, notably streptococci. At the same time, however, it provided a starting point for the production and trial of a large series of compounds of the sulphonamide group, and many of these were found—by workers in several countries—to have useful actions against different spectra of infections. An early and notable instance was sulphapyridine, which extended the range of sulphonamide therapy to cover pneumococcal infections. This valuable advance was made by the research department of the pharmaceutical firm of May & Baker Limited of Dagenham, Essex, under the direction of Dr A. J. Ewins (a former member of the Council's staff); and it became known to the public by the brand initials of the firm, with doubtless gratifying commercial results. The further development of 'sulfa drugs', as they were called in America, need not be considered here; they remain an important part of the medical armamentarium, even if they have been superseded to a large extent by antibiotics (see later).

Later developments in chemotherapy
The sulphonamide breakthrough, originating from Domagk's discovery of the effect of prontosil in experimental infections and clinically established by Colebrook and colleagues, added weight to the Council's proposals for an intensive programme of research in

chemotherapy. These had already been framed, and it was at the annual dinner of the Royal Society on 30 November 1936 that the Chancellor of the Exchequer, Mr Neville Chamberlain, took the opportunity of announcing the Government's intention of providing the Council with an additional £30 000 per annum specifically for this purpose, as recorded in the Report for 1935–36. In the following year the Committee of Privy Council gave its approval of the scheme, which now included the removal of the National Institute to a new and larger building at Mill Hill in order to provide room for the expansion (Volume One). Before this was ready the Second World War had intervened.

After the war, the scientific situation had substantially changed, as related in the Report for 1948–50:

> In the necessarily long interval that has elapsed between the taking of the decision and the final occupation of the new building, the whole subject of chemotherapy has been revolutionised by the introduction of the antibiotic drugs, of which penicillin was the first in a long succession. As a result, the orientation of chemotherapeutic research has somewhat changed, but the subject remains one of cardinal importance, and still forms and will continue to form one of the most prominent parts of the Council's programme. The greatly improved facilities in the new National Institute have made it possible to expand chemotherapeutic research in both the chemical and the equally important biological aspects.

In its Report for 1953–54 the Council referred to the celebration, at Frankfurt, of the centenary of the births of Paul Ehrlich and Emil von Behring. In retrospect it seemed that the need for close collaboration between chemists and biologists had for surprisingly long been overlooked, largely owing to the absence of any underlying theory; large-scale, semi-empirical screening of new synthetic compounds had then appeared to offer the best chance of success. From these reflections, the Council proceeded to take stock of progress in its own research programme:

> Two principal factors have contributed to the very different outlook on chemotherapeutic research that prevails today. One is the great broadening of the field of application of chemotherapy that has resulted from Domagk's discovery of the antistreptococcal action of prontosil and the consequent development of the sulphonamide drugs, and from the discovery of the antibiotics. The other is the increase in knowledge of the biochemistry of microorganisms and the realisation that this subject is important for the understanding of the way in which drugs act on pathogenic bacteria—advances due in large measure to the work of the Council's former Bacterial Chemistry Research Unit under the direction of Sir Paul Fildes. By patient investigations over many years the workers in this Unit had acquired extensive knowledge of the factors important in bacterial growth and metabolism. It was this work that paved the way for discovery by Dr D. D. Woods, of the staff of the Unit, that the sulphanilamide derivatives exercised their antibacterial effect by interference with an essential bacterial metabolite closely similar in chemical constitution to sulphanilamide itself—namely p-aminobenzoic acid. On the basis of this observation Sir Paul Fildes advanced what was in fact the first satisfying theory

of chemotherapy; according to his hypothesis an effective chemotherapeutic agent will be a substance that interferes with some essential metabolic reaction of the pathogenic microorganism, and such a substance should be sought among compounds having close chemical similarity with those normally utilised by the organism in its metabolism. The Woods-Fildes theory is in reality a special application of the generalisation that emerged from the much earlier work of Dr J. H. Quastel and of the late Dr Marjorie Stephenson (also of the Council's scientific staff), in which it was shown that enzymic reactions are inhibited by compounds that are chemically very similar to those in which the enzymes normally produce a change; its development is thus an excellent example of the way in which an academic biochemical research can lead to an idea of practical importance in medicine.

These considerations led on to the general conclusion:

In any effective consideration of chemotherapy it is necessary to avoid adhering too rigidly to the original simple conception of a chemotherapeutic agent as one that is damaging to the parasite and harmless to the host. The parasite is, after all, dependent on the metabolism of the host's defence mechanisms; one can therefore conceive of the existence of drugs which would arrest the course of an infection not by direct action on the parasite, but by so altering the metabolism of the host that the parasitic environment became unfavourable, or by raising the normal defence mechanisms of the host to a higher level of effectiveness. . . . Chemotherapy has travelled a long way since the days when it amounted to little more than the empirical selection and biological testing of organic compounds, whether already known or specially prepared for the purpose.

Another new factor was the vastly increased interest and effort of the British pharmaceutical industry in chemotherapeutic research. The quest for new synthetic drugs was now being conducted by the manufacturing firms on a much larger scale than could be contemplated by the Council. The approach from the organic chemistry angle was in good hands in the research departments of these concerns, although it was in large measure due to the earlier work of the Council that chemotherapy had at last become well established as a subject of industrial research in Britain. As a result of this change, the emphasis of the Council's programme at the National Institute fell increasingly on the study of the biological problems of chemotherapy, such as the mode of action of drugs and the causes of resistance to them; these questions in turn implied the need for a fuller understanding of the metabolism of the parasites themselves and of the effect of metabolic factors on host–parasite relationships. The purely chemical approach was largely left to industry.

Nevertheless, as Sir Charles Harington said in a memorandum to the Council in 1957, its chemists should still "feel themselves under an obligation to be on the alert for any new idea in chemotherapy that may emerge and eager to develop any such idea as it comes within the range of their skill". Examples from the National Institute were Dr J. Walker's synthesis of pyrimethamine, leading to a method adopted for commercial use; and (earlier) Dr H. King's discovery of a series of diamidine compounds, on the basis of which the laboratories of a pharmaceutical firm developed a drug useful in the treatment of kala-azar.

Furthermore, it was considered that various studies of the biochemistry of bacteria, although not promoted with this end particularly in view, might at any time provide valuable clues in problems of chemotherapy. Several of the Council's research units have for long been engaged in such studies from different angles; and there has been work at the National Institute on such subjects as the biochemistry of the cell wall and bacterial interference. Work on bacterial genetics, also, is directly relevant to the important and intractable problem of drug resistance (see p. 110).

From bacteria, the chemotherapeutic attack has latterly been extended to viruses. Here the approach was seen to be intrinsically more difficult, since the multiplication of a virus depends on the metabolic processes of the normal cell which it invades; to inhibit or destroy the virus without damaging the host cells thus presents a formidable problem. Once again the hope lies in acquiring greater basic knowledge of the natural processes concerned; for instance, as the Report for 1962–63 put it, "the study of the biochemistry of viruses in tissue culture might well reveal features of cell metabolism that are favourable or unfavourable to virus growth".

Chemotherapy of cancer

This account of chemotherapy would not be complete without a brief mention of work on cancer, certain lines of which have been supported by the Council, notably at the Institute of Cancer Research, as described in the Report for 1962–63. Research on the fundamental chemical and biological processes of both malignant and normal cells, and the effects of specific drugs on them, is laying the foundations for a more rational approach to treatment which is thought to have greater promise of ultimate success than the empirical screening of compounds for anti-tumour activity. The now well established value of oestrogenic hormones in the control of certain kinds of cancer has been mentioned in an earlier section. An important contribution of the Council in this field, as in others, has been—and continues to be—the organisation of controlled clinical trials of different treatments, including various combinations of established drugs and other therapeutic agents. 'Immunotherapy' is a promising new approach but is still at an early stage of development (see Annual Report for 1972–73).

Antibiotics: penicillin

As Chain has pointed out, knowledge of the fundamental phenomenon of antagonism between different microorganisms goes back to Pasteur and Joubert in 1867. Many examples of this have been observed in academic laboratories; and occasional attempts were made to use it as a basis for preparing bactericidal agents against infections. The most notable instance occurred in 1929, when Professor (later Sir) Alexander Fleming of St Mary's Hospital, London, reported that as a result of an accidental contamination of a staphylococcal culture with a mould, he had observed dissolution of the bacteria by some product of the mould. He had then cultivated this mould—*Penicillium notatum*—on broth, which after a few days proved capable, even in high dilution, of preventing the growth of a number of bacterial species. He called this broth 'penicillin', a name since applied to the active principle which it contained. It was shown that the broth could be injected into animals without undue reactions; Fleming indeed noted that this was the first antiseptic in his experience that was substantially more harmful to bacteria than to tissue cells.

Fleming suggested that the penicillin broth might be useful for local application to infected wounds; these were at that time relatively uncommon in hospital wards but some patients were so treated, with favourable although not striking results. Work by Fleming himself and by others, during the next few years, showed that penicillin was difficult to manipulate chemically, and eventually the thought of producing a valuable therapeutic agent was discarded. As the Council's Report for 1939–45 says, "the idea of antibacterial chemotherapy was much less familiar in 1929 than it became later as a result of the introduction of the sulphonamides". As Hare (1970) has made clear, however, there is no good foundation for the suggestion of a novelist biographer that Fleming's abandonment of the quest was partly due to opposition by Almroth Wright as head of the laboratory.

Ten years after the initial discovery, the subject was reopened at the Sir William Dunn School of Pathology, University of Oxford; this was in 1939, but before the outbreak of the Second World War and without any direct relation thereto. A plan was drawn up by Dr E. B. (later Sir Ernst) Chain and Professor H. W. (later Sir Howard, eventually Lord) Florey for a comprehensive investigation, both chemical and biological, of some of the antibiotics known at that time. The products of three microorganisms were chosen for the first studies, but the work was soon concentrated on the product of *Penicillium notatum*. The problem, as left by Fleming and others some years before, was to purify a very unstable chemical substance to an extent, and in a form, that would enable it to be used as a therapeutic agent; and then to determine its efficacy and safety in that role.

The early promise of this new research on penicillin led to the gradual assembly of a team of workers for the various phases of the plan. They were named in the Council's Report for 1939–45 as follows: Professor Florey, Dr Chain, Professor A. D. Gardner, Dr N. G. Heatley, Dr E. P. Abraham, Dr M. A. Jennings, Dr Jean Orr-Ewing, Dr A. G. Saunders—and later, for the clinical work, Dr C. M. Fletcher and Dr M. E. (later Lady) Florey. The project was supported throughout by substantial grants from the Council, with contributions also from the Rockefeller Foundation of New York and the Nuffield Provincial Hospitals Trust.

The mould had first to be cultivated in adequate quantities; and under wartime conditions even such practical matters as the need for several hundred suitable culture vessels presented difficulty. (At one stage it was suggested that porcelain bed-pans might be admirable for the growing moulds, and when the point was explained at a meeting of Council one of the non-scientific members misheard 'moulds' as 'moles'; the mental picture thus evoked—rows of industrious little animals sitting in their appointed vessels making penicillin —was altogether too much for the gravity of the august body.)

A simple biological test was devised whereby the results of the chemical procedures could be followed. Then by a series of steps the penicillin was extracted and eventually prepared as a stable dry powder. This was found to be capable, in dilutions of one part in a million, of inhibiting growth *in vitro* of staphylococci, streptococci, gonococci and various other pathogenic bacteria. Yet, in the light of later knowledge, these early crude extracts contained only a minute proportion of the active substance.

The next phase was to test the bactericidal effect of injected solutions of penicillin on infections in the body. Favourable results in animals were reported in 1940—so rapidly had the work progressed—and in human beings in 1941. Penicillin was shown to be a true systemic chemotherapeutic agent that could, when absorbed into the blood stream after administration, arrest a distant or a generalised infection without itself harming the host. Different phases of the programme had been undertaken concurrently, so that by this time much was already known about the behaviour of penicillin in the body, including its absorption from various tissues and its excretion. Also, a unit of potency had been defined, so that the strength of different preparations could be compared; later this 'Oxford Unit', widely adopted, was replaced by an official International Penicillin Unit of approximately the same value.

The evidence of clinical success, however, was as yet based on the treatment of only a few patients, owing to the pitifully inadequate supplies of penicillin that the laboratory could provide. Under wartime conditions it was impossible to get any of the resources of commercial firms diverted to the project without more evidence of its importance; and without more penicillin the evidence could not be obtained. In this situation, everything possible was done to increase the production of the laboratory, by improvements in technique and by raising the scale of operation. In giving some account of this phase the Council's Report for 1939–45 said:

> The months spent in increasing the output, with all their disappointments and difficulties, are not likely to be forgotten by those involved. Undoubtedly the possibility that the drug might be of value in treating war injuries provided by this time a powerful stimulus to persevere. . . . All the early work was

HCMR—E

dominated by the struggle to accumulate a few hundred milligrammes of the impure material.

In the summer of 1941 Professor Florey and Dr Heatley went to the United States to secure the cooperation of manufacturers there, with their large resources. The American firms showed enterprise and energy in undertaking production; and by the middle of 1942 British firms were beginning to make such contribution as they could under the stress of war.

As somewhat larger amounts of penicillin became available, the scope of therapeutic trials could be increased. So long as the drug remained in short supply, however, the policy was to give priority to the treatment of infected war wounds. The clinical work thus developed in collaboration with the Army, and of it some account is given later (Chapter 15). With greater supplies subsequently, the trials were extended to other conditions. This phase was coordinated by the Council's Penicillin Clinical Trials Committee, under the chairmanship of Professor H. R. Dean; it had a distinguished membership, which included both Fleming and Florey. Eventually, in wide experience following successful commercial development of methods of production by deep culture, penicillin became firmly established as a chemotherapeutic agent of the first importance.

From an early stage, the experimental and clinical work was complemented by parallel investigations of the chemistry of penicillin. The object was to determine the chemical structure of penicillin, with a view to a possible synthetic method of production. To this end the Council appointed a Penicillin Synthesis Committee under the chairmanship of Professor Sir Robert Robinson. On it there were both academic workers and representatives of the research departments of manufacturing firms which had been invited to collaborate. This programme was later integrated with that of a similar consortium in the United States, under arrangements of which some account is given later (Chapter 11). The scientific results of the chemical work, on both sides of the Atlantic, were subsequently published in book form under international editorship (Clarke et al., 1949).

Fleming's discovery of the bactericidal effect of penicillin was even more fortuitous than has until recently been supposed. This has been brought out in a book by Professor Ronald Hare (1970), a worker in the department at the time, giving an account of a retrospective investigation of the circumstances. As he says, if the bactericidal effect of contamination by the mould could have become apparent on any bacterial culture plate put aside, the discovery would have been made while Fleming was still a child. He himself made attempts to reconstruct the phenomenon that gave him the essential clue, but always without success. The effect, indeed, becomes manifest only when a particular combination of favourable conditions is present; these relate to such factors as the maturity of the bacterial colonies and the ambient temperature prevailing. Furthermore, it seems likely that the timely arrival of airborne spores of the particular species of mould was due to the fact that some quite unrelated work with *Penicillium notatum* happened to be in progress in another laboratory on the floor below. Nothing in this, of course, in any way affects the importance of the discovery; nor does it appear either to augment or diminish the merit of Fleming's hand in it.

The general public, led by the popular press, has no doubt gone too far in regarding Fleming as the sole 'discoverer' of penicillin— as in a purely literal sense he was—and in being impatient of the qualification that he did nothing effective to bring his finding to practical fruition. At the opposite extreme are those who discount the merit of a purely accidental discovery, thereafter left to others to exploit by planned and laborious investigations. In fact, Fleming was, by temperament and experience, just the man to strike gold in this field. He was essentially a lone worker, a little man with a soft Scots voice, and unassuming even though he latterly blossomed in the rays of fame. During the First World War he worked for the Medical Research Committee, first at St Mary's Hospital and then at Boulogne (Chapter 14); he made special studies of various groups of chemical antiseptics, for which he obtained quantitative values both of bactericidal efficiency and of toxic effects upon body cells. Then in 1922, back in his post at St Mary's, he discovered lysozyme by observing the rapid clearing of a turbid suspension of bacteria on addition of a drop of nasal mucus, and he found it to be an enzyme which catalytically promotes lysis of bacteria; it is now known to be one of a group of such enzymes occurring in a wide range of secretions of animal and plant origin. The finding found no practical application, but is evidence of a mind attuned to appreciate such phenomena. If this and the later discovery were purely accidental, then Fleming was accident-prone! The great Pasteur had an analogous stroke of good fortune in making one of his discoveries and made the comment (1854) that *"Dans les champs de l'observation, le hasard ne favorise que les esprits préparés"*.

When the work of Florey and his colleagues eventually brought penicillin as a boon to mankind, Fleming rightly received his share of the scientific and public acclaim, and of the many honours that this brought—Nobel Prize, knighthood, and much else. He thoroughly enjoyed—and why not?—this late phase of his working life; and he travelled widely to receive honorary degrees and other awards.

Howard Walter Florey, who died in 1968, was born in Australia in 1898 and came to Britain as a graduate of the University of Adelaide. He held a succession of academic posts and had to his credit a long series of distinguished researches, planned with care and pursued with vigour. He received a Nobel Prize and a knighthood simultaneously with Fleming. Later he attained other high

honours—President of the Royal Society, the Order of Merit, Chancellor of the National University of Australia, a Life Peerage. His
principal colleague, Chain, now Sir Ernst Chain, who also received
a Nobel Prize, has latterly held a chair at the Imperial College of
Science, London.

Other antibiotics

The next phase was acclaimed by the Council in its Report for
1945–48:

> The British discovery, during the war, of the remarkable effect of penicillin in
> preventing and curing many acute and chronic infections has had an impor-
> tance going beyond its own contribution to the saving of life and limb. For
> penicillin has proved to be only the first of a whole series of naturally occurring
> antimicrobial agents, now known as antibiotics, and its successful application in
> medicine has opened a new and most hopeful era in chemotherapy.

There was room for alternatives to penicillin in dealing with resistant strains of bacterial species usually sensitive to its action; and
there remained a need for antibiotics effective against species outside
its range, such as the tubercle bacillus and the intestinal bacteria of
the coliform group.

The American discovery of streptomycin in 1944 introduced a
therapeutic agent that was of substantial value in the treatment of
tuberculosis, although subject to serious drawbacks. Some account
of the trials of it organised under the Council's auspices is given
later (Chapter 11).

In the first generation of post-penicillin antibiotics there were also
chloromycetin, aureomycin and terramycin—all mould products of
American origin. Of these and others the Council said in its Report
for 1949–50:

> All the new antibiotics have a useful range of activity against pathogenic
> bacteria. Still more significant, however, is the fact that they are also effective
> against rickettsial diseases, such as typhus and scrub-typhus fevers, and even
> against some virus infections. They have therefore opened up a new field of
> chemotherapy and have resolved the doubt, frequently expressed on theoretical
> grounds, whether diseases caused by these infective agents could be susceptible
> to chemotherapeutic attack. Rickettsiae and viruses must resemble very closely
> in their requirements the cells of the host and it is therefore surprising to find
> that chemical compounds exist which can destroy the infective agent and at the
> same time have little or no ill effect on the infected organism.

Meanwhile the search for still other antibiotics had passed the stage
of "holding out suppliant Petri dishes", as Florey himself pic-
turesquely put it, and was involving soil surveys on which the
pharmaceutical industry, especially in the United States, was spending large sums.

The Council's own later programme included much work in the
search for new antibiotics, and in determining their value and
limitations. Florey and his co-workers at Oxford remained especially

active in this field, and among other things were responsible for all the cephalosporins. It was largely for the production of newly discovered substances of this kind, in quantities adequate for testing on more than a laboratory scale, that the Council acquired, and for some years maintained, premises and plant at Clevedon, Somerset, for an Antibiotics Research Station. This scheme was eventually abandoned in favour of contracting out 'semi-scale' production to the Microbiological Research Establishment of the Ministry of Defence at Porton, Wiltshire.

Chapter 4
Curative Medicine: Therapeutic Agents (Physical)

Radiotherapy: radium sources—Radiotherapy: machines—Biological effects of radiation—Non-ionising radiations—Instruments and appliances—Oxygen chambers and breathing machines—Hearing aids—Diagnostic equipment—Biological engineering

Radiotherapy: radium sources
The entry of the Medical Research Committee into research on radiotherapy, particularly of cancer, was largely due to the availability of a quantity of radium at the close of the First World War. The circumstances are recounted in the Committee's Report for 1918–19:

> The Ministry of Munitions, through their Optical Munitions Department, offered to deposit with the Committee under agreed conditions a few grammes of radium salt, which, for this substance, is a very large quantity, during the period between its collection from innumerable gun-sights, watch dials, and other instruments of war, and its final disposal for other purposes. The Committee gratefully accepted this modern instance of turning swords into ploughshares.

The story and the metaphor are pleasing—but illusory! The radium had not been recovered as salvage, as at first believed, but was in fact stock awaiting use when the war came to an end. In the event, the radium was not merely lent but was transferred to the ownership of the Committee, from the Disposal Board of the Ministry, for a sum of £72 500 specially provided by HM Treasury—a 'book transaction' (Volume One).

The quantity was nearly 5 grams of radium bromide, equivalent to about $2\frac{1}{2}$ grams of radium; in these early days amounts were customarily expressed in terms of salt, although later in terms of element. This, according to the Report already quoted, was about ten times as much as any amount previously available for similar work. And in its Report for 1919–20 the Committee made this comment:

> Hitherto the opportunities of inquiry have been closely limited by the high cost of radium; radium made available by private benefaction has not always been distributed with a view to scientific use, and the effects produced by it have not always been recorded or recorded completely. There has been little systematic study of its curative properties, and empiricism still in large part governs radio-therapy.

Formal ownership having been transferred, the next step was to gain physical possession of the valuable and dangerous material; and for a
58

short while this proved to be unexpectedly difficult. The Ministry of Munitions was in the throes of dissolution; and the present writer (on one of his earliest assignments) had the experience of being referred from one to another of its offices scattered over London, each in the process of closing down. Eventually the radium was located in a chemist's shop in Clapham (South London) owned by Mr F. Harrison Glew. This remarkable man had apparently been acting as broker in the purchase of radium for the Government; he also personally manipulated the material in his own laboratory, filling it into such containers as might be required. He continued for some years to perform this latter office for the Council, but he developed a neoplastic condition of the hands; in respect of this disability, the Council was able to procure for him a small Civil List pension. Mr Glew died in 1926.

There was also, at the outset, some difficulty in effecting insurance cover against loss of the material. The companies were unwilling to quote, owing to lack of experience of insuring radium and to ignorance of its properties. Lloyds underwriters eventually wrote a policy which excluded loss by explosion or spontaneous combustion; these 'non-risks' were gladly accepted by the owners!

It was decided that the whole quantity should in the first place be used at the Middlesex Hospital and be placed under the control of Professor W. S. Lazarus-Barlow, Mr C. R. C. Lyster and Professor Sidney Russ—the last named being a physicist and for many years the Council's chief technical adviser on radium. A report on this phase of the work was published in 1922; and in its own Report for 1922–23 the Council said:

> One of the principal conclusions drawn in this preliminary report is that for progress in the treatment of malignant disease by radium therapy it is essential that the investigation should be directed towards the quantitative determination of the means which give particular results.

This was an important consideration, as it was known that too little as well as too much radiation might worsen the patient's condition. The actual therapeutic results in this phase of the investigation inevitably reflected the limitation that in the main only surgically inoperable cases, many in an advanced stage of the disease, were treated with radium.

The next phase began with the distribution of fractions of the radium among a number of centres selected on the basis of schemes submitted—University College Hospital, St Bartholomew's Hospital, the Middlesex Hospital, King's College Hospital, the London Hospital, and the Radium Institute—all in London; the General Hospital, Birmingham; the King Edward VII Hospital (later the Royal Infirmary), Cardiff; the Royal Infirmary, Aberdeen; and the Council for Public Health for Ireland, Dublin. Within the next few years further centres were added: St Peter's Hospital, the Marie Curie Hospital and St Mark's Hospital, in London;

and the Royal Infirmary, Manchester. Each portion was filled into a number of minute needles of platinum for interstitial treatment, these being temporarily inserted in the growth by a surgeon; a few flat applicators were also filled for surface treatment. The Irish fraction was placed in solution in the laboratories of the Royal Dublin Society as a source of radium emanation, containers holding the latter being issued for treatment.

The whole scheme was coordinated by the Radiology Committee, set up by the Council with Sir Cuthbert Wallace as its first chairman and Professor Russ as secretary. Later, this Committee also regularly advised the British Empire Cancer Campaign and was regarded as jointly appointed. The Committee received annual reports from the treatment centres and prepared a summary. The summary for 1922 was printed for private circulation to those taking part in the work, but thereafter the summaries were published in the Council's series; that for 1938 was the seventeenth and last. Latterly, by courtesy of the Radium Commission, King Edward's Hospital Fund for London, and the British Empire Cancer Campaign, the reports covered all patients treated at the participating centres, irrespective of the ownership of the radium used.

In 1924, a grant from the British Empire Cancer Campaign enabled the Council to buy an additional $\frac{1}{2}$ gram of radium salt for extension of the work in certain directions considered to be urgently desirable. Another grant from the Campaign covered the initial and current cost of an emanation service established by the Council at the Middlesex Hospital; about one gram of radium salt belonging to the Council was there put into solution as a source of emanation ('radon'). Around this time, the Council was also promoting experimental work on the biological effects of irradiation, notably by Dr T. S. P. Strangeways, Dr Malcolm Donaldson, Dr R. G. Canti and Professor F. L. Hopwood at the Research Hospital, Cambridge (later the Strangeways Research Laboratory).

Although successful treatment of a malignant growth by irradiation had been reported as long ago as 1899, the physical properties of the radiation used were not well enough understood, and the apparatus for producing it was not sufficiently reliable, for much progress to be made. Work with radium such as that promoted by the Council, and paralleled in other countries, was now gradually transforming the outlook. In its Report for 1927–28 the Council said: "As radium treatment has won its way from inoperable to operable and earlier cases, its successes have multiplied and the growth of faith in it has been both justified and accelerated." There was thus an increasing demand for radium, and in the same publication the Committee of Privy Council for Medical Research, over the signature of the Earl of Balfour, stated the position as follows:

It has become obvious that the present supply of radium is wholly insufficient for the needs of the population, having regard to the known incidence of cancer in its various forms. In view of the results already achieved, and the high probability that these are only the beginning of still further gains, the claims of the people for an increased supply of radium become paramount.

The Committee of Privy Council went on to record that the Committee of Civil Research had in 1928 appointed a Radium Sub-committee under the chairmanship of Lord Rayleigh; this included representatives of the departments interested in adequate provision of radium for military and civil purposes.

In the following year the Committee of Privy Council was able to record that, on the recommendation of the Subcommittee of the Committee of Civil Research, the Government had decided to establish a National Radium Trust. This chartered body included both ministerial and other members, with the Lord President as chairman. Its function was the acquisition and formal ownership of radium; and it had an official of the Ministry of Health as its secretary. Under it was a Radium Commission "to make arrangements for the custody, distribution, and use of the radium acquired by the Trust". To this working body the Council appointed one commissioner—in the first place the present writer, and later Dr F. H. K. Green. The Commission's office, demolished by a bomb during the Second World War, stood on part of the site in Park Crescent (London W.1) now occupied by the Council's own headquarters. Eventually, the functions of Trust and Commission passed to the National Health Service; but meanwhile, the Cancer Act 1939 had provided for expenditure of public funds on making radium therapy more widely available—although without provision for the control by parallel research that the Council believed to be necessary (Volume One).

By 1933 developments abroad, especially in Stockholm and Paris, had shown the need for further work on the use of gamma rays from massive quantities of radium—known as 'radium beam therapy' or 'teleradium therapy', the rays being directed on the growth as a beam from a radium source external to the body. To this end was created an organisation curiously styled 'The Radium Beam Therapy Research', controlled by an unincorporated 'governing body' purporting to represent the Council, the Department of Scientific and Industrial Research, the Royal Society, the Royal College of Surgeons of England, the Royal College of Physicians of London, the Radium Commission and the Radium Institute, London. The constitution and nomenclature were the invention of Lord Dawson of Penn, to whose energy and diplomacy the cooperative effort was largely due. The scheme was made administratively feasible by the adoption of the governing body as a joint Research Board of the Council and the Department, the former exercising the main responsibility.

For this work, 8¾ grams of radium element were lent to the Council by the Union Minière du Haut Katanga, the important mining company operating in what was then the Belgian Congo. A further one gram was lent by the Royal College of Surgeons; and the total available was about 10 grams (in terms of element). Grants towards the cost were made by the Royal Colleges and by the British Empire Cancer Campaign, and there were also donations. The Radium Institute provided accommodation for patients and nursing staff. The team was directed by Dr Constance Wood.

At first much time was necessarily given to developing methods of dosage measurement and control, and for the protection of patients. A few inoperable growths of the mouth, tongue, pharynx and larynx were treated, and after four years the results were sufficiently encouraging to warrant further exploration of the possibilities. The Council's Report for 1937–38 mentions a proposal to compare the effects of the 10-gram radium beam with those of high-voltage X-rays, for which apparatus had now been developed. (A report by Wood and Boag on this comparison, in respect of oral cancer, was published in the Council's series in 1950.) The Report also refers to a "looming" need for work on the effects of a neutron beam, and on those of temporarily radioactive substances such as radiosodium; these new possibilities followed the invention and developments of the cyclotron by Lawrence at Berkeley, California (where Dr F. G. Spear of the Council's staff was sent to acquire information).

Then came the Second World War, and work with radium had to be greatly restricted owing to the risk that a high-explosive bomb might dissipate quantities of radioactive dust. The material was kept at the bottom of boreholes, 50 feet deep, that had been prepared at various hospitals in London. The Radon Centre at the Middlesex Hospital was moved to a deep cave at Barton-in-the-Clay, Bedfordshire, as also was the London Hospital radon plant and, later, a 'Hospitals Radon Centre'; there all three operated together under the general direction of Professor Russ. In 1941 the Council assumed full control of the Radium Beam Therapy Research, which became its Radiotherapeutic Research Unit, with Dr Constance Wood as Director; and in 1942 the radium lent by the Union Minière was acquired by the National Radium Trust and left at the Council's disposal.

Radiotherapy: machines
Just as the availability of a supply of radium left over from the First World War had provided the opportunity for the Council's entry to this field of research, so did the existence of much new physical knowledge after the Second World War afford a basis for major developments of the programme. As the Council said in its Report for 1939–45:

> The access of knowledge of nuclear physics in recent years, made manifest in the atomic bomb, has created new possibilities in the application of physical methods to the study of medical and other biological problems, and the development of research on this subject has been one of the Council's most important post-war tasks. There is, in the first place, the further study of radiations as

curative agents in cancer and other diseases. Secondly, there is need to determine the toxic and lethal effects of radio-active substances and to devise methods for protecting the body against these. Thirdly, the use of radio-active or stable isotopes of various chemical elements as 'tracers' is of great value in the elucidation of biological function and provides new methods for the study of many fundamental problems of physiology and biochemistry. Before long, isotopes also found a place in the clinical diagnosis of disease, and to a limited extent in treatment.

To exploit this situation as fully as possible, the Council in 1945 appointed a strong Committee on the Medical and Biological Applications of Nuclear Physics, with Sir Henry Dale as chairman. This worked chiefly in three subcommittees, concerned with the three divisions of the field mentioned in the foregoing quotation; these subcommittees had as their respective chairmen Lord Horder, Sir Ernest Rock Carling and Sir Charles Harington.

On the therapeutic side this was the dawn of the era of the giant machines—as one might say, 'the age of the dinosaurs'. Of these, the Council said in its Report for 1945–48:

> Physical research has led to the development of machines which accelerate electrons to extremely high velocities and are therefore capable of generating very penetrating X-radiation. . . . It would be expected that the X-radiation generated somewhere between 10 and 50 million volts would give the radiotherapist the greatest scope for securing the desired distribution of dose round a cancerous growth.

These costly monsters all had different characteristics; for all of them claims of potential value in therapy could be made; and, where the stake was so high as in the fight against cancer, all had to be put to the test.

In 1949 it was decided to equip the Council's Radiotherapeutic Research Unit at Hammersmith Hospital with an 8-megavolt linear accelerator as a powerful source of X-rays. The machine was made for the Council by Metropolitan Vickers Limited, at a cost of £68 000, and became operational in 1953. In the Unit also, in the period 1950–57, a 45-inch cyclotron was built at a cost of £86 000. This was not at first for the treatment of patients but was for experimental work on the biological effects of its beam of alpha particles and deuterons, and also for the production of radioactive substances for purposes of research. Its operation involved the services of an engineering staff, and it had to be housed in a specially designed building with elaborate precautions against radiation hazards to persons in the vicinity; while in action it was under remote control. Since 1962 it has been in the hands of a Cyclotron Unit providing short-lived radioactive substances and radiation for collaborative research. Since 1965 the neutron beam has been used for clinical trials of fast neutron therapy.

The Council also provided, at a cost of £78 000, two 30-megavolt synchrotrons made by the English Electric Company Limited.

These were installed at the Institute of Cancer Research, London, and at Addenbrooke's Hospital, Cambridge; they became operational in 1949 and 1950 respectively. In 1953 the Council instituted a Betatron Research Group (later Unit) under the honorary direction of Professor Ralston Paterson at the Christie Hospital and Holt Radium Institute, Manchester; the object was to explore the clinical application of radiation from a 20-megavolt betatron presented by the makers, Metropolitan-Vickers Ltd. All of these machines, especially the synchrotrons and the betatron, presented frequent technical difficulties; and in time the giants had had their day.

It was eventually concluded that the future of radiotherapy lay with the linear accelerator, but not necessarily of such high voltage. It was in fact 4-megavolt linear accelerators that were made available through the National Health Service for routine treatment. At this stage, radiotherapy largely passed out of the field of intensive research into that of hospital practice. The Radiotherapeutic and the Betatron Research Units were disbanded in 1962.

Biological effects of radiation
Another post-war development was a greatly increased effort in research directed towards a fuller understanding of the biological effects of irradiation. New knowledge was clearly required both to guide the medical use of radiations and to devise protective measures against radiation hazards of all kinds. The keystone of this programme was the Radiobiological Research Unit established by the Council in 1947, with Dr J. F. Loutit as director, at the Atomic Energy Research Establishment at Harwell in Berkshire—but outside its security perimeter. The general subject is the action of ionising radiations on living cells; and particular attention is being paid to fast neutrons, X-rays and gamma radiation (now under the direction of Dr R. H. Mole).

Investigations of a similar kind but with a direct bearing on radiotherapy—and indeed made in close association with the Radiotherapeutic Research Unit—were undertaken by an Experimental Radiopathology Research Unit; this was established by the Council at Hammersmith Hospital in 1953, with Dr G. J. Popjak as the first director. What later became the Clinical Effects of Radiation Research Unit at the Western General Hospital, Edinburgh, was set up by the Council in 1956 under the direction of Dr W. M. Court Brown. The work was particularly concerned with the delayed effects of radiation exposure in man, with human cytogenetics, and with the application of experimental virological techniques to the study of human tumours.

Reference to the Environmental Radiation Research Unit and to the Radiological Protection Service is made later (Chapter 6).

The Council's early work on the use of isotopes in experimental studies was mainly centred on the National Institute for Medical Research, but later the use of the techniques was widespread. What became the Bone-seeking Isotopes Research Unit, under the honorary direction of Dame Janet Vaughan, was established by the Council at the Churchill Hospital, Oxford, in 1959. The diagnostic and therapeutic use of radioisotopes was a special interest of the Council's Department of Clinical Research at University College Hospital, London; its director, Dr E. E. (now Sir Edward) Pochin, was a pioneer of the treatment of thyroid cancer with radioiodine.

The Council's Report for 1968–69 included a special review by a Radiobiology Committee, appointed for the purpose, under the chairmanship of Professor W. D. M. Paton. This summarised the current situation with regard to radiation protection, radiotherapy, and the mechanics of radiation injury, and made recommendations for future policy.

Non-ionising radiations

At the beginning of 1922 the Council appointed a Committee on the Biological Actions of Light, with Professor Sir William Bayliss as chairman. Its function was to advise and assist the Council in "more active promotion and better coordination of the scattered inquiries into the actions of light upon the human body in health and disease which have recently been undertaken in various directions". The latter included the sunlight treatment of tuberculosis. Investigations were initiated into the specific effects of light and its constituent rays on the body fluids and tissues, and their simpler components, and also on bacteria and protozoa both inside and outside the human body, and on blood *in vitro*. Much of the work was done at the National Institute for Medical Research, particularly in Dr (later Sir) Leonard Hill's department. There was also grant-aided work on the effect of sunlight on blood platelets at Montana, Switzerland; and work at the Lister Institute of Preventive Medicine and by the mission sent to Vienna in these early post-war years (Chapter 5).

In 1925 Professor F. A. Lindemann (later Lord Cherwell) became chairman of the special committee. Two subcommittees were appointed—one to determine simple and accurate methods of measuring the energy of ultraviolet rays of different wave-lengths, whether in sunlight or from artificial sources, and the second to study therapeutic and other biological effects. In its Report for 1927–28 the Council (after discussing liver treatment for pernicious anaemia) opened a review of the therapeutic aspect as follows:

Another new mode of therapeutic treatment, very different in its sanctions, has lately come widely into use in this country with a rapidity not hitherto common even for the best attested therapeutic novelties. This is medical treatment by artificial ultraviolet light (as distinguished from sunlight), which is now advocated and used, as all know, in a great variety of serious or mild disorders. Great sums of private and public money are being expended upon it and large new commercial and professional interests are involved.

Meanwhile, the cult of ultraviolet radiation had received a fresh impetus from the discovery, at the National Institute for Medical Research in 1927, that the rays could convert the substance ergosterol into a potent form of vitamin D, as described later. The Report already quoted proceeds as follows:

> The discovery of this powerful intervention of sunlight in nutrition led naturally to the suggestion, and even to the expectation, that it might act beneficially in other unrevealed ways. Since the invisible rays of ultraviolet 'light' were found to hold the nutritive properties of sunlight, it was natural to suspect that artificial lamps, rich in ultraviolet rays, might be an effective substitute for the missing sunshine in our cities. It was hoped that it might have other beneficial effects on child life besides its indirect value in supplying a vital food constituent. Heavy expenditure was soon incurred in the provision of lamp treatment in many schools and institutions. Since the children under treatment varied much in their states of nutrition, the results reported were in general, as was to be expected, widely conflicting or uncertain.

The question had therefore to be put to scientific test. In 1925 the Council provided statistical help in a controlled trial, organised by the British Medical Association, of the effect of ultraviolet treatment on children of subnormal physique in the East End of London. In the winter of 1927–28 Dr Dora Colebrook, of the Council's external staff, made a similar controlled trial on school-children in Willesden (north-west London), with the approval of the Board of Education and the Borough Council. The results of both these trials were wholly negative; and the Council's review sums up as follows:

> The Council are aware of no properly controlled experiments which have been made elsewhere to set against these two series. The last report of the Chief Medical Officer of the Ministry of Health shows that the results collected from Artificial Light Centres provided by local authorities exhibit much variation of opinion, as we should expect for the reasons just given; but no objective evidence is provided that results have been achieved that could not have been far more cheaply gained by proper food, and if that be so it is obvious that exercise and fresh air are greatly preferable to indoor sessions around a lamp.

The point was further pressed home with the economic argument:

> The use of artificial light to supply only what the right food can give is merely wasteful. It commonly costs three or four shillings to give by light an effective supply of vitamin D that would cost less than a penny if given by the mouth in the form of cod-liver oil or otherwise.

Then, sweeping up the debris of ultraviolet radiation therapy, the Report concluded:

> The only other medical uses of 'light' radiations which have already a basis in physiology depend upon their power of exciting a local inflammatory reaction in the skin, the severity and extent of which can be controlled and graded with some precision. . . . Moreover, exactly the same effects for good or evil follow inflammation of the skin blood-vessels inflicted by heat or by other irritants than light. There is no present reason to know that artificial light can do more in this way than a mustard plaster, which is indefinitely cheaper.

That "mustard plaster" stung! The phrase was seized upon by the press; and, predictably, there were angry reactions from vested interests and from devout slaves of the lamp. But nobody today would question that a salutary exercise in 'debunking' had been effectively performed.

Later, Dr Colebrook made further trials of 'artificial sunlight' in three working environments—an office, a factory and a coalmine— where the natural light of day was deficient or lacking. Regular treatment of some subjects by mercury vapour lamps was controlled by the exposure of others to apparently similar lamps from which no ultraviolet rays were in fact emitted, as well as by the records of still others who received no treatment at all. The results, again quite negative, were published as a report of the Industrial Health Research Board in 1946. Still later, an Air Hygiene Committee appointed by the Council returned to the question, seeing that negative results are not necessarily valid over a wide range of conditions. In this investigation, of which a report was published in the Council's series in 1954, it was found that ultraviolet irradiation of school classrooms reduced the numbers of airborne bacteria, but that any effect of this reduction on sickness absenteeism was insufficient to justify recommending widespread use of the method.

Scientific interest in ultraviolet and other non-ionising radiations was not confined to this aspect. It seems somewhat ironical, however, that attention gradually veered from their putative benefits to their possible hazards. In 1944 the Council approved a proposal for initiating and coordinating quantitative studies of the non-ionising radiations, with particular reference to their medical applications. A special committee for the purpose was set up under the chairmanship of Professor H. Hartridge. In 1948 this body decided to meet in two separate divisions, one dealing with infrared and ultraviolet radiations and the other with radiofrequency. It was disbanded in 1951. In 1958 a Committee on the Possible Hazards of 'Microwave' Radiations was appointed, under the chairmanship of Professor G. Payling Wright; and in 1966 it was reconstituted as a Non-Ionising Radiations Committee, with Professor A. R. Currie in the chair, specifically to advise on safety standards and to stimulate research to that end. The Committee has been studying the hazards involved in the diagnostic and industrial uses of microwaves (e.g. lasers) and ultrasonics.

Oxygen chambers and breathing machines
The study of some medical problems of chemical warfare during the First World War led to important new investigations in the physiology of respiration, and especially of the effects of deficiency in the oxygen supply to the body; and at Cambridge Mr (later Sir) Joseph Barcroft and others studied the effects of oxygen administration to patients with damaged lungs. Two oxygen chambers that had been installed by the Medical Research Committee at the North Staffordshire

Infirmary, Stoke-on-Trent, were used for the treatment of industrial workers who had been accidentally gassed, and for patients
suffering from pneumonia and pernicious anaemia. This scheme was
brought to completion soon after the war, but in 1920 the Council
provided part of the expense of installing an oxygen chamber in a
ward at Guy's Hospital, London, and made grants for various other
projects. This programme was coordinated by a Clinical Uses of
Oxygen Committee set up by the Council under the chairmanship
of Professor T. R. Elliott. It was brought into relation with an
Oxygen Research Committee appointed by the Department of
Scientific and Industrial Research to deal with the chemical, physical
and engineering aspects of the problems of oxygen use, as without
further progress in these fields the medical uses of oxygen would
clearly be restricted.

In 1938, following a request from the Ministry of Health for
guidance, the Council appointed a Committee under the chairmanship of Professor L. J. Witts to advise on the best type of breathing
machine for use in cases of respiratory paralysis. The report of this
Committee was published by the Council and in it were discussed
the advantages of the different types of machine available, the kind
of assistance required for their operation, and the policy to be adopted
in order to meet sudden demands for supply.

Britain's first large epidemic of poliomyelitis, in 1947, gave further
impetus to the quest for more satisfactory respirators, or breathing
machines, than the 'iron lung' introduced much earlier in America
and used in various conditions, or than the lighter model devised in
Australia. In the early part of the century poliomyelitis had been
chiefly a disease of childhood, with paralysis usually limited to the
limbs; the respiratory form, especially in adolescents and adults,
was a more recent phenomenon, of which there was insufficient
experience.

The upshot was a great burst of invention of new or improved
forms of respirator and of ancillary equipment. Some machines were
cabinet respirators, others were cuirass respirators allowing the
patient some mobility; some made use of negative pressure, as
before, and some of intermittent positive pressure, while others made
use of the rocking-bed principle. To all this the Council's workers
made a substantial contribution, and much of the effort was centred
on its Electro-medical Research Unit at Stoke Mandeville directed
by Dr R. B. Bourdillon of its staff. An account of the programme is
given in the Report for 1956–57, concluding as follows:

The part played by the Council in research on the design of respirators to meet
important and increasing needs may be briefly summarised as follows. A
preliminary assessment of the situation by a Council Committee in 1939 was
followed by the 1950 Special Report to the Council which pointed the way to
exact measurement of respiratory factors, and led to a standard performance
specification for new respirators. The principles so elucidated ultimately led,
with assistance from other sources, to the development in this country of

unsurpassed models of new respirators and ancillary equipment. Although the results in the treatment of respiratory poliomyelitis cannot yet be precisely measured, it is gratifying to note that the mortality from this form of the disease has shown a steady fall over the past 10 years, and in the last year or two has reached record low figures.

The medical uses of oxygen again became of concern to the Council in 1964, when it called a conference to consider hyperbaric oxygen therapy. It was concluded that the technique of using oxygen, or air, under high pressure—for example in operative surgery or in respiratory disorders of the newborn—needed careful evaluation and further experiment, with due regard also to the hazards of hyperbaric chambers. To keep this rapidly developing subject under continuous review, a standing advisory committee was set up by the Council in 1966, with Professor (later Sir) Hedley Atkins as chairman—shortly succeeded by Sir John McMichael. The Council also has a Radiotherapy and Hyperbaric Oxygen Working Party.

Hearing aids
In 1943, with the new National Health Service in prospect, the Ministry of Health consulted the Council on the question of hearing aids for the large number of people, estimated at over a half a million in England and Wales, handicapped by some substantial degree of deafness. The Council had for long promoted research on the advice of its Committee on the Physiology of Hearing, and this body had produced several reports including one on the use of hearing aids. The Council then took further steps.

Firstly, an Otological Research Unit was established at the National Hospital for Nervous Diseases, London, and Mr C. S. Hallpike—already a member of the Council's staff—appointed as its Director. Secondly, the former Committee was replaced in 1944 by a group of three interlocking committees to assist in planning and coordinating investigations, in the Unit or elsewhere, into the prevention, treatment and relief of deafness. These consisted of experts in the different disciplines involved, and they dealt respectively with electro-acoustical questions, with medical and surgical problems, and with the educational treatment of deafness.

The Electro-Acoustics Committee was asked by the Council, at the instance of the Ministry of Health, "to advise upon the design, performance and application of electro-acoustic equipment used in the investigation and alleviation of deafness", and if possible to devise a hearing aid of standard performance which could be used with advantage by a large proportion of the deaf people in the country. In this special task, the Committee and Unit had the help of the Post Office Engineering Research Station and of the National Physical Laboratory, and also of the Department of Education of the Deaf in the University of Manchester. After two years of intensive work, the Committee was able to recommend a new type of hearing aid of high efficiency and light weight, capable of being produced

HCMR—F

cheaply in large quantities and expected to help a good proportion of the deaf population. The Committee's report, which also gave performance specifications for pure-tone audiometers for the assessment of deafness, was published in the Council's series in 1947. Thereafter, arrangements for the manufacture of the instruments were made by the Ministry of Health and the Ministry of Supply, the former also undertaking the distribution and servicing of the aids (to which the identifying name 'Medresco' was given); the Electro-Acoustics Committee remained available to advise. Free issue of the aids through the National Health Service began in 1948. Other work on hearing is mentioned later (Chapter 6).

Diagnostic equipment
Other instruments which the Council has been concerned in developing have been diagnostic rather than directly therapeutic in their purposes. To give a single example, support was given to a project concerned with the design of a mass spectrometer suitable for respiratory investigations; this was in the department of Professor (later Sir) John McMichael at the Postgraduate Medical School of London, and began in 1952. The requirement was a means of readily determining the continually fluctuating process of gaseous exchange in the lungs without the use of bulky apparatus. To quote the Council's Report for 1955–56, "the practical difficulties . . . compared with the simplicity of collecting blood or urine for liver or kidney function tests, may well explain the relative neglect of lung function studies in clinical medicine". The spectrometric analysis of a mixture of gases by separating the different molecules according to their mass was by no means new, but the available apparatus was unsuited to clinical use. The new project, after five years of design and trial, resulted in a fully engineered prototype of a mobile machine well adapted to the particular purpose.

Biological engineering
As the Council said in its Report for 1961–62, "the unlovely labels 'bioengineering' and 'biological engineering' have been attached to an activity which is concerned with the application of engineering techniques to medicine and the biological sciences"; the term 'biomechanics' has also been used. The subject has come into prominence in recent years with increasing need for its service. According to the same Report, "the ultimate boundaries of scientific research and of scientific practice will always be set by the availability of instruments, techniques and apparatus".

For long the medical research worker's needs for special equipment could be met largely by his own ingenuity and the help of a workshop technician and glassblower. Latterly, however, instrumentation has become more complicated, mainly owing to the growing use of electronics. The biologist's taste for 'gadgetry' thus ceased to be adequate for ancillary tasks of increasing sophistication, and it was in any event more economical of his time to provide him with specialist aid in the exploitation of new technical developments for the purposes of his particular research. It thus became the Council's policy to create special departments for the development of new techniques of instrumentation; these differ from the old-style workshops in having one or more members of staff who themselves have the status of senior scientific workers, and who have had some biological training in addition to their engineering qualifications. The function of such a department is to advise on the choice of commercially available equipment; to design new apparatus; to arrange for the commercial exploitation of any such new items as may seem to have general utility; and to apply "a measure of informed criticism" to the demands of the biologists.

The Council maintains two main laboratories fulfilling this sort of function: the Engineering Division of the National Institute for Medical Research and the Division of Bioengineering of the Clinical Research Centre (formerly of the National Institute). Many of the Council's other establishments have extensive workshops serving their specialised needs. The National Institute also had a Laboratory for Human Biomechanics, concerned with research work of its own rather than with providing a service for others.

In the Council's programme, the recent developments of instrumental design have followed two main directions—apparatus for the investigation of biological systems of ever decreasing size; and apparatus allowing measurements to be made on the intact animal or man under, as nearly as possible, the conditions of normal life. An example of the latter type is the radio pill—a subminiature radiotransmitter with a self-contained power supply and transducer, the whole small enough to be swallowed. Pills can be made sensitive to pressure, to temperature or to acidity–alkalinity levels. They are used clinically for diagnostic purposes, as well as in experimental work. On a very different physical scale is a version of the whole-body plethysmograph, an instrument which measures cardiac output without any direct contact with the circulation.

The subject has its place in this chapter because many of the devices have diagnostic or therapeutic as well as experimental uses—others that relate to the social environment rather than to the human body are mentioned later. On the purely experimental side, however, mention may be made of the construction of analogues—physical models in which biological processes can be simulated, with ready means of changing particular variables until the results match those obtained from biological experiment but less easily interpreted in that context. In such a model condensers may be substituted for tissue spaces, resistances for diffusion barriers, short circuits for excretory channels, and electricity for an injected substance; more sophisticated components also play various roles.

The replacement of a lost limb or other part by an artificial prosthesis goes back historically to the peg leg and the iron hook. Up to almost the present time, however, the most elaborate artificial limb had no equivalent of muscles within itself; any movement of joints had to be produced at the attachment or by external means. Members of the Council's staff, among others, have been concerned in the development of limbs containing pistons performing the function of muscles; these are operated by compressed carbon dioxide from small cylinders carried by the wearer, the movements being controlled by valves activated by some intact part of the body. (Pneumatic 'muscles' can also be applied externally to reinforce an intact natural limb weakened by paralysis.) The main technical difficulties in design are to achieve a favourable power-to-weight ratio and a sufficiently smooth control.

In reviewing this whole field of biological engineering, in its Report for 1961–62, the Council said:

> Plastic valves for the heart, aids for the blind, artificial kidneys and heart-lung machines could all be said to fall within the province of prostheses in so far as they replace, temporarily or permanently, even if imperfectly, the function of a part of the living body. The subject is in its infancy and has many possibilities; for instance, greater miniaturization should make it possible to produce implantable systems with the complexity necessary for replacing a lost sensory organ. Improvement in materials which the body will accept, and which will wear only slowly, would make a mechanical heart feasible. There is no doubt that of all the advances which are likely to result from the application of engineering principles to biology those concerned with prostheses will be among the most exciting.

Expansion of work in this field, near the end of the period covered by this history, was marked by the Council's establishment of a Neurological Prostheses Unit at the Institute of Psychiatry, London, and a Physical Aids for the Disabled Unit at Edinburgh.

Chapter 5
Preventive Medicine: Nutrition

The scope of preventive medicine—Nutrition research between the wars—
Vitamin studies—Rickets as a deficiency disease—Mission to Vienna—Artificial
vitamin production—A dietetic trial—Mineral constituents of diet—Wider
aspects of nutrition—National dietaries—Nutrition research since the 1939–45
war—Dental disease

The scope of preventive medicine

Preventive medicine, as distinct from the treatment of disorders
already existing, is concerned with the conditions of healthy living
and with defence against inimical external influences. It has an
individual aspect, in that a man's way of life is important—the
proper use of his functions, his personal hygiene, his own nutrition;
but it has a larger community aspect, in that many of the conditions
and defences are matters for public provision or control.

There has nevertheless been some discouragement to research
efforts in the preventive field, successful though they have been
in many instances, because of the relatively greater difficulty
experienced in the practical application of results. This may be
less true today than it was when, in its Report for 1937–38, the
Council discussed the question of achieving in practice "the improved level of health of civilised communities made possible by
the access of knowledge won by medical research". On the one hand,
new methods of diagnosis and treatment were eagerly adopted by
the medical profession, while new specialist services for their administration were provided by the hospitals as soon as possible; the
pharmaceutical industry, for its part, was quick to develop production of the preparations required. On the other hand, there tended
to be delay in implementing discoveries in the field of preventive
medicine:

> Everybody will agree that, of the two types of knowledge, that which leads to
> the eradication of disease is much the more important to the community. Why
> then should there be great delay in its application? No simple answer can be
> given to this question. Prophylaxis against disease does not depend solely on
> the alertness of medical men or of Government departments to procure rapid
> application of new knowledge. Just as important is enlightenment of the public
> as to the merits of a particular discovery, since these applications of medical
> science often require direct action on the part of individuals. The public, however,
> cannot understand the merits of such very technical subjects unless they are clearly
> expounded and the meaning of the results driven home. Again, successful cure
> of disease is always dramatic, and brings with it intense relief both to patients
> and their friends. There is, however, nothing dramatic about the disappearance

73

of disease. It is here to-day and gone to-morrow, and the very success of prevention of disease is measured by forgetfulness. Whoever thinks nowadays of the decimation once caused in this country by plague, cholera, typhus and other diseases now eliminated from our midst? The relative lack of dramatic interest in the prevention of disease, as compared with that in its cure, is partly responsible for the difference in rates with which their advantages are obtained by the public. A third cause of delay is the fact that preventive medicine mostly concerns children, and it is curious that illness and death in the young do not, apparently, impress themselves on the public mind with the emphasis associated with disease in the adult.

It is becoming every day more clear that these difficulties in matters of health and disease, especially when the co-operation of the public is necessary, will remain so long as there is no means of educating and giving them the requisite guidance. It does not seem to be anybody's business in the country to undertake this task. Only too often are the public dependent for information and guidance on advertising propaganda, exaggerated and false as it so often is, financed by those with something to sell. Others who are most assiduous in publicity are those who believe that advances in medical knowledge, especially when of great practical value in public health, are snares and delusions, and who by extensive propaganda mislead in every conceivable way and hinder the process of application.

Sir Edward Mellanby, Secretary of the Council, made the same point in 1947 in giving evidence to the Select Committee on Estimates at the House of Commons.

Nutrition research between the wars

From the beginning, the Council attached the highest importance to nutrition as a subject for research. Practical problems of malnutrition had presented themselves in time of peace mainly as a concomitant of poverty and conditions of special hardship; the question of adequate feeding tended to be considered in quantitative terms, and therefore as largely economic. Experience during the First World War had accentuated the problem and aroused interest from fresh angles. Moreover, research into qualitative aspects of diet had received a great stimulus through the discovery, by Hopkins at Cambridge in 1912, of a fat-soluble 'accessory food factor' (vitamin A), which was essential, albeit in minute amounts, for the normal growth of young animals. It was on all grounds plain that a much greater and more certain basis of knowledge was a prime necessity for effective practical action.

There were outstanding questions about the required amounts and proper balance of the primary nutrients (proteins, carbohydrates and fats), both as substances entering into the composition of the body and (in terms of calories) as sources of energy. A greater gap in knowledge related to essential food factors (vitamins and mineral constituents) that are accessory to the primary nutrients. There was thus abundant scope for a full programme of research in human nutrition, but the subject also impinged on matters outside the Council's ambit.

During the First World War, the role of the Medical Research Committee in the nutrition field was largely to assist the Food (War) Committee of the Royal Society in its task of collating information and conducting inquiries for the guidance of the Government in the administration of the food resources of the nation. After the war, the Food Committee prepared a memorandum expressing the opinion that the science of nutrition had been insufficiently studied, and that there was an urgent need for a central institute or organisation to promote investigations into the connected problems of human and animal nutrition, and of the utilisation of agricultural products so as best to serve the national health and economy. This was transmitted by the Royal Society to the Development Commission, the Medical Research Committee and the Department of Scientific and Industrial Research, and resulted in a conference of the various bodies. Research on the production of food was (at that time) a matter for the Commission, research on its processing and preservation for the Department, while research on human nutrition itself was clearly in the medical field. Standing arrangements were made for the coordination of these three lines of activity, and it was eventually found that no *ad hoc* organisation was needed.

The Council's Report for 1934–35 discussed the application of modern knowledge of nutrition, referring to its own programme of research on rickets, dental disease, vitamin standardisation, and nutritional anaemia. The Report for 1935–36 commented on the growing public interest in nutrition: "Perhaps the most significant action which emphasises the new importance attached to nutrition is the recent announcement that his Majesty's Government is determined to regard the improvement of physical fitness as a fundamental point of policy." An advisory committee on nutrition had been set up by the Health Departments. The Economic Advisory Council had appointed a committee on problems of nutrition in the Colonial Empire. The Health and Economic Sections of the League of Nations had jointly appointed technical and 'mixed' committees on nutrition—with Sir Edward Mellanby as chairman of the Technical Committee.

Vitamin studies
In 1918 the Medical Research Committee and the Lister Institute of Preventive Medicine jointly appointed an Accessory Food Factors Committee under the chairmanship of Professor F. Gowland (later Sir Frederick) Hopkins, and with Dr (later Dame) Harriette Chick as secretary. This body, which included the leading active workers on this subject in this country, continued to advise the Council on a wide range of questions for many years. It also rendered a special service by its preparation of a review of the existing state of knowledge of vitamins, edited by Professor (later Sir) Arthur Harden;

this valuable work of reference was originally published in the report series in 1919, revised and enlarged editions appearing in 1924 and 1932.

Much of the research work on vitamins was done at the Lister Institute, by members of the staff there and by workers supported by the Council. Among the latter, for many years, was Dr S. S. Zilva of the Council's external scientific staff, working on vitamin C (the antiscorbutic factor, later chemically identified as ascorbic acid); he also worked with Dr J. C. (later Sir Jack) Drummond, assisted by a grant, on the nutritive values of different commercial oils and fats, including cod-liver oil. Another centre of work on vitamins was formed in 1926, when the Council established the Dunn Nutritional Laboratory at Cambridge (Volume One). Work at Oxford by Professor R. A. (later Sir Rudolph) Peters and others on the vitamin B complex—as it proved to be—was assisted by grants from the Council. Work on the antirachitic factor is discussed in succeeding sections below.

Of vitamin research in general, the Council said in its Report for 1920–21:

> This new development of physiology originated in this country, but its progress was crippled at the beginning and for several years by the inability of Universities and other private institutions to provide the necessary funds. The Government grant-in-aid for medical research has in recent years allowed more rapid and fruitful increase in knowledge to be gained by workers in this country, after a period in which it seemed that the whole subject must pass, after its origination here, to development in other countries. The present situation is a very curious one, upon which posterity will probably look back with great interest. We still have almost no knowledge of the nature of these elusive food substances or of their mode of action, but we have gained empirical knowledge already of the greatest practical value for the prevention of scurvy and of other grave diseases and for the promotion of health and beauty in the population. If the war services alone of this kind of work be reckoned, it has repaid very many times over all that the State has spent upon it. Its great economical value in time of peace is becoming almost monthly more apparent, affecting as it does at a thousand points the food of the population, its choice, its preparation in manufacturing processes and in the kitchen, and its production by agriculture. To agriculture it has its own importance, too, for the nutrition of livestock. Though this practical harvest has already begun to be reaped, pure science is still waiting for its share of the benefits. Nevertheless, it seems certain that in the early future great, if unforeseen, advances in knowledge will come as the clue to the real nature and mode of action of these substances in the body is gained.

It is of interest that, since the foregoing passage was published, all the vitamins—a substantially greater number than was then realised —have been chemically identified. In thus ceasing to be enigmatic biological factors, they have lost no whit of their practical importance.

Rickets as a deficiency disease
It is only with hindsight that one places rickets under the heading of nutritional disorders, but this can now be done very firmly indeed.

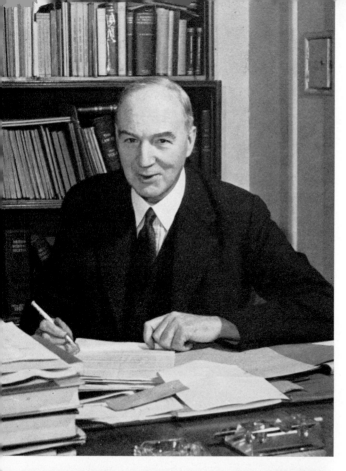

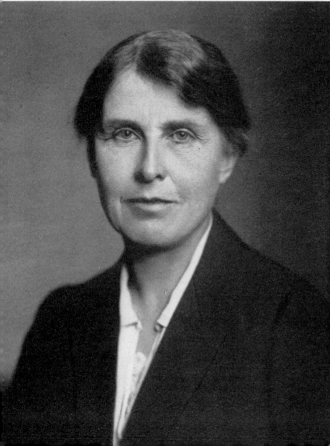

1 Two nutritional scientists:

Sir Edward Mellanby, GBE,
KCB, FRS (Secretary of the
Council 1933–49—see p xi)

Dame Harriette Chick, DBE
(late Lister Institute of
Preventive Medicine),
who celebrated her 100th
birthday in 1975

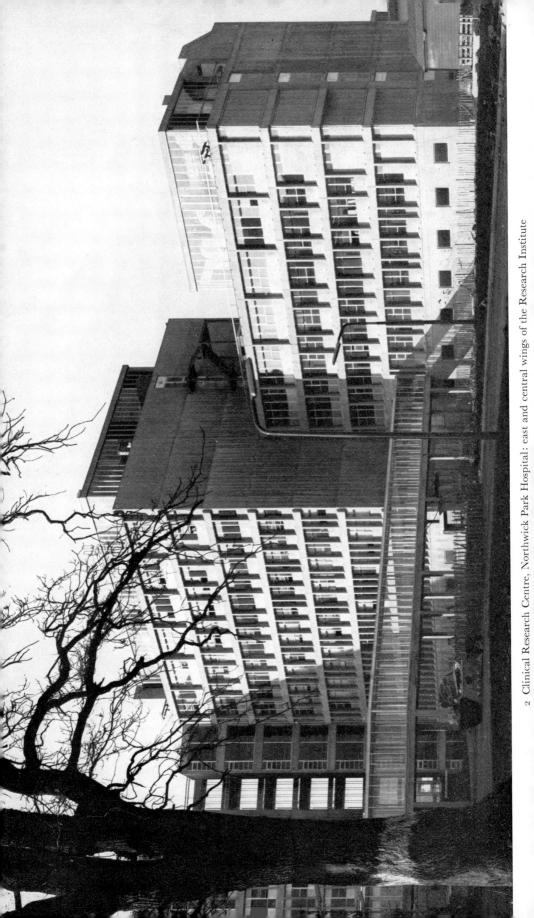

2 Clinical Research Centre, Northwick Park Hospital: east and central wings of the Research Institute

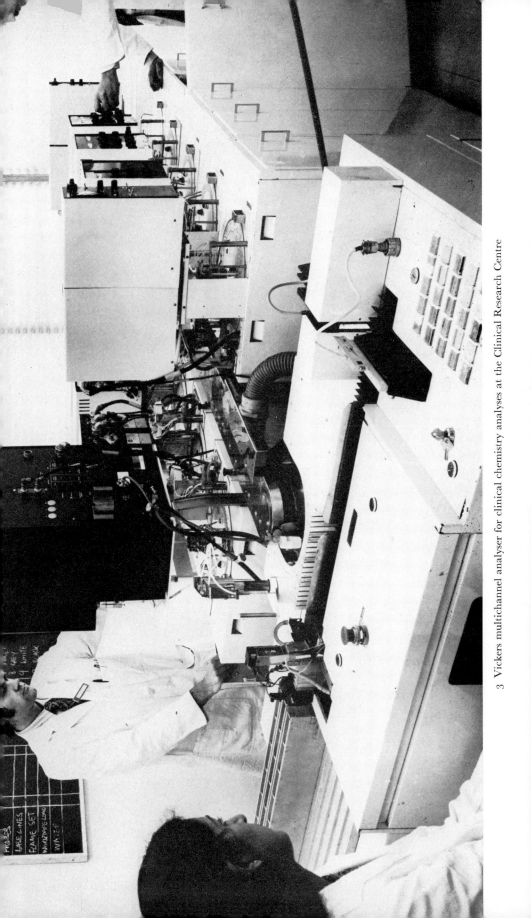

3 Vickers multichannel analyser for clinical chemistry analyses at the Clinical Research Centre

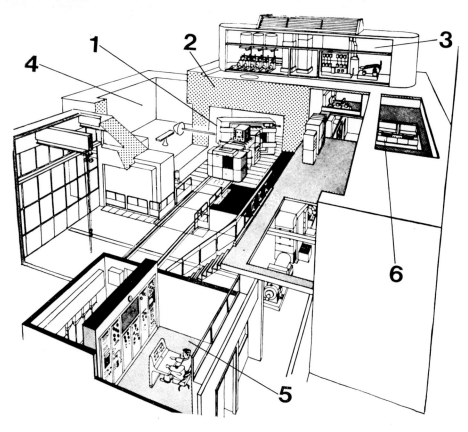

4 MRC cyclotron at Hammersmith Hospital: (*Above*) Layout of laboratory area: 1 cyclotron; 2 shielding concrete 6 ft thick; 3 auxiliary plant; 4 neutron therapy treatment room; 5 cyclotron control room; 6 radioisotope production laboratory (*Below*) A patient being set up for fast neutron therapy

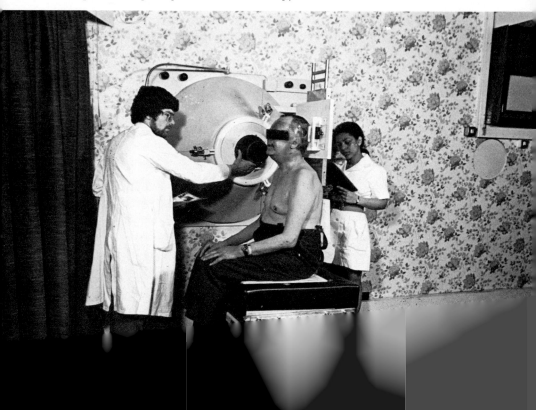

The Medical Research Committee gave rickets a prominent place in its original Research Schemes, and did so rightly, seeing that this permanently bone-deforming disease of growing children was notably prevalent among the urban poor in Britain. The cause was unknown or disputed, so that there was no guiding principle for prevention or treatment. The Committee, therefore, planned an attack from a variety of angles—experimental, observational, bacteriological, biochemical. The Report for 1916–17 gave the first announcement of Dr (later Sir Edward) Mellanby's finding, in experiments with puppies, that rickets was due to deficiency of a component of the diet (a fat-soluble vitamin) and could be produced or prevented virtually at will. He had been working for the Committee in London since 1915, and at the Cambridge University Field Laboratories from 1917. This result, at first somewhat narrowly based, was not at once generally accepted. In the Report for 1917–18, side by side with a further account of Mellanby's work, appears a summary of contrary conclusions reached by a group of workers in Glasgow, also supported by the Committee, under the leadership of Professor D. Noel Paton. Their studies of rickets in children had yielded no evidence supporting ideas that rickets was related to dietetic deficiency, or to inheritance; the cause was considered to lie in social conditions, such as bad housing, lack of open-air life, and inefficient parental care. In the following year experiments in Glasgow with dogs were reported as showing that lack of exercise was a likely cause. The opponents of Mellanby's view kept the subject in the field of controversy for several years; and the dispute engendered a degree of personal bitterness that is happily unusual between divergent schools of thought in scientific research. From an early stage, however, there was in the minds of most judges little doubt who was right.

A full account of Mellanby's experiments was published in the Council's series in 1921, and a further report in 1925 dealt with the interaction of different dietetic and environmental factors in aetiology. A report in 1922 by Dr H. Corry Mann, working for the Council in London, assessed the importance of dietetic and environmental factors from a clinical standpoint; while a report in 1922 by Dr V. Korenchevsky, working with rats at the Lister Institute, discussed the aetiology and pathology of experimental rickets, his results supporting Mellanby's thesis. Korenchevsky was one of a number of distinguished 'White' Russian exiles who received grants from the Council at about that time; some of the others proceeded to posts in Canada, Egypt and elsewhere, while another met an untimely death by falling down a lift-shaft at University College London.

The practical outcome eventually stilled all controversy on the main point. As the experimental results carried conviction, the simple prophylactic measure of administering cod-liver oil to children on poor diets was widely adopted, and fresh cases of rickets gradually ceased to occur in Britain except in a few pockets of resistance to new knowledge. (The findings were also applied in other parts of the world; the Council's Report for 1937–38 records that, at the Children's Hospital in Toronto, a case of rickets caused such surprise that a meeting of staff and students was summoned to examine the baby.) The story of the antirachitic vitamin is continued in the next two sections.

Mission to Vienna

This knowledge of fat-soluble vitamins had developed largely in Britain during the years of war and had scarcely penetrated to enemy countries. The economic collapse of these countries at the end of hostilities thus found them badly placed to deal with the appalling conditions of malnutrition, especially among growing children, that supervened in some areas. The state of affairs reported from Austria was particularly bad, and although the international relief organisations were doing what they could to meet the sheer quantitative lack of food the medical profession of the country, even in such a famous centre as Vienna, was not equipped with the latest knowledge for combating qualitative deficiencies. In these circumstances, on the recommendation of the Accessory Food Factors Committee, the Council and the Lister Institute decided to send Dr Harriette Chick of the Institute's staff and Dr Elsie Dalyell (Beit Memorial Research Fellow) to Vienna in September 1919, to study the deficiency diseases reported to be so prevalent there. As the Report for 1919–20 says, "They found a condition of qualitative malnutrition worse even than had been expected, and the amount of material for research was almost overwhelming." The Council provided the expenses of the mission, and early in the following year added Miss E. M. Hume to the team. Help was received from the relief organisations, and cooperation from all Austrian quarters.

The results of the first winter's work were summarised in the Report for 1919–20:

> Many interesting and confirmatory facts have been collected with regard to infantile scurvy, and the antiscorbutics which had been recommended for infants as the result of animal experiments were given extensive trials with extremely satisfactory results. Highly encouraging and suggestive results were obtained from the treatment of nursing mothers with butter or cod-liver oil and antiscorbutics; in many cases their infants, who had failed to thrive before the treatment of their mothers, made instant improvement, which was maintained. The weight of the babies who had previously been far below normal at once began to approach the normal. Cod-liver oil gave better results even than butter. Children, so backward that at three years of age they could not even sit alone, were themselves given butter and lemon juice. In a few weeks they began to shake off the lethargy in which they had lain for months, in many cases even for years, and in six months all could stand and many could walk.

Still younger children with arrested development were also studied towards the end of the period, and during the winter a disease known as 'hunger osteomalacia' in adults of both sexes.

The work was resumed in the winter of 1920–21 on a larger scale, with Dr Helen Mackay (Beit Memorial Research Fellow) and Sister H. Henderson Smith added to the personnel. And in its Report for that year the Council commented that the conduct of the investigation on scientific lines had been made possible by Professor C. Pirquet's well organised system by which the composition of hospital diets was controlled with quantitative accuracy. A comparison of two different dietetic treatments, the results of one controlling those of the other, was thus being made under the equivalent of experimental conditions.

The full results were published in the Council's series in 1923, and in its own Report for 1922–23 the Council referred to them as follows:

> The change of view which these have brought about is perhaps more easily seen abroad than at home where the change has been more gradual. An expression of this is given in the Preface which Professor Pirquet has most generously contributed to the Report of Miss Chick and her colleagues, and there is probably no scientific man or clinician to whose words would be given greater weight in Europe and America upon this subject. Professor Pirquet writes with characteristic frankness and magnanimity:—
>
> 'When Dr Chick and her colleagues on behalf of the Medical Research Council and the Lister Institute began their work in my Klinik in 1919, I had little expectation that it would lead to results of much practical value. At that time I was of the opinion that a vitamin deficiency in our ordinary diet was a very exceptional occurrence, as, for example, in case of infantile scurvy (Möller–Barlow disease). With regard to the etiology of rickets I held the view that it was an infectious disease, widely prevalent in this part of Europe, producing severe symptoms only in case of those children who possessed special susceptibility as the result of an inherited tendency, of a faulty diet, or of defective general hygiene. I imagined rickets to be a disease comparable to some extent with tuberculosis.'
>
> After critical discussion of the Report he concludes as follows:—
>
> 'The crucial experiment was thus successfully made. The British workers succeeded with the accuracy of a laboratory experiment, in a city where rickets is extremely prevalent, in maintaining a large number of artificially-fed babies free from the disease, and further, in the same wards, were invariably successful in healing children admitted with rickets already developed.
>
> 'With this the chain of evidence appears to me to be complete that animal experiments upon rickets are applicable to man, that rickets is a disease of nutrition, and that deficiency of fat-soluble vitamins in diet is an essential cause of the disease.'

Artificial vitamin production

Workers in several countries contributed, but the development of further understanding of vitamin D was very largely due to British investigators supported by the Council; the story illustrates the programme that was being promoted. Mellanby's wartime experiments with puppies had shown, as already noted, that rickets was due to deficiency of a fat-soluble vitamin; and this had been amply confirmed for human rickets by the addition of the vitamin (usually as a constituent of cod-liver oil) to the diet of children, and not least in the Council's mission to Vienna mentioned above.

It had also been noted that the deficiency was in some obscure way counteracted by the effect of summer sunshine on the children; and while the Vienna work was in progress it was shown by Dr K. Huldschinsky in Berlin that rachitic children could be cured by irradiation of their bodies with a quartz mercury lamp. Many experiments were made to elucidate this phenomenon, and Professor H. Steenbock of Wisconsin showed that many types of food would yield the antirachitic vitamin on irradiation; this was even made the subject of a patent (Chapter 11). Meanwhile, workers in America first drew a distinction between Mellanby's anti-rachitic vitamin (D) and the other fat-soluble vitamin (A) earlier shown by Hopkins to be necessary for growth; and it was vitamin D alone that was produced by the irradiation of foodstuffs. Thereafter, practically simultaneously in America and in Britain, it was found that cholesterol—a substance widely distributed in the body and in various foodstuffs—produced vitamin D on irradiation, although not in large or regular quantities.

At this point Dr Otto Rosenheim and Mr T. A. Webster at the National Institute for Medical Research showed that specially purified cholesterol did not give this result, and that the effect was due to another sterol commonly associated with cholesterol and not readily separable therefrom. With the collaboration of Professor A. Windaus of Göttingen, the crucial substance was identified as ergosterol. This was an important result, as ergosterol was a readily available source and yielded an enormously potent preparation of vitamin D on irradiation. Further researches, in which Miss Hume and others working for the Council played a part, led to the conclusion that the preventive and curative effects of sunlight on rickets, or of ultraviolet light from an artificial source, were due to the production of vitamin D from ergosterol present in the grease of the skin.

A further advance came a few years later, in 1931, when Dr R. B. Bourdillon and others at the National Institute for Medical Research succeeded, by irradiating ergosterol under special conditions, in producing a crystalline compound which had an astonishingly intense biological activity; it was chemically characterised and called 'calciferol'. Weight for weight this substance was 400 000 times as potent as a good sample of cod-liver oil in preventing or curing rickets; a solution of a single ounce, according to calculation, could provide the daily dose necessary to protect more than a million children. Vitamin D was thus, among all the vitamins, the first to be chemically identified.

A dietic trial

During the period 1922–25 the Council was able to promote a comparative trial of diets for groups of boys of school age in an institution, described as a model colony, not far from London. Every boy received, throughout, the basic diet of the institution—one that was considered adequate in the light of existing knowledge and apparently confirmed as such by the uncontrolled practical results. Various additions to this diet were provided for different groups of boys, and the group in which each boy received a daily pint of milk showed the greatest physical improvement as compared with boys continuing to receive only the basic diet of the institution. The trial was conducted for the Council, with meticulous care, by Dr H. C. Corry Mann; and a report by him was published in 1926. In the Council's preface to this, the following comment summed up the most significant findings:

> The investigation described shows clearly that the nutritive value of a dietary which was originally chosen with every regard for the welfare of the children to be reared upon it could be strikingly improved by additions which in a quantitative sense were small. It is startling to learn, as we now do, for instance, that the addition of one pint of milk a day to a diet which by itself satisfied the appetite of growing boys fed upon it could convert an average annual gain of weight of 3·85 lb. per boy into one of 6·98 lb., and an annual average increase of height from 1·84 inches to 2·63 inches. This unmistakable betterment in nutrition was proved by trial to be due, not to the relatively small increase in the fuel value of the dietary, not to the extra protein supplied in the milk, but rather to more specific qualities of milk as a food. Quantitative results of this sort, established as they have been by rigid evidence, show that the real adequacy of a dietary cannot be determined without close scrutiny of its qualities. The nutritional influence of its constituents is not to be measured by their value as fuel or building material alone. It is desirable at the present moment to accept the objective facts won by these studies without attempting to decide upon what precise factors the striking effect of various additions to the basic diet depends. We may come to attribute it to vitamins, but it may be due to other factors.
>
> It is of the first importance to notice that the improved gains in weight and height, taken as the measurable characters in this inquiry, were found to be accompanied regularly by improved general health and by improvement in what may perhaps be called 'spirit'.

Mineral constituents of diet

In the period between the wars, considerable attention was also paid to those inorganic substances—mineral elements and their salts—which are essential components of diet, if again often in very small amounts. Among investigations in this field promoted by the Council was the work of Dr Helen Mackay, as a part-time member of the staff, on the role of iron in relation to nutritional anaemia in infancy; a report was published in the Council's series in 1931.

In respect of iodine, in 1929 the Council published a review of existing knowledge concerning the place of this element in nutrition, the authors being Dr J. B. Orr (later Lord Boyd-Orr) and Dr

Isabella Leitch, both of the Rowett Research Institute near Aberdeen; and in 1934 a report by Dr Orr on iodine supply and the incidence of endemic goitre. A further report on this latter theme, published in 1936, was the work of a special Committee on Iodine Deficiency and Thyroid disease. In the course of these studies the Council arranged with the Government Chemist for a member of his staff to devise a new method of estimating iodine in biological substances; and an account of this was published in the Council's series in 1935. Later, in 1948, some practical guidance on thyroid enlargement and other changes related to the mineral content of drinking water was given in one of the Council's Memoranda.

The Council's Report for 1936–37 referred to work on the role of common salt (sodium chloride) in relation to certain conditions—a deficiency being associated with 'miner's cramp', heat stress and certain diseases, while there is an excess in some other diseases. Dr R. A. McCance and Miss E. M. Widdowson, then working with support from the Council at King's College Hospital, London, made experiments on normal volunteers which threw light on the physiological mechanisms involved in controlling the volume of the blood and extracellular fluids.

Wider aspects of nutrition

A certain early preoccupation with purely qualitative problems of nutrition did not preclude consideration of wider aspects, and soon the programme in this field began to broaden out. In the Report for 1926–27 the Council said:

> These studies of vitamins are but one part of the nutritional science of which indeed we are now only seeing the dawn. Modern studies of the nutritional value of inorganic elements or their salts are indicating that here again, as with the vitamins, we are concerned with another science of the 'infinitely little'. Vitamin actions are found to be related in vital ways to subtle factors of balance between them, and again between them and other factors in diet. New knowledge is coming of constituents of diet which appear able to nullify the action of vitamins. Qualitative problems of all these kinds are linked, of course, with the quantitative problems of nutrition. . . . But indeed the knowledge we have so recently gained only serves to illuminate the darkness of our present ignorance. In hardly more than a dozen years disorders believed to be specific diseases, such as beri-beri, scurvy, and rickets, have become assignable to dietetic errors. We cannot guess what new relations to diet of disease, or of liability to disease, are waiting to be revealed. In many of the simplest matters no physicians, or surgeons, can give advice based on scientific knowledge, even if they hazard opinions based on earnest but uncontrolled observations. It is not yet scientifically known, for instance, how much water a man should drink in the day, or what is the best kind of bread to eat.

The report at the same time recorded the Council's recent appointment of a small Human Nutrition Committee to coordinate the different lines of study with a view to framing a comprehensive programme of research. The six members were leaders drawn from both the qualitative and the quantitative schools of investigation; Professor E. P. Cathcart, of Glasgow, was chairman. The Committee was reported as "attempting to frame, in cooperation with the agricultural interests, a chemogeographical survey of the inorganic constituents of diet available in different parts of the country and their relation to the distribution of disorders in health, human or animal". On the quantitative side, the Committee considered the validity of the existing formulae for referring dietetic estimates to a single 'man value' standard, allowing for age and sex. A similar problem related to the accepted standard for the energy requirement of an average adult man. Associated with the latter was the question of 'luxus' consumption—the biological value, if any, of food taken in excess of actual needs in terms of energy expenditure.

National dietaries
Earlier, the Council had had a separate Committee on Quantitative Problems of Human Nutrition which produced a report, published in the Council's series in 1924, on the nutrition of miners and their families. The Council's Report for 1927–28 referred to the importance of the study of national dietaries; an indispensable datum in considering the wider problems of nutrition is knowledge of what the people do in fact eat. Particular reference was made to an investigation, by Cathcart and others, of the diet of the inhabitants of St Andrews, taken as a type of a non-industrial, rural town. The diet of 139 households, of all classes, was studied for a week; and in 35 of them the work was repeated six months later. The Council's comment was that "this is the largest investigation of the dietaries of a single place which has yet been made, and it is believed that it is the most complete". Similar studies were afterwards made in two other urban areas of different types, Cardiff and Reading. Reports were published in the Council's series in 1931 and 1932. There followed in 1940 a report on the diets of families in the Highlands and Islands of Scotland, living in highly contrasted environmental conditions.

Methodological refinements of such surveys of family shopping are exemplified by reports in the Council's series in 1936 and 1947 respectively. In the one, again by the Cathcart team, a dietary survey was described in which the actual consumption of foodstuffs was recorded. The other, by Dr Elsie Widdowson, was a study of the diets of individual children. In 1952 there was a report by Garry and others comparing the energy expenditure and food consumption of Scottish miners and clerks.

Surveys in terms of commodities purchased or consumed may not give sufficiently precise information about the nutrients contained in the diets. For this and other reasons greater knowledge was required of the composition of different foodstuffs. The research undertaken resulted in a number of reports, by McCance and others, in the Council's series: on the carbohydrate content of foods, especially in relation to diabetic diets (1929); on the chemistry of flesh foods and their losses in cooking (1933); and on the nutritive value of fruits and vegetables (1936). These were followed in 1940 by a comprehensive monograph by McCance and Widdowson, with tables showing the chemical composition of foods, to which fuller reference is made elsewhere (Chapter 15); a revised edition was published in 1960. Information about the vitamin content of foods was given in the special publication mentioned earlier; and the composition of foods used mainly in tropical countries was considered separately (Chapter 10).

Nutrition research since the 1939–45 war
During the Second World War the Council played an active and prominent part not only in promoting research on nutrition but also in advising on, and assisting, the practical applications of scientific knowledge on the subject. An account of this wartime work is given elsewhere (Chapter 15).

Sir Edward Mellanby, Secretary of the Council, had taken an important personal role in this research programme, working in the Nutrition Building which the Council had specially provided for him on the Mill Hill site of the National Institute for Medical Research. While in office he could of course only give his spare time; but Lady Mellanby (see later) and their assistants worked there throughout the week, as he himself did when he had retired. After his sudden death in 1955, the Council allocated the accommodation to its Human Nutrition Research Unit, which had been formed during the war under the direction of Professor B. S. Platt; the work of the Unit related mainly to the nutrition of populations in the tropics and is discussed later (Chapter 10).

Mellanby had been led back (actually before the war) to a former theme, the interaction of cereals with fat-soluble vitamins. When the war came, this had an important relation to the increased extraction rate of flour used for making bread, and led to the addition of extra calcium to counteract an effect antagonistic to that of vitamin D. Earlier work, including Mellanby's, was likewise the basis of the Council's advice that led to the compulsory fortification of margarine with fat-soluble vitamins.

These and similar lines of thought persisted after the war, as indeed did some of the practical problems for several years. The Council's Report for 1945–48 includes an essay on 'the sophistication of food', of which the opening may be quoted:

> The preparatory treatment of ingredients of diet by chemical substances, either to make them more palatable or to preserve them, has become a very extensive practice in western civilisation. There are, of course, some foods, such as milk and butter, to which the addition of chemical substances is forbidden by law. On the other hand, in the case of certain foodstuffs of equal or greater importance, considerable licence is allowed to manufacturers to add chemicals in order to increase the palatability or the keeping qualities of the products. One

of the outstanding articles of consumption in this category is flour and, indeed, cereals in general. In this country flour for human consumption may have been 'improved' by treatment with oxides of nitrogen, benzoyl chloride, chlorine dioxide, potassium bromate, nitrogen trichloride or 'agene', and ammonium persulphate.

It is not always easy to understand why many consumers prefer to have bread and related products so treated, but probably the best generalisation is that, when the chemical treatment of such foods makes them lighter in texture and in colour, and more easily masticated, then that is regarded as a preferable condition. In the case of bread, for instance, this means that, within limits, bread which contains more air and more water is more popular than bread in the more solid form. If this were the end of the matter there would be little reason for discussing the subject as a medical problem, but we have to take account of the possibility of harmful effects from these chemical admixtures.

The Report then proceeded to recount the then recent discovery, by Mellanby, that feeding dogs with bread or dog-biscuits made from agenised flour induced 'canine hysteria' (or 'running fits'), an unexplained condition of which outbreaks had been for long familiar to dog-owners and veterinarians. Other species of animals reacted in different ways; and although definite toxic effects were not demonstrated in humans, it was difficult to believe that the substance could be entirely harmless over long periods. Thus "there seems a good *prima facie* case for abandoning a method of flour 'improvement' which is known to be associated with the production of serious and often fatal disease in animals". And again: "On the wider question, it is clear that here is a warning, not to be disregarded, on the possible dangers associated with the chemical treatment of food."

Just as Austria had provided an exceptional occasion for the study (as well as, of course, for the massive relief) of malnutrition after the First World War, so did Germany after the Second. The selected place was the Wuppertal, an industrial valley of the Ruhr, and here a team from the Department of Experimental Medicine worked during 1946–49 under the direction of Professor R. A. McCance of the Council's staff. A comprehensive report was published in the Council's series in 1951, sections being contributed by various members of the team and by others with special interests who had been temporarily associated with the mission. The subjects included the significance and aetiology of hunger oedema, the effects of undernutrition on different organs and systems of the body, the absorption and excretion of certain elements, and water metabolism.

There were also separate reports on certain special investigations in the Wuppertal. One of these, by Widdowson and McCance (1954), described studies of the nutritive value of bread and the effect of variations in the extraction rate of flour on the growth of undernourished children. Another, by Dr R. F. A. Dean (1953), dealt with the use of plant proteins in the feeding of children, a subject in which the author continued his interest while working for the Council in East Africa (Chapter 10).

In the Report for 1953–54 it was pointed out that the young

science of nutrition had had three phases. First there had come the study of the chemical nature and energy values of the main nutrients. Second, between the world wars, had come the era of intensive vitamin research with its emphasis on qualitative factors essential in small amounts; and this had introduced into medicine the concept of deficiency diseases, in breach of earlier dogma attributing all ill-ness to positive agents such as infections or poisons. Third, there was the development of a more complex view of the interplay of various nutritional and other factors. This involved a renewal of interest in the basic foodstuffs, with "the realisation that for the inhabitants of a large part of the world the first problem is how to get enough to eat, and the second how to get an adequate supply of protein". The world problem of nutrition had in fact become the supply of protein of good biological value.

Two years later, in the Report for 1955–56, protein deficiency in man was selected for special discussion, as a subject that was attract-ing world-wide investigation. Within the Council's organisation a substantial research effort was being made in that field; it involved, among others, workers at the National Institute for Medical Research and in the Human Nutrition Research Unit, while field studies were being made in the Council's establishments overseas.

The Department of Experimental Medicine at Cambridge ceased to be one of the Council's Units in 1966 on the retirement of Profes-sor McCance from his chair in the University. Other members of the staff were transferred to the Dunn Nutritional Laboratory, also in Cambridge, to form a Division of Infant Nutrition Research there. And in 1968 an extension was opened which approximately doubled the accommodation of the Dunn Laboratory and provided facilities for which the need had not earlier been foreseen. In 1967 the Human Nutrition Research Unit at Mill Hill was closed down on the retire-ment of Professor Platt from the Council's service. The establish-ments in East Africa and the West Indies maintained their pro-grammes.

Dental disease

This subject may conveniently be included in this chapter, as the orientation of so much of the research has been to the nutritional aspect.

The Council has always regarded research on dental disease as falling within the scope of its responsibilities; no professional distinc-tion between 'medical' and 'dental' has relevance from the scientific point of view. In 1921 the Council appointed a special Committee for the Investigation of Dental Disease; the first chairman was a distinguished physiologist, Professor W. D. Halliburton, while the other members were drawn partly from the dental profession and partly from various scientific disciplines that could be brought to bear on the subject, such as pathology, bacteriology, biochemistry and nutritional studies.

From 1923 the newly formed Dental Board of the United Kingdom (later General Dental Council) provided the Council with £3000 per annum for an extended programme of dental research. The Board nominated a member to serve on the special Committee and received periodical reports on the progress of the work, but the conduct of the scheme was left to the Council. This arrangement continued until 1939.

The Council supported various lines of attack on the problems of dental and periodontal disease—histological, biochemical, and bacteriological. Under the last head, for two years from 1923, Dr J. Kilian Clarke held a whole-time grant from the Council for experimental work at St Mary's Hospital, London, on the role of certain infective organisms in the production of dental caries. His findings appeared to incriminate especially an organism which he named *Streptococcus mutans*; and this has since come to be regarded by some as an important clue.

The Council had already evinced a particular interest in the relation between the structure of the teeth and their liability to caries, and thus in the dependence of normal structure on proper nutrition. The Report for 1918–19 contains the first announcement of the discovery by Professor and Mrs Mellanby that the calcification of the dental enamel, like that of the skeleton (see above), depended on an adequate supply of a fat-soluble vitamin, as well as calcium, in the diet. This preliminary indication was followed up by Mrs (later Lady) Mellanby during a life-time of research assisted by the Council.

The evidence of Mrs May Mellanby's findings was eventually presented in three reports in the Council's series. The first (1929) covered the influence of nutrition upon the development of the jaws and teeth in dogs; the second (1930) dealt with dental structure in other animal species, and with nutritional factors concerned in periodontal disease in dogs; and the third (1934) discussed the structure of human teeth and the part played by diet in determining their resistance to disease.

Other research work on dental structure was likewise aided by the Council. In 1922 a report by Mr J. Howard Mummery, writing as a dentist on the structure of the teeth in relation to disease, was published in the Council's series. In 1932 there was one by Miss C. Smyth and Dr Matthew Young (of the Council's staff) on facial growth in children with special reference to dentition; and in 1940 one by Mr J. Thewlis (of the National Physical Laboratory, by arrangement with the Department of Scientific and Industrial Research) on the structure of the teeth as shown by X-ray examination.

In its report for 1925–26, the Council discussed the importance of Mrs Mellanby's experimental findings, and the Committee for the Investigation of Dental Disease, under the chairmanship of Sir Norman Bennett, decided to follow them up with a practical dietetic trial on groups of children. This was made in institutions in Birmingham, by arrangement with the local authorities, the variations in diet consisting wholly of additions to that ordinarily provided. This enterprise was largely due to the initiative of Dr H. C. T. Langdon of the Board of Education, as secretary of the Committee. The final results, published in the Council's series in 1936, supported Mrs Mellanby's findings. The Council's reference to this, in its Report for 1935–36, included the following comment:

> It was impossible in a test of this nature to apply all modern knowledge of nutritional influences to the production of perfect teeth or the suppression of dental decay in children; nor was it possible to test the whole theory of nutritional influence, as advanced by Mrs Mellanby, in its several aspects. The object was of a more limited nature, namely, to test the effect of adding a single factor to the diets of children and to see whether the incidence of dental decay was altered. . . . If it were confirmed that the supply of a minute fraction of the general diet in the form of vitamin D exerted an undeniable influence in inhibiting dental caries, the establishment of Mrs Mellanby's thesis in one important instance would not only support the whole; it would also orientate the minds of those practically concerned with dental caries to this aspect of the problem, and thus lead to more promising methods of eliminating this form of disability.

In 1940 a report by Dr J. D. King on dental conditions in the island of Lewis, in the Outer Hebrides, was published for the Council. It was already known that there was locally a relative absence of obvious dental complaints, but a more precise assessment was desirable. Further, King was able to make a dental study of some of the families whose diets were being investigated by Cathcart and others (see above); he also made comparative examinations, using the same standards, of families on the mainland of Scotland (Wester Ross) and in England. He was able to confirm that the teeth of the inhabitants of the rural areas of Lewis (but not of Stornoway town) were markedly superior, in their freedom from carious disease, to those of the inhabitants of most parts of Great Britain; it was not a matter of a narrow statistical margin, but a striking contrast. Moreover, the lower susceptibility to decay was associated with a greater freedom from minor structural defects in the teeth. There were also strong indications that the better dental state of the country children was associated with a greater proportion of natural produce (richer in fat-soluble vitamins and mineral salts) in their diet, and a lesser dependence on bought foodstuffs. A new dental survey of children on the Isle of Lewis has more recently been carried out under a Council grant, showing that a deterioration had taken place.

Periodical attempts were made to test a widely held view, unsupported by scientific evidence, that there is a relation between caries and the consumption of carbohydrates, especially refined carbohydrates such as sugar—particularly, eating sweets. In 1928 a trial, which involved adding treacle to the diet of children, was organised by the original Committee for the Investigation of Dental

Disease, but the results were inconclusive; a small trial made in 1946 by King also gave no positive answer. So when a new Dental Research Committee was appointed in 1947 it decided to undertake a trial on a larger scale. Various forms of carbohydrates were added to the basal diets of young children—diets of good nutritional standard —in residential homes in London, Liverpool and Sheffield; these children, in control groups, were kept under observation for up to two years by four members of the Committee. The evidence was published in the Council's series by King and others in 1955, and of it the authors said: "It certainly points to the practical conclusion that, provided a child is fed on a diet as good as that of the average children's residential institution in England, a substantial increase in the amount of sugar in the diet will not affect the child's liability to dental caries within a period of at least two years." As the preface pointed out, however, "The investigation cannot be said to prove that sugar, however distributed and however eaten, will never affect the teeth." In fact, in the years since 1946 evidence that refined carbohydrates are cariogenic has come to be widely accepted, as a review article on the early lesion of dental caries in the Report for 1960–61 makes clear. A symposium on the significance of sucrose in relation to dental caries was organised by the Council in 1968 and the summary of its proceedings, referring to the study just mentioned, concludes: "The present unanimity in incriminating sucrose as a powerful cariogenic substrate is in striking contrast to the earlier uncertainty."

The Council had been anxious to have an establishment of its own for dental research, in or near a dental school and with clinical opportunities; this would not only provide facilities for research but, it was hoped, also attract to it young workers with dental or other relevant qualifications. A suitable director was eventually found in Dr J. D. King, a qualified dentist whose participation in work for the Dental Research Committee has already been mentioned. So in 1946 the Council was able to establish its first Dental Research Unit at Kings' College Hospital, London. This promising venture was unhappily cut short by the death of Dr King in 1953, and the Unit had to be disbanded; two relatively junior workers who had been appointed to the Unit were placed, as members of the Council's staff, in the School of Dental Surgery at Birmingham and in Guy's Hospital, London, respectively. Other investigations continued to be supported by grants at the Dental Surgery School in Liverpool, the Dental School in Sheffield, and elsewhere. It was not until 1961, however, that a new Dental Research Unit could be formed; this was established, under the honorary direction of Professor A. I. Darling in the Dental School of Bristol University.

An article in the Report for 1960–61 discusses one line of attack that was being followed in the new Unit, namely the origin and prevention of the early lesion in the enamel that gives caries its entry, whatever may be its causative agent. This involved histological, chemical and physical studies of both normal and carious enamel, with observations of the mode of spread of what is "probably the most prevalent disease in man." Factors such as the protective hardening effect of traces of fluorides in the drinking water were also taken into account. It is perhaps a sign of changed times that no other mention of the dependence of dental structure on nutrition was apparently considered necessary.

A once more reconstituted Dental Committee held its first meeting early in 1967, under the chairmanship of Professor B. Cohen, and a year later submitted a memorandum to the Council urging the creation of further research units in the subject and the expansion of career opportunities for investigators with various qualifications. Shortage of research personnel and a piecemeal approach to the problem were believed to be retarding progress.

A Dental Epidemiology Unit, directed by Professor G. L. Slack, was set up in 1970 in the Dental School of the London Hospital Medical College.

Chapter 6
Preventive Medicine: Age and Environment

Paediatrics—Obstetric medicine—Geriatrics—Physical exercise—Vision and hearing—Climatic influences—Air hygiene—Toxicology—Alcohol—Tobacco—Hazards of Radiation—Mental health

Paediatrics

Several of the subjects covered in this chapter, particularly those related to ages of life, have therapeutic as well as prophylactic aspects, but the latter have predominated in the research work which the Council has supported.

Much of the research on nutrition and dental disease, discussed in the preceding chapter, has special relevance to the health of growing children. Other work again has been directly orientated to that subject. The original Medical Research Committee appointed a Child Life Committee, which became particularly active in the years immediately following the 1914–18 war. This in fact consisted of two committees, one in London and the other in Scotland. Of the work to be done, the Report of the Medical Research Committee for 1918–19 carried the following statement:

> The Committee from the beginning of their work have had in view the early organization of a widespread inquiry into the chief factors contributing to infant mortality, both antenatal and postnatal. Much of the present high mortality is obviously due to general preventible causes like maternal ignorance, urbanization and improper housing, and to imperfect feeding. But while available knowledge is already far ahead of effective administrative action in these respects, there are many factors contributing to a high infant death-rate which are at present quite imperfectly understood. It is clear, moreover, that our knowledge of the causes of many dead births and premature births is lacking, and chiefly for the want of organized scientific work. Dead and premature births in enormous numbers have gone almost wholly unexamined, and it is probable that there are important problems to be faced in this respect which have not yet been even stated, in the absence of carefully recorded systematic examinations. Provision for examinations of the kind, and for their scientific analysis, is likely not only to contribute to the immediate object of diminishing child mortality but also to give information about disorders in the balance of chemical changes or in the rates of embryonic development which may throw new light upon general physiological and pathological processes.

The London Committee, under the chairmanship of Dr G. F. Still, had a predominantly pathological programme; it was indeed once cynically suggested that a better name would have been 'Child Death Committee'. The investigations reported upon in the Council's series dealt with the effects of maternal syphilis, with the estimation of foetal age, and with the causes of foetal death, dead birth and neonatal death.

The Scottish Committee in Glasgow came under the immediate chairmanship of Professor D. Noel Paton, who was also chairman of the combined Committee, and had Dr Leonard Findlay as its senior clinical member. It had a more definitely postnatal outlook, and it was enabled by the Council to employ assistants in the investigation of social factors. The results of a comprehensive study of children in cities and rural districts of Scotland—with poverty, nutrition and growth as the main theme—were published in a long report in the Council's series (Paton, Findlay et al. 1926). An early report in the series, also from Glasgow, had been on infant mortality (Chalmers, Brend, Findlay & Brownlee 1917).

Over many years, Dr Helen Mackay was a part-time member of the Council's external staff, working at the Queen's (later Queen Elizabeth) Hospital for Children, London. Her subjects of research included anaemias of infancy, iron metabolism, serum protein levels, and comparison of results of breast feeding and various forms of artificial feeding on the health of infants. A monograph on these subjects by Dr Mackay and others was published in the Council's series in 1959.

Another example of work bearing on the health of infants related to renal function. Whereas, within wide limits, adults are enabled to keep their body fluids stable by the action of the kidney and other organs and can eat and drink what they like without unduly straining the mechanism, infants cannot do so. A study of the reason for this was made by Professor R. A. McCance and his colleagues in the Council's Department of Experimental Medicine at Cambridge; and they showed that infants are less well able than adults to concentrate waste products in the urine, and particularly to excrete urea or salt. Among other points, it was found that the kidney of the newborn is relatively unresponsive to the antidiuretic hormone of the posterior pituitary gland. The recognition of these limitations of renal function in very early life has helped towards explaining certain established facts, and also towards improving the management of infants, especially when sick. It follows, for instance, that growth and diet play a more important part than the kidneys in maintaining the stability of the body fluids in infancy; and this is a consideration which, to quote the report for 1955–56, "has special significance when an infant or newborn animal is fed on a food which has not been provided for it by nature, and which is therefore almost inevitably unbalanced in some respect".

In the 1940s an eye disease in premature infants, first described in America under the name of retrolental fibroplasia, came into prominence as a cause of total and permanent blindness. It suddenly appeared in epidemic form in nurseries for premature infants attached to hospitals in the United States, Great Britain and other countries. In 1952, accordingly, the Council convened a conference under the chairmanship of Sir Stewart Duke-Elder to correlate investigations into the nature and cause of this condition; statistical and pathological studies were set in train. At the same time the Ministry of Health initiated an inquiry into the eye condition of all premature infants born in England and Wales in 1951. Eventually all the evidence, including dramatic results of experimental work by Dr N. H. Ashton and others at the Institute of Ophthalmology in London, showed that the cause was damage to the retinal circulation from the use of too high concentrations of oxygen in rearing these infants through their most difficult stage. This discovery led directly to prevention by reducing the concentration of oxygen, and in reviewing the investigation in its Report for 1953–54 the Council concluded:

> It is probable that some other factors may enter into the causation of the disease, and that sporadic cases may occur in the future as they did before 1942; but it seems clear that retrolental fibroplasia as a common and tragic disease has already virtually disappeared as dramatically as it appeared a little over a decade ago. Seldom has a disease, so apparently enigmatic in its causation, so intractable to treatment and so tragic in its effects, been so rapidly brought under control.

Obstetric medicine

In 1954 the Council considered how it could best aid the advancement of knowledge in obstetric medicine, so-called in distinction from the surgical aspects of obstetrics and gynaecology which have dominated practice in this field and the training of specialists to work in it. The research approach through surgery having been largely exploited, the problems pressing most urgently for investigation were those requiring the point of view and methods of the physician. Toxaemias of pregnancy, premature labour, stillbirths and disordered lactation presented perplexing questions of this kind.

During the preceding sixteen years, an integrated plan of research had been built up by Professor (later Sir) Dugald Baird as head of the Department of Midwifery in the University of Aberdeen and its associated hospitals. Under this scheme, investigations were pushed back into the community to seek possible causes of the difficulties later encountered in hospital. The method was to use a social medicine team as a reconnaisance unit to break down broad problems into smaller and more clearly defined subjects for intensive study. Some of the investigations lay in the field of epidemiology, social medicine and nutrition, some in that of reproductive physiology, and others in that of clinical obstetrics. The Council had assisted this project and had provided a team of six workers as a detachment from its Social Medicine Research Unit in London.

In agreement with the University and other authorities, the Council decided to consolidate the position by establishing an

Obstetric Medicine Research Unit in Professor Baird's department and under his honorary direction. Dr Angus Thomson, then also holding an academic appointment, was Honorary Deputy Director but later joined the Council's staff. The detachment from the Social Medicine Research Unit became part of the new Unit; and the provision of a suitable building was financed by the Scottish Hospital Endowments Research Trust.

This arrangement proved to be very fruitful in research, and it was maintained until Sir Dugald Baird's retirement in 1965. Part of the staff, under Dr Thomson, was then moved to the Princess Mary Maternity Hospital, Newcastle upon Tyne, where it became the Council's Reproduction and Growth Research Unit. The rest of the staff remained in Aberdeen as the Medical Sociology Research Unit; this is under the honorary direction of Professor R. Illsley, a member of the original Unit, who had been appointed to a chair of sociology in the University.

There were of course, over the years, various other investigations in the obstetric field. For instance, in the period immediately preceding the Second World War, Dr Matthew Young of the Council's staff, working in the Institute of Anatomy at University College London, had collected observations for a combined radiological and clinical investigation of the influence which minor variations in the form of the pelvis had on foetal presentation and labour. This was done in collaboration with Dr J. G. Hastings Ince of the Obstetric Unit in University College Hospital. Among other conclusions, a classification of pelvic form which had recently been strongly recommended was shown to be not only unscientific but cumbersome and of no practical value.

Reference has been made earlier (Chapter 3) to a useful collaboration between Dr A. S. (later Sir Alan) Parkes of the National Institute for Medical Research and Dr J. (later Sir John) Hammond of the Animal Nutrition Institute at Cambridge, in studies of stimulating and controlling female reproduction potential. The work began with an investigation by Dr Parkes into the effect of horse pituitary extracts on the fertility of rabbits. It was extended by Dr Hammond to sheep, of which a small flock was maintained at Cambridge. It was found that fertility could be increased by the method—a result which might obviously have high agricultural importance. There was the further possibility of practical application to the human female in certain circumstances; but there was in any event a demonstration of interplay between veterinary and human physiology.

Investigations of puerperal infection ('childbed fever'), and the success of chemotherapy in dealing with this dangerous condition, are mentioned elsewhere (Chapter 3).

Geriatrics
The Council's chief project in geriatrics was the Unit (originally Group) for Research on Occupational Aspects of Ageing, set up

in 1955 and directed by Dr Alastair Heron, and subsequently by Professor L. S. Hearnshaw, in the Department of Psychology, University of Liverpool. This was disbanded in 1970.

The problem of mental disorders in old age was discussed in the Report for 1960–61. A field study had been made in the north of England by the Department of Psychiatry of Durham University, where the Council thereafter set up a Research Group on Mental Disorders (later the Research Group on the Relation of Functional to Organic Psychiatric Illness) under the honorary direction of Professor (later Sir) Martin Roth. Contributions to the subject, in the same period, were also made by Dr J. A. N. Corsellis, receiving a grant from the Council at Runwell Hospital, Wickford (Essex), and by the Council's Clinical Psychiatry Research Unit at Graylingwell Hospital, Chichester (Sussex). From 1966 the Council supported a Research Group on the Biology of Ageing, under the direction of Dr Alex Comfort, at University College London.

Experiments in senescence have recently been undertaken, on microorganisms, at the National Institute for Medical Research. The object has been to test a theory, put forward in the literature, that ageing is due to an accumulation of errors of protein synthesis brought about by biochemical accidents affecting the transcription or translation of genetic information. Theories of senescence have been reviewed in the Reports for 1966–67 and 1971–72.

Physical exercise

In its Report for 1937–38, the Council made comment on the Physical Training and Recreation Act 1937, which gave effect to the Government's previously announced intention of providing increased facilities for the promotion of physical exercise and recreation:

> The powerful instinct in all healthy young and adolescent human beings to take exercise, and the feeling of well-being that usually accompanies and follows it, are well recognized. In addition, however, to these immediate effects of exercise, there is the larger problem of its ultimate effect on physique and health. . . . In view of such beneficial effects it is surprising how little is known as to the physiological basis, either of the processes underlying the feeling of well-being or of the mechanism of improved physique and health. Even less study has been given to the optimum nature and amount of exercise for individuals differing in physique and mental outlook. Training in various exercises and sports is still largely based on empiricism, and the undoubtedly deleterious effects which may result from too arduous and otherwise unsuitable forms of physical activity for some individuals require careful analysis.

The Council then referred to the relation between physical exercise and nutritional state, concluding that there was need for scientific inquiry, and also for providing scientific advice on how best to use the opportunity presented by the Act for studying the combined effects of exercise and food on the body.

In these circumstances, the Council gladly accepted an invitation from the (then) Board of Education to advise on certain aspects of the subject, including the kind of provision needed at the proposed National College of Physical Training for teaching the elements of the sciences on which the art of physical training rests. The Board also sought the Council's advice about research into the effects of effort, repose, diet and growth. For this purpose the Council appointed a Physical Exercise Research Committee and liaison was established between this and the National Advisory Council on Physical Training and Education under the Viscount Dawson.

The outbreak of war put an end to that scheme for the time being; but in the 1960s both the Division of Human Physiology in the National Institute for Medical Research and the Council's Environmental Physiology Research Unit worked on problems of exercise physiology, using athletes as subjects. The creation of the Sports Council in 1965, and subsequent plans for the development of research facilities at the Crystal Palace National Recreation Centre, provided an opportunity for taking this interest further. As an initial step a caravan fitted as a mobile laboratory was provided by the Central Council of Physical Recreation (who managed the centre) for the use of Council staff interested in physiological research of this kind. The relation of leisure exercise to health and disease (particularly cardiovascular) has been the subject of prospective studies by the MRC Social Medicine Unit.

Vision and hearing

The prevention of blindness and deafness, or of lesser defects in vision and hearing, may appropriately be considered in this chapter, although there are of course also purely clinical problems in relation to diseases of eye and ear. Basic physiological and psychological questions are involved in the full understanding of these vital senses, and in both cases the Council's programmes of research began at that level—apart from applied studies of illumination and noise prevention (Chapter 9).

The appointment in 1924 of the Committee on the Physiology of Vision, under the chairmanship of Sir John Parsons, led to the promotion of numerous investigations, mainly experimental, on its advice. Many of the results were embodied in the fourteen reports of the Committee published in the Council's series in the period 1926–35. These were contributed by individual authors and dealt with such subjects as illumination and visual capacity, dark adaptation (review of literature), adaptation in relation to flicker, peripheral vision, measurement of visual acuity, psychology of reading, and (four reports) various problems of colour vision. At a later stage, from 1957, the Council's series included a number of reports by Professor Arnold Sorsby and others, chiefly on questions of refraction. Sorsby was also the author of a Memorandum, issued by the Council in 1950, on the causes of blindness in England and Wales.

In 1944 the Council had established a Vision Research Unit under the direction of Dr Hamilton Hartridge at the Institute of Ophthalmology in London. On the retirement of Dr Hartridge in 1951, this became the Group for Research on the Physiology of Vision, under Dr L. C. Thomson. On the untimely death of the latter in 1955, the Group was absorbed by the Council's Ophthalmological Research Unit, which had been set up at the same centre in 1948 under the part-time direction of Sir Stewart Duke-Elder. When he retired in 1962, the Unit was transferred to the Institute of Ophthalmology, except for one division retained by the Council as a new Vision Research Unit under Dr H. J. A. Dartnall, now attached to the University of Sussex. From 1954 till 1966 the Council was also enabled to maintain a Wernher Group (later Unit) for Research in Ophthalmological Genetics, under Professor Sorsby, at the Royal College of Surgeons of England.

As expressed in the Report for 1950–51, the great blinding diseases of the past had dwindled in importance as the general infections to which they were due had been largely mastered; but progress in dealing with diseases peculiar to the eye itself, such as cataract and glaucoma, was hampered by ignorance of the fundamental physiology of the organ. This applied especially to the fluid which fills the eye and in which the tissues function. Research on the circulation and pressure within the eye, with special reference to glaucoma, was therefore a main preoccupation of the unit directed by Sir Stewart Duke-Elder; the subject was reviewed in the Report for 1959–60. The Unit also studied the metabolism of other tissues of the eye, notably the lens and cornea, while on the clinical side the applicability of antibiotic and cortisone therapy received much attention. The work of the Trachoma Research Unit, falling within the field of tropical medicine, is mentioned elsewhere (Chapter 10).

The Committee upon the Physiology of Hearing, appointed by the Council in 1928 under the chairmanship of Professor T. Graham Brown, sponsored a number of investigations, and five reports contributed by various authors appeared in the Council's series in the period 1932–37. These dealt with the localisation of sound, hearing and speech in deaf children, and the use of hearing aids.

Towards the end of the Second World War, the position with regard to the prevention and relief of deafness had greatly improved. Chemotherapy with sulphonamide drugs and penicillin had proved efficacious in dealing with middle ear and mastoid infections, in children the commonest causes of loss of hearing. New surgical procedures of great refinement could relieve certain types of deafness. Better methods of educating the deaf had been devised. Miniature electronic equipment had been developed, primarily for military purposes, that was capable of incorporation in hearing aids of higher efficiency and greater convenience than those previously available.

The Council's work for the Ministry of Health on hearing aids (considered as therapeutic appliances) has been mentioned earlier; and, in that connection, also the establishment of the Otological

Research Unit in 1944, and the appointment of three related committees in the same year. On the retirement of Dr C. S. Hallpike in 1965, the Unit continued for a further two years under the honorary direction of Sir Terence Cawthorne. A Hearing and Balance Unit, under Dr J. D. Hood, later took its place. From 1949 to 1965 the Council had, in addition, its Wernher Research Unit on Deafness at King's College Hospital, London, under the direction of a physicist, Dr T. S. Littler. At the end of the period of this history deafness was designated by the Council as a priority area for research.

Climatic influences
Reference is made elsewhere to the research work undertaken for the Services, during the Second World War, on protection against the effects of climatic extremes, both of cold and of heat (Chapter 16). Work on this subject was maintained by the Council after the return of peace, for civilian purposes as well as for the continuing requirements of the Services. Apart from the analogy with artificial conditions met with in certain industries, there are practical applications to life in the tropics (on the part of unadapted people) and to the rigours of exploratory expeditions (Chapter 10).

The expanding post-war facilities for research of this kind were provided by several of the Council's establishments, old and new. The Environmental Hygiene Research Unit, the Applied Psychology Research Unit and the Department of Experimental Medicine at Cambridge all played a part. In addition, a Climate and Working Efficiency Research Unit was established at Oxford, a Division of Human Physiology (with climatic chambers for studying the effects of extreme temperatures on human performance) was formed in the National Institute for Medical Research, and a Tropical Research Unit was set up jointly with the Admiralty at Singapore (Appendix C); and on the advice of the Colonial Medical Research Committee the Colonial Office established a laboratory near Lagos, in Nigeria.

Air hygiene
Measures under this head aim at the maintenance of adequate standards of purity, temperature, humidity and movement of air breathed by human beings, particularly in enclosed spaces and built-up areas; and in respect of purity it is necessary to consider not only the absence of an excessive proportion of carbon dioxide but also reasonable freedom from contamination by airborne micro-organisms, noxious gases and deleterious particles in the form of dust. Such measures must be based on knowledge both of the natural human requirements and of the mechanical means of securing them. Mention is made elsewhere of research undertaken by the Council, more particularly in respect of industrial premises, tropical conditions and the special needs of the Services (Chapters 9, 10, 15).

From the beginning, the Medical Research Committee had a Department of Applied Physiology in the National Institute for Medical Research. This was under the direction of Dr (later Sir)

Leonard Hill, who made a special study of air hygiene from the physiological point of view. A main tool in the investigations was his 'katathermometer', which could be used with either a dry or a wet bulb to measure the cooling and evaporative power of the atmosphere; it worked on the principle of measuring its own rate of cooling at approximately body temperature. Hill's monograph, issued in two parts as special reports, not only gave the results of his own work but constituted a textbook of the physiological information then available on ventilation and open-air treatment. The first part (1919) dealt with the cooling and evaporative power of the atmosphere in relation to heat loss of the body in still and moving air, and also with heat loss in water. The second (1920) dealt with radiations in the atmosphere and the action of light on the body; with the effects of exercise, sweating and diet, and with the causation of heat-stroke; with the purity or impurity of the air in various respects, and more generally with the relation of health to the environment; and with open-air treatment, including treatment at Alpine altitudes. Nor was clothing forgotten, and the following counsel was given to Europeans in respect of life in the tropics: "Custom and fashion should not forbid white women to secure in their dress sufficient exposure and ventilation of the body surface"— which advice would latterly appear to have been taken.

Later work by Sir Leonard Hill and Dr J. Argyll Campbell had special reference to life at high and low atmospheric pressures. Work on the 'decompression' of divers was undertaken for the assistance of the Deep Diving Committee of the Admiralty.

After Hill's retirement, the subject—so far as the Council's programme was involved—became largely the concern of external scientific staff, working mainly in an industrial context. After the Second World War there was again a division of human physiology at the National Institute for Medical Research, as mentioned in the preceding section, and from this there has more recently been derived a Laboratory of Field Physiology (see final section of this chapter).

Further work on the pollution of urban air was stimulated by dense fog persisting for four days in the Greater London area in December 1952. This led to an exceptionally high concentration of pollution in the lower atmosphere, to which some 4000 deaths from bronchitis and pneumonia were attributed; there was also a heavy mortality among animals entered for the Smithfield show. A special subcommittee of the Council's Social and Environmental Health Committee was charged with investigating the nature of such pollution and its effects on health. Afterwards, in 1955, an Air Pollution Research Unit was set up by the Council at St Bartholomew's Hospital, London, with Dr P. J. Lawther as Director, and a Group for Epidemiological Research on Respiratory Diseases (Air Pollution) under Dr J. Pemberton in the University of Sheffield. Investigations were made into the composition of 'smog' (smoke/fog); into both acute and chronic effects of breathing this polluted air; and into methods of protection, particularly for the sick and aged. Epidemiological inquiries were also undertaken into the relation of the intensity and composition of pollution to the incidence and severity of various forms of respiratory disease. Meanwhile, in parallel, a nation-wide survey of these conditions was organised by the Department of Scientific and Industrial Research. The Clean Air Act 1956 was intended to diminish the nuisance but could be implemented only gradually. By the early 1960s, however, a striking improvement in smoke concentrations could be demonstrated in London, and there is evidence that this has had a beneficial effect from the point of view of respiratory disease. This subject is discussed in a review article on bronchitis in the Report for 1967–68. Research on bacteriological contamination of air is mentioned in the next chapter.

Toxicology

Modern manufacture has introduced many poisonous substances into human use for a variety of purposes, or into man's environment more or less incidentally; and new possibly harmful compounds are constantly being added. The study of the effects of such substances, and the assessment of the risks involved in different degrees of exposure to them, form an important subject for research in preventive medicine. The experimental approach is handicapped by the wide variations in the responses of different animal species. And although acute toxic effects may be relatively simple to determine, the possibility of long-term damage—especially if the substance accumulates in the tissues—is much harder to assess; the familiar difficulty of proving a negative is apt to be experienced.

In so far as the risks arise in the course of making these substances, or of using them in other manufacturing processes, the subject falls within the particular sphere of industrial medicine and is considered later (Chapter 9). The risks to the public at large may be more limited in kind although they obviously have a wider incidence. One channel of danger has been mentioned in the preceding chapter, namely the addition of various substances to foodstuffs as preservatives or 'improvers'; this use is strictly controlled by law, but regulations have to be based on secure knowledge.

Another hazard to the general public lay in the widespread and increasing use of pesticidal chemicals, particularly in agriculture, a question discussed in the Council's Report for 1952–53. Many of these are highly toxic, although the specially dangerous group of organophosphorus compounds has been banned in the United Kingdom and elsewhere. It is surprising that others, such as the widely used and long-persisting chlorinated hydrocarbons, have so far not been shown to have deleterious effects on the human population comparable with the damage done to wildlife, but constant vigilance is clearly required. The risk to industrial workers manufacturing toxic substances can be controlled, but where the pesticides are excessively or carelessly applied, as by some farmers and domestic users, the chances of serious exposure cannot be discounted. There is also the danger inherent in the contamination of human foodstuffs as the result of application either to growing crops or to stored products.

The Council's chief instrument of research in all these matters is its Toxicology Unit, set up in 1947 with Dr J. M. Barnes as Director. It was at first housed in the Chemical Defence Experimental Establishment at Porton, Wiltshire, by arrangement with the Ministry of Supply; but it was moved in 1950 to the MRC Laboratories, Carshalton, of which it is now the largest component. The original purpose was defined as being to assist in the solution of toxicological problems referred to the Council by other bodies, and to do research on fundamental problems arising from the routine work. The need was due to the increase in the number of requests from the chemical industry for information about the toxicity of new compounds. The aim was later described as being to establish the basic concepts necessary for explaining at the molecular level the mechanisms of toxicity and of chemical and physical injury to the tissues, and thereby to further the understanding of physiological processes. The work includes assessment of the acute and chronic toxic effects of various substances; elucidation of the biochemical mechanisms by which such substances act in the body; and the experimental pathology of trauma. The Unit is recognised by the World Health Organisation as a Reference Centre for Evaluation and Testing of New Insecticides. A review of toxicological research was included in the Report for 1968–69.

Alcohol
During the First World War, the Medical Research Committee promoted work on the physiological effects of alcohol at the request of the Central Control Board (Liquor Traffic), and was represented on a committee which prepared a booklet summarising knowledge of the subject. As mentioned in Volume One, the Council subsequently took responsibility for preparing later editions (1929, 1938) of the book, reconstituting the special committee for this purpose. Scientific accounts of the investigations were published in three special reports: by Dr Edward Mellanby on the absorption of alcohol into the blood and its disappearance therefrom under different conditions; by Dr H. M. Vernon on the influence of alcohol on manual work and neuromuscular coordination; and by Professor J. McDougall and Dr May Smith on the effects of alcohol and some other drugs during normal and fatigued conditions. Dr Smith, for many years a member of the Council's staff, was herself the subject of many of the dotting machine tests and all the better for her innocence of the uses of alcohol in ordinary life.

In 1932 a report was published in the Council's series giving the results of a long and laborious experiment conducted by Miss

F. M. Durham at the National Institute for Medical Research with the statistical collaboration of Miss H. M. Woods. The results gave no support to the alarming findings in a similar experiment that had been made in America on the effects of alcohol on the fecundity of guinea-pigs and on the quality of their offspring, when administered daily in quantities just sufficient to produce visible intoxication. The American results had seemed to show that alcohol caused a fall in the number of births, an increased liability to stillbirths, and the production of weakly and defective offspring; and, more seriously, that these tendencies were inherited, so that without further exposure of the stock to alcohol the proportion of weakly or deformed animals continued to be high in subsequent generations, implying injury to the germ cells and permanent deterioration of the stock. That no such effects were observed in repetition of the work was an important negative finding, although the reason for the discrepancy remained a matter for speculation; there was possibly some undetected dietetic or genetic factor in the earlier work, but further experimentation on an adequate scale and over many years was impracticable.

At a much later date, attention became strongly directed to the serious social problem of the effect of alcohol on the drivers of motor vehicles and the extent to which the toll of road accidents was increased thereby. In 1959 a Memorandum was issued by the Council giving the results of experiments by Professor G. C. Drew and others on the effect of small doses of alcohol on a skill resembling driving. In 1961 the Council sponsored an investigation into the comparative reliability of different methods of measuring alcohol in the breath, including the use of an apparatus developed at the National Institute for Medical Research, and into the value of the measure as an indicator of blood alcohol levels (Begg *et al.* 1964). And in 1965, at the request of the Home Office, the Council commented on the association between the consumption of alcohol and impairment of skill in driving a motor vehicle. The Council's statement, of which the substance was given in a Government White Paper in the following year, supported the findings of a committee of inquiry appointed by the British Medical Association.

Tobacco

As regards tobacco, in 1947 the Council convened a conference to discuss the possible causes of the great increase in mortality from cancer of the lung that had been noted in the United Kingdom and other countries; and among the possibilities was the habit of smoking, which had also much increased. Professor (later Sir Austen) Bradford Hill and Dr (later Professor Sir) Richard Doll of the Council's Statistical Research Unit undertook an investigation, and they were able to publish a preliminary paper in 1950. This indicated a relation between lung cancer and smoking, and no comparable association was found with any of the other possible factors studied.

This first investigation was retrospective, ascertaining the histories, with respect to smoking and other factors, of some 700 patients with carcinoma of the lung and more than twice that number of hospital patients with other conditions. The lung cancer group was found to contain a much smaller proportion of non-smokers than did the control group, and also a larger proportion of heavy smokers. The importance of this finding was so obvious that secondary investigations were initiated at thoracic centres in different parts of the country; another was undertaken independently in the United States. All produced very similar results.

The final paper (1952) covered about double the number of patients, and as the Council's Report for 1955-56 said: "Analysis of the histories and habits of the patients with various diseases revealed only one striking contrast—the difference in the smoking habits of those with and those without lung cancer". The smoking of cigarettes was particularly incriminated, as compared with tobacco in other forms. The same Report reviewed the great spate of work on the subject that had developed, both under the Council's aegis and in other countries. The British statistical evidence had been greatly strengthened by a paper (Doll and Hill 1956) giving the results of an inquiry, prospective rather than retrospective, in which over 40 000 replies were received to a questionnaire sent to all members of the medical profession in the United Kingdom asking for brief particulars of their smoking habits. The subjects were classified in broad groups, and information was collected during the next four-and-a-half years about the deaths occurring among them. The Report said:

Analysis of the data relating to men has shown a marked and steady increase in the mortality from lung cancer as the amount smoked increases. Thus, at ages 35 and over, the death rate per year rose from 0·07 per 1000 in non-smokers (based upon the observation of one death only) to 0·47 per 1000 in smokers of 14 grams a day, to 0·86 per 1000 smokers of 15 to 24 grams a day and finally to 1·66 per 1000 in smokers of 25 grams a day (one gram of tobacco is approximately the amount contained in one cigarette). The death rate of the heavy smokers was therefore some 20 times the rate in the non-smokers. In cigarette smokers the rate was substantially higher than in pipe smokers, while the rate for smokers by both methods fell in between. Among men who had given up smoking within the previous 10 years the rate was lower than among men who, at the time of completing their questionnaire, were continuing to smoke, and among men who had given up smoking for more than 10 years it was lower still. It follows that the highest mortalities were found among men who were continuing to smoke cigarettes, and among heavy smokers in this group the death rate was nearly 40 times the rate among non-smokers (that is an *annual* rate of 2·76 per 1000 against an annual rate of 0·07 per 1000).

No adequate explanation of the statistical evidence has been advanced other than that smoking is indeed the principal factor in the causation of lung cancer. Nor is it difficult to interpret this, theoretically, in terms of physics and chemistry. To obtain direct proof by experiment is another matter, and the complications have not been successfully overcome in spite of much work on the subject (in which the possible role of other factors, such as certain industrial hazards and particular forms of atmospheric pollution, was not neglected). In financing its programme in this field, at a number of centres, the Council was helped by a benefaction from a group of British tobacco manufacturers (Volume One).

It has been mentioned in Volume One that the subject provided the occasion for one of the Council's rare essays in public information, a statement issued in 1957 entitled *Tobacco smoking and cancer of the lung*. Research on addiction is mentioned later (Chapter 9).

Hazards of radiation
The Council has been involved in research on many other carcinogenic hazards, arising from a very diverse range of sources, often in an occupational context. Moreover, new substances are constantly being introduced into the environment and into the medical armoury—and these must be monitored by means of both experimental investigations and epidemiological surveys. A particular concern of the Council has been with the hazards of ionising radiations, which include both cancer and genetic mutation.

Protection against the hazards of radiations has indeed become an additional task of preventive medicine. Exposure to ionising radiations may arise from natural sources, which is inescapable, and from medical and industrial applications—and of course fallout from nuclear weapon tests. The relative magnitude and significance of these different types of exposure have been a matter of prolonged and detailed study, in which the Council has played a prominent part.

Mention has been made in Volume One of the Council's role in advising HM Government on the subject. In 1955, following debates in Parliament, the Council accepted responsibility for preparing a White Paper on the medical aspects of nuclear radiation, including the genetic aspects, and appointed a committee to undertake the task; this was presented to Parliament, under the title *The Hazards to Man of Nuclear and Allied Radiations*, in 1956. A second White Paper with the same title was published in 1960 to take account of the most recent developments, and two shorter reports were later published (see below). In 1957 the Prime Minister, through the Lord President, asked the Council to appoint an independent committee to comment on the health and safety aspects of a report, by a committee chaired by Sir William (now Lord) Penney, on an accident at the nuclear energy station at Windscale, Cumberland; these comments were quickly provided. In 1964 the Council received a report from its Committee on Protection against Ionising Radiations on *The Exposure of the Population to Radiation from Fallout*, and this was published as a pamphlet by Her Majesty's Stationery Office.

In 1965, the Council submitted a memorandum to the Department of Education and Science giving a reassessment of certain aspects of the problem; this was published by the Stationery Office in the following year under the title *The Assessment of the Possible Radiation Risks to the Population from Environmental Contamination*. Reference was made in Volume One to the series of Monitoring Reports, also issued by the Council, on the concentrations of strontium-90 in human bone. The subject is, of course, one of concern to all countries, and latterly Sir Edward Pochin and Dr J. Vennart of the Council's scientific staff have been Chairmen of the standing International Commission on Radiological Protection under the auspices of the International Congress of Radiology. The report of a special Council Committee on Radiobiology was published in the Annual Report for 1968–69.

The Council has several establishments engaged in research in this field. In 1947 the Council set up its Radiobiological Research Unit, under the direction of Dr J. F. Loutit, alongside the Atomic Energy Research Establishment at Harwell. This project originated from a request from the Ministry of Supply that the Council should appoint a medical director of research at Harwell to study the hazards to health from work in nuclear physics. The Unit in the event developed a wide programme related to radiological protection and became, while the need was greatest, virtually an institute, with divisions of biophysics, chemistry, genetics, cytogenetics, and experimental pathology. Eventually, Dr Loutit and his immediate assistants were transferred to the External Scientific Staff, while still working at Harwell, and the Unit continued with less wide terms of reference under the direction of Dr R. H. Mole.

Another establishment was set up at the Western General Hospital, Edinburgh, in 1956, as the Group for Research on the General Effects of Radiation—later the Clinical Effects of Radiation Research Unit, and, when the scope of the work had widened, renamed the MRC Clinical and Population Cytogenetics Unit. The Director, until his death in 1968, was Dr (later Professor) W. H. Court Brown. Originally, the aim was to ascertain the incidence of leukaemia in patients who had been treated with X-rays for ankylosing spondylitis. Subsequently the main theme was the study of radiation-induced tumours in man, and this led the Unit to play a leading role in the development of human cytogenetics, including investigation of the chromosome constitution of malignant cells and chromosome aberrations in people who had been irradiated. A Registry of Abnormal Karyotypes was set up, for prospective studies on people with congenitally abnormal chromosomes, and a Special Report by Court Brown and his colleagues on abnormalities of the sex chromosome complement was published in 1964. Professor H. J. Evans became Director of the Unit in 1968.

The work of the Experimental Radiopathology Unit at Hammersmith Hospital, London, set up in 1953 under Dr G. J. Popjak (succeeded by Dr T. Alper), was also directed to the effects of radiation on living organisms, but with emphasis more on the clinical side in relation to radiotherapy.

In 1959 the Council set up an Environmental Radiation Research Unit under the honorary direction of Professor F. W. Spiers in the University Department of Medical Physics at the General Infirmary, Leeds. The aim was to assess the dose received by human tissues from environmental ionising radiations and to consider its biological significance. Apart from direct relevance to practical problems of radiation protection, the results have had potential clinical applications and much scientific interest. Before its disbandment on the retirement of Professor Spiers, the Unit had developed extremely sensitive whole-body radiation counters, and enclosures with exceptionally low background levels for their use; it has also employed thermoluminescence dosimetry for the direct measurement of the radiation delivered to the marrow cells in animal bone by isotope deposits.

From 1953 the Ministry of Health and the Council jointly maintained a Radiological Protection Service, which acted as a central organisation for the control of radiation hazards; it collected and disseminated information, and it engaged in monitoring and advisory services. Its research work was mainly of a physical nature. The Director, Mr W. Binks, had headquarters at Sutton, Surrey; and there were regional centres at Birmingham, Leeds, Manchester and Glasgow, the last maintained jointly with the Scottish Home and Health Department. In 1971 the service, hitherto administered by the Council, was amalgamated with the Radiological Protection Division of the UK Atomic Energy Authority and became the responsibility of a new National Radiation Protection Board set up under the Radiological Protection Act 1970.

In 1959, the World Health Organisation's Expert Committee on Radiation urged the importance of obtaining data on the consequences of prolonged exposure to low doses of radiation in the world's few areas of high natural radioactivity. In 1961–62 Professor H. Grüneberg, Honorary Director of the Council's Experimental Genetics Research Unit, went to one such area—Kerala, in southern India—to make a study of local populations of the black rat. Skeletal and dental material was brought back for examination, measurement and statistical treatment, in which several additional workers took part. A report published in the Council's series shows that no positive evidence of any genetic effects of radiation was found. At the other extreme, two members of the Council's staff already mentioned, Court Brown and Doll, took part in studying late effects of radiation among survivors from the dropping of atomic bombs on Nagasaki and Hiroshima in 1945.

Mental Health
Research on mental disorders has already been discussed as a branch of clinical science; and certain basic physiological studies are men-

tioned later. It remains to say here that the maintenance of positive
mental health is an aspect of preventive medicine, and that the
eventual fruits of research into the causes of its impairment are likely
to have importance for prophylaxis as well as for treatment. This
may be especially true of research into the influences of the social
environment, including occupational stresses, as discussed later. The
special problem of mental disorders in old age has already been
mentioned, in this chapter.

With regard to the scientific basis for the study of mental health
and disorder, Sir Harold Himsworth has summarised the position
as follows, in a memorandum in the annual report for 1967–68:

> It would be idle to pretend that there is any part of this field in which we can
> operate with anything like the confidence that we feel in practically all others.
> Yet there is undoubtedly a stirring of interest among men of ability such as
> normally presages advance. On the biological wing research into many aspects
> of brain function is starting up widely. Behaviour and learning studies are
> developing significantly over the range from clinical and epidemiological studies
> to the biochemical and pharmacological laboratory. Psychopharmacology both
> on human subjects and on animals has made significant moves. On the psych-
> iatric side, review and analysis are introducing a new definition into the subject.
> Collaborative work with sociologists is probing the influence of environment.
> At present we can claim to be doing no more than nibble at the perimeter, but
> opportunities are reappearing and we cannot afford to neglect any.

In 1968 the Council set up a special committee to review the field
of biochemical research in relation to psychiatric disorders and to
make recommendations. The report of this committee was published
in 1970, and since then the Council has established a new unit, the
Neurochemical Pharmacology Unit under Dr L. L. Iversen; the
work of the new Clinical Pharmacology Unit, directed by Professor
D. G. Grahame-Smith, is also pertinent.

Chapter 7
Preventive Medicine: Infections and Infestations

Microbiology and parasitology—Research in bacteriology—Epidemiology—
Bacteriology of tuberculosis—Tuberculosis in cattle—Intestinal infections—
Viruses—Canine distemper—Influenza—The common cold—Poliomyelitis—
Viruses and cancer—Fungal infections—Protozoology—Metazoan parasites
and vectors—Immunology—Drug resistance—Cross-infection and air hygiene

Microbiology and parasitology

An important part of preventive medicine consists in defence against
infections and infestations by living organisms of various kinds.
This involves a study of the natural history of the organisms in
question; it is necessary to know one's enemy. There has thus grown
up a group of secondary sciences that are ancillary to medicine—
and sometimes to agriculture or industry. Under the general head
of microbiology are the branches of science concerned with bacteria
(bacteriology), viruses (virology), fungi (mycology) and protozoa
(protozoology). There is also the study of the metazoan parasites,
external or internal, such as insects and arachnids (entomology and
acarology) and different classes of 'worms' (helminthology). It is
likewise important to have some understanding of animals that act
as vectors of disease, either by the mechanical transmission of infection or by serving as intermediate hosts of parasites with complex
life-cycles; here again insects and arachnids are of outstanding significance, but a part is played by molluscs (malacology) and vertebrates of various classes.

The purely medical aspect is the study of the manifestations of
infection in human beings; and this may involve not only preventive
but also curative considerations. This leads on, notably in respect of
bacteria, to the study of the specific biochemical reactions that take
place between certain components of the infecting organism and
the human or animal host. On this is based the science of immunology, with the preparations that it has made available to both
preventive and curative medicine—vaccines, sera, antitoxins and
the like.

Research in bacteriology

Bacteriology has always had an important place in the programme
of the Council and its predecessor Committee; and the Report for
1917–18 referred to the significance of the subject in the First World
War:

> In the actual field of war the work of the bacteriologist must always be pro-
> minent; it has only been some developments of that science, new almost within
> a single generation, that have defended the armies now engaged from quite

108

unimaginable loss of life. In all previous European wars, and in all wars fought elsewhere by our troops in the past, the deaths from the infecting organisms of disease have greatly exceeded those caused by weapons of war in battle. If this relation, this previously normal experience in war, had not been reversed by bacteriological science and its applications, we can find some measure to estimate, but hardly the imagination to grasp, the volume of added suffering that would have overwhelmed Europe during these years. But happily some of the largest preventive problems had been solved in time, and analogy, where knowledge is still wanting, has allowed further success to administrative and sanitary organization.

In its Report for 1923–24, however, the Council expressed its view that the position and recent progress of pathology and bacteriology in the United Kingdom could not be regarded as satisfactory. In particular, repeating from the Report of 1918–19, attention was drawn to the compulsion on university departments of pathology and bacteriology to earn money by engaging largely in routine examinations for public health authorities, hospitals and medical practitioners, while the pathologists of the teaching hospitals had to earn much of their living in private practice. Subsequently, the development of hospital laboratory services relieved university departments —at some centres more rapidly than at others—of the burden of routine. From the Second World War onwards, too, the new Public Health Laboratory Service not only greatly improved the provision for routine examinations in the preventive sphere but itself became an important instrument of research (Chapter 13). The Service, which was directly under the Council's control during the formative period, not only provided well staffed and equipped bacteriological laboratories throughout the country, but by its very nature gave full access to a field of study into which the Council had earlier found it difficult to obtain entry.

The reason for the difficulty was that public health administration was mainly in the hands of local authorities, which were not only numerous but varied widely both in their own effectiveness and in their readiness to cooperate with a central agency such as the Council. It was largely in the hope of surmounting this obstacle that the Council in 1939 appointed a Preventive Medicine Committee under the chairmanship of Sir Wilson Jameson, then Professor of Public Health at the London School of Hygiene and Tropical Medicine and later Chief Medical Officer of the Ministry of Health. The Second World War supervened before the efficacy of this arrangement had been fully tested; afterwards it was scarcely required, and the Committee was disbanded in 1949.

The Council's own organisation for microbiological research has always been headed by a strong department or division of the National Institute for Medical Research. This was successfully directed by such eminent bacteriologists as Sir Almroth Wright, Captain S. R. Douglas, Sir Patrick Laidlaw and Sir Christopher Andrewes; latterly the subject has been increasingly subdivided among different sections. For many years, also, the Council was advised by a Bacteriology Committee with wide terms of reference; among other things, it prepared some notable works published for the Council (Volume One). An earlier committee had dealt with pathological methods, especially the standardisation of serological diagnostic tests for certain diseases.

Research units have been set up to work in special parts of the field. In addition to those named in other sections of this chapter, a Microbial Genetics Research Unit was established at Hammersmith Hospital in 1957 under the Direction of Dr W. Hayes; this later moved to Edinburgh, when Dr Hayes was appointed to a chair of molecular biology, and was subsequently called the Molecular Genetics Unit. The object was the use of bacteria and viruses as model systems for studying the molecular basis of cellular processes. A Microbial Systematics Unit was set up at Leicester in 1965 with Dr P. H. A. Sneath as Director. Mention is made elsewhere of the National Collection of Type Cultures of microorganisms, set up in 1920 as a trustworthy source of authentic strains of recognised bacteria and protozoa for use in scientific work, and of the Standards Laboratory for serological reagents (Chapter 12).

Epidemiology
Another approach to the study of infective diseases is the epidemiological one—the incidence of the diseases in relation to geographical, meteorological, social or other possible factors, and the apparent mode of spread. One method of investigation is purely statistical, making use of official figures. Such work has been part of the programme of the Council's staff from the beginning; one of the major early undertakings of the kind, Dr John Brownlee's investigation of the epidemiology of pulmonary tuberculosis, has been mentioned earlier. More intensive studies of particular outbreaks were made by bacteriologists and clinicians, making use of statistical methods: in the Council's series there are reports of work of this kind relating to such diseases as cerebrospinal meningitis, food poisoning, encephalitis, influenza, diphtheria and infective hepatitis. An unusual item was a study by Major-General Sir Leonard Rogers of smallpox in India in relation to climate, with indications for forecasting epidemics (1926). Latterly, as already mentioned, epidemiological studies have been largely a function of the Public Health Laboratory Service.

Of special interest is an experimental approach to the subject that was supported by the Council for many years. This was made by Professor W. W. C. Topley and his assistants at the University of Manchester and later, with the collaboration of Professor Major Greenwood, at the London School of Hygiene and Tropical Medicine; a summary of the results was published in the Council's series in 1936. The work was based on the assumption that, apart from the characteristics of the particular infection and the mode of its transmission, the epidemiological picture must depend on a number of variable conditions in the population at risk; these include the size and density of the community, the degree of segregation into groups, the rate at which new entrants are being received, the ratio between immune and susceptible individuals at each stage of the epidemic, and the extent to which immune individuals are carriers of the infection. In natural epidemics in man the phenomena tend to be obscured by complex variations of many factors at the same time; the experiment with a captive community of mice, maintained under controlled conditions, was accordingly designed so that the effect of a single variable could be studied while the others were kept constant.

A complementary study was made of infectious illnesses in the more or less closed communities presented by boarding-schools. The data were collected by a special committee, appointed by the Council, under the chairmanship of Sir George Newman of the Ministry of Health. Among the diseases studied, measles, scarlet fever, mumps and influenza figured prominently. These, which are all spread by minute droplets expelled from the nose and mouth of the patient and inhaled by contacts in the neighbourhood, were of particular interest to Dr J. A. Glover, who was conducting the inquiry, because of his previous observations on the same mode of spread in cerebrospinal meningitis during the First World War. Scientific reports were published in the Council's series in 1938 and 1950.

Earlier, in 1923, the Council had been able to include in its series the first of three reports by Surgeon-Commander S. F. (later Vice-Admiral Sir Sheldon) Dudley, RN, on the epidemiology of diphtheria and other infections in the semi-isolated community presented by the pupils of the Greenwich Hospital School. This put forward a hypothesis of the 'velocity of infection', by which the characteristics of the epidemic spread can be explained in terms of the rate at which the specific pathogenic agent is received by an exposed individual and the rate at which the defences of the body can deal with it. The value of a later study was enhanced through the acceptance by the authorities, midway, of preventive inoculation against diphtheria; this made possible a close comparison of such natural immunity as is acquired by a closed population in which diphtheria was endemic with the condition of artificial immunity induced by inoculation.

Epidemics can thus be studied in the human population at large, in semi-isolated human communities where the conditions are relatively stable, and in animal communities under strict scientific control. To these methods may be added the observation of epidemics in communities of wild animals living free. This last is exemplified by work near Oxford by Mr C. S. Elton and others on epidemics among wild rodents, particularly field-mice. These animals are subject to periodic fluctuations in numbers, which rise over a few years to a maximum and are then sharply reduced by a supervening epidemic, after which the build-up of the population begins afresh.

The periodicity is often remarkably regular, and a close study of the conditions makes it possible to forecast epidemics with considerable accuracy. Apart from the general interest of the mechanism involved, there is the practical possibility of a connection between human and animal epidemic diseases (as, for example, between the occurrence of bubonic plague in the house-rat and that in human beings). The investigation was grant-aided by the Council from 1936.

Bacteriology of tuberculosis

Before the Medical Research Committee came into being, the Royal Commission on Tuberculosis was particularly concerned to determine what part the bovine type of tubercle bacillus played in human infections. Dr A. Stanley Griffith worked for the Royal Commission on this subject, and later for many years continued his studies at Cambridge as a member of the external staff of the Medical Research Committee and successor Council. After his retirement in 1940 the work was carried on by others under the auspices of the Agricultural Research Council, as the residual problems seemed to be predominantly of veterinary interest. From the Report for 1914–15 onwards there have been references to other work, assisted by grants, on the tubercle bacillus; in later years the changing objectives have reflected the development of knowledge of the subject.

In 1923 Professor Georges Dreyer published an account of work in the School of Pathology at Oxford which the Council had been assisting with grants for some years. This related to the preparation of a vaccine for the treatment of tuberculosis, by means of a new method devised to make the tubercle bacillus (and, in principle, some other organisms) more amenable to the purpose. The underlying assumption was that the apparent feebleness of the antigenic properties of the bacilli was due to hindrance by their fatty covering or contents, which were not removed by the reagents ordinarily used for extraction. This difficulty seemed to be overcome by the use of formalin, followed by repeated extraction with acetone, and the resulting vaccine was termed 'diaplyte' (meaning 'washed through and through'). After *in vitro* and animal tests, supplies of diaplyte vaccine were issued to a number of centres for clinical trial. The results were disappointing, the vaccine proving to have at most a very limited value. A restrained account of the episode was published in the Council's Reports for 1922–23 and 1923–24; but it is recalled that at the time there was much over-optimistic talk and undesirable press publicity.

Later, in the same department at Oxford, Dr A. Q. Wells of the Council's staff produced a vaccine made from the bacillus causing tuberculosis in voles (the subject of an epidemiological study mentioned in the preceding section). This was eventually found to have useful prophylactic properties, similar to those of the better known BCG vaccine.

Tuberculosis in cattle

The evidence showing the substantial role of bovine tuberculosis as a source of human infection opened up several lines of work that clearly had medical importance. In 1920 the Council appointed a Tuberculin Committee to investigate the diagnostic and possible therapeutic value of tuberculin preparations in human medicine. In 1922 this body's terms of reference were widened to include tuberculin testing of cattle, and its membership was increased by the addition of veterinary and agricultural experts. This was done at the suggestion of the Ministry of Health, to which representations had been made by some leading stock-owners about the anomalous and confusing results obtained by the methods currently in use. The Agricultural Research Council had not at this time been established, and the initiative was taken wholly on the medical side.

The results of the Tuberculin Committee's investigation were published by the Council in 1925. They showed that an intradermal test, done with tuberculin of proved high potency, constituted a satisfactory method of detecting the presence of infection in cattle; and this conclusion was confirmed by an analysis of practical experience published in 1928.

There was then an interesting development, which the Council could probably not have undertaken but for having at its disposal a substantial private benefaction for tuberculosis research. This was a field experiment to determine the practicability of eradicating bovine tuberculosis. An area of 9 square miles in Ayrshire, Scotland, was chosen for the purpose and 30 (out of 37) farms therein cooperated over a period of three years, being given free tuberculin testing and expert advice. M. L. Jordon's report on the results was published by the Council in 1933. In short, the number of farms free from tuberculous infection increased from 8 to 20 while others showed a substantial reduction in the numbers of reactors, and there was a general improvement of stock.

In 1933, by an agreeable act of interdepartmental cooperation, the Council was enabled to include in its series of reports one by the Department of Health for Scotland on tuberculosis infection in milk.

Intestinal infections

Another large group of bacteriological studies has throughout been that relating to gastrointestinal infections, mainly due to micro-organisms ingested with food or water. During the First World War the Medical Research Committee was much concerned with enteric and dysenteric infections. A few landmarks in the Council's general programme may be mentioned.

In 1925 the Council included in its series two reports on food poisoning by organisms of the *Salmonella* group, contributed by Dr W. G. Savage, Medical Officer of Health for Somerset, and Mr P. Bruce White, a bacteriologist then working in the University of

Bristol but later on the Council's staff at the National Institute for Medical Research (where he became, among other things, an authority on the causative vibrios of cholera). In 1933 the Council issued a report, by Professor C. H. Browning of Glasgow University and others, on enteric carriers and their treatment; the investigation of this medical and social problem had been undertaken by the Council at the request of the Department of Health for Scotland.

From time to time the Council has supported special bacteriological investigations of gastroenteritis in children, a highly lethal disease at early ages and apt to occur in epidemic form in institutions. There has also been continued interest in outbreaks of food poisoning. In these and other conditions, however, the work has latterly been mainly in the hands of the Public Health Laboratory Service, which is well placed and specially equipped to deal with such problems. In its Report for 1951–52 the Council said:

> When the history of food poisoning during the last ten years is reviewed, it is gratifying to consider how much of the new knowledge gained can be ascribed to the Public Health Laboratory Service. The large-scale distribution of spray-dried egg by the Ministry of Food in 1942 formed the starting point of a fresh investigation into salmonella food poisoning that resulted in the discovery of a number of new types of this organism, and led to the establishment under Dr Joan Taylor of a Salmonella Reference Laboratory which now serves most of the British Commonwealth.

Important systematic studies of certain groups of microorganisms, aimed at their better classification and readier identification, were undertaken between the wars by staff members and grant-holders, the findings being published in the Special Report Series. The subjects included the serological races of the Flexner group of dysentery bacilli, the meningococcus, and the aerobic and anaerobic members of the *Actinomyces* group (see Appendix A).

Viruses

Very early in its history, shortly after the First World War, the Council turned its attention to the group, as yet little understood, of infective organisms that had been named viruses. The adjective 'filter-passing' (or 'filterable') was at that time usually attached, a characteristic of viruses being their ability to pass through the fine pores of a filter that would keep back microorganisms of the more familiar kinds. In general, their dimensions appeared to lie between those of the smallest bacteria and the largest chemical molecules. In terms of the equipment then commonly available, they were ultramicroscopic. Their presence could therefore be demonstrated only by their effects, especially by their producing a particular disease in an animal of a susceptible species. There were thus formidable obstacles to research, calling for new techniques which could be only gradually developed; but as viruses were known or suspected to be the causal agents of many important infectious diseases of man and animals, the need for research was pressing.

Dr M. H. Gordon of the Council's external staff was already working in this field at St Bartholomew's Hospital, London, on the causative agents of vaccinia and variola (smallpox). As a result, a much needed laboratory test was made available for the rapid diagnosis of smallpox; a report was published in the Council's series (1925).

In 1922, however, the Council took a policy decision that had far-reaching effects, namely to initiate a major effort to promote research in what later came to be called virology. Sir William Leishman was prominent among the members urging this step. The proposal was warmly welcomed by the senior members of the staff of the National Institute for Medical Research, which would clearly have to be the main focus of the programme. They presented a memorandum to the Council on the additional requirements in personnel and equipment; and they stressed the need for developing new methods.

Although it had certain disadvantages canine distemper seemed to offer the best opportunity for the initial research. Two things soon happened to clinch this choice: one was an offer of financial support from dog-owning interests, and the other was the successful outcome of the Council's search for a site for farm laboratories as an extension of the facilities of the National Institute at Hampstead. The development and successful outcome of the distemper project are the subject of a separate section below.

With regards to methods, the bacteriologists at the National Institute had the collaboration of Mr J. E. Barnard's department of applied optics, where the use of ultraviolet microscopy was being developed for the photographic study of objects of dimensions below the powers of resolution of visible light. Later, after Barnard's time, this was superseded by the electron microscope, which in the hands of Dr A. S. McFarlane and others eventually became a major weapon in the Institute's armament.

At the outset another method was developed in the department by Dr W. J. Elford, who had been added to the staff with this in view. Ultrafiltration, for separating out particles which passed through the pores of an ordinary bacteriological filter, was achieved by means of collodion membranes, and eventually Elford produced a series of such membranes of various degrees of porosity ('gradocol' filters) which permitted the differential filtration of viruses of different particle sizes.

The subject was again reviewed in general terms in the Council's Report for 1928–29, where one notes that the term 'virus' was still indefinite, the nature of the agents unknown, and their part in the aetiology of many diseases uncertain.

No part of the work directly promoted by the Council has greater biological interest at the present time, or more vital practical importance for the cure and prevention of disease, than the inquiries now being made into various diseases in animals and man caused by the so-called 'viruses'. . . . . No detective story has ever offered more puzzling features than this to the curious mind. The reward for the solution of the present mysteries will certainly be immense in the new control it will bring over diseases that kill by the million, and another kind of reward will almost certainly be found in the new illumination that discovery of the laws governing the structure and behaviour of these virus bodies will give within the unknown territory between living and non-living matter. Our present almost complete impotence in face of such deadly diseases as measles, yellow fever, and encephalitis, among many others, and of such ruinous plagues among live stock as foot-and-mouth disease, swine fever, and rinderpest—and to these may be added destructive diseases affecting potato, tobacco, and banana crops—is such as to justify and indeed to demand an army of skilled workers.

A modified method of cultivating viruses in the developing egg of the domestic fowl—to be precise, in the chorioallantoic membrane of the embryo chick—was devised and used by Dr F. M. (later Sir Macfarlane) Burnet, partly in his own laboratory in Melbourne and partly during a visit to the National Institute for Medical Research. An account of the work was published in the Council's series in 1936. The principle of egg-membrane culture had been applied before with limited success, but this improvement was an important advance in research technique; earlier, as viruses would not grow on the artificial culture media used for bacteria, maintenance of an organism under study had depended on constantly repeated passage from animal to animal.

It still remained difficult to study the mechanism of virus infection, because the salient characteristic of viruses is that they grow only within the living cells of the host. Although this is true also of some bacteria and many protozoa, viruses are even more dependent; lacking the enzymatic equipment and metabolic processes necessary for growth and multiplication, they must use those of the host cells which they inhabit.

In these circumstances, and largely under the stimulus of work in America, attention became drawn to the value of bacteriophages in the study of viruses generally. These virus-like organisms are parasitic—often more or less specifically—on bacteria and are in many instances lethal for them. This action was discovered in 1915 by Dr F. W. Twort in London and independently in 1917 by F. H. d'Hérelle in France, and was at one time commonly known as the Twort-d'Hérelle phenomenon. Essentially, it was much simpler to experiment with agents that are parasitic on unicellular organisms rather than on cells forming more complex structures. As recounted in the Council's Report for 1953–54, the clue was followed up by investigators in many countries, including various workers supported by the Council in the United Kingdom and also by Burnet's team in Australia.

As time went on, an increasing number of virus diseases came under study at the National Institute. Separate sections below deal not only with canine distemper, already mentioned, but also with influenza, the common cold, poliomyelitis and certain kinds of tumour. A veterinary pathologist, Mr I. A. Galloway, also had the facilities of the National Institute in laboratory work for the Ministry of Agriculture and Fisheries on the virus of foot-and-mouth disease and on the viruses of certain diseases affecting domestic fowls.

General progress in the virological field may be gauged by comparing some of the earlier statements, quoted or mentioned above, with a review of the situation in the Report for 1952–53. That the problem of treatment remained relatively intractable may be seen from the comment that the new sulphonamide drugs and antibiotics were powerless against any but a few of the largest viruses.

Mention is made of the valuable additional resources, for diagnosis and research, provided by the new Virus Reference Laboratory under the direction of Dr F. O. MacCallum at the Central Public Health Laboratory at Colindale, London. And it is stated that "The Council's plans for further work in this field include attempts to investigate, especially by the newer techniques of *in vitro* cultivation in growing tissues, including human tissues, the common cold, poliomyelitis, hepatitis and measles and others of the more elusive viruses which cannot be studied by simpler means."

The Council further strengthened its resources for work in this subject in 1955 by placing a Virus Research Unit in the London School of Hygiene and Tropical Medicine (moved later to Carshalton, Surrey); in 1956 by creating a Virus Culture Laboratory in the MRC Laboratories at Carshalton; and in 1957 by establishing an Experimental Virus Research Unit under the direction of Professor M. G. P. Stoker in a new Institute of Virology, University of Glasgow, for which funds had been provided by the Scottish Hospital Endowments Research Trust. The Council's Laboratory of Molecular Biology at Cambridge has investigated the fine structure of virus particles, a subject reviewed in the Council's Reports for 1958–59, 1965–66 and 1970–71. About this period there was also collaboration with the Virus Research Unit of the Agricultural Research Council, working particularly on virus diseases of plants.

The phenomenon known as 'viral interference' was first unequivocally demonstrated, in 1937, by Dr G. M. Findlay and Dr F. O. MacCallum, the latter receiving a grant from the Council. Infection with one virus can protect against infection with another, not necessarily related, and in a manner found to be quite different from an ordinary immunity reaction. Six years later, American workers showed that an inactivated virus can produce the same inhibitory effect. The possibilities thus opened up were explored by many investigators.

In 1957, Dr A. Isaacs and Dr J. Lindenmann at the National Institute for Medical Research showed that the inhibition was probably mediated by a previously unknown substance produced by the host tissues; and to this substance the name 'interferon' was given. This further clue was actively followed up not only by its discoverers but by others elsewhere. It was clear that interferon provided a valuable tool for virus research; and there seemed to be a possibility that it might be developed as a therapeutic agent against a wide range of infections. The work at the National Institute was helped by the preparation of sufficiently large batches of interferon at the Microbiological Research Establishment at Porton, Wiltshire; and, with a view to possible large-scale production for practical use, the cooperation of industry was secured, the Council entering into an agreement with the National Research Development Corporation and three pharmaceutical firms. Much of scientific interest has emerged, but as yet the hopes of important practical applications have not been realised.

Meanwhile, world-wide studies were bringing to light additional viruses infecting the respiratory tract (including the 'adenoviruses') and the intestinal tract ('enteroviruses'), and also arthropod-borne viruses ('arboviruses'—transmitted by the bites of insects or arachnids). Some of the rickettsia bodies, midway between the viruses and the bacteria, are mentioned later (Chapter 15).

(Virology has also had its seamy side, and the intangible or indirect nature of much of the evidence for its phenomena lends itself to hoax or fraud—to which scientific workers are particularly vulnerable, because the last thing that they expect to encounter among their fellows is bad faith. There was the case, in 1927, of a young woman highly recommended as an investigator, who received a small grant from the Council for a study of the cerebrospinal fluid in disseminated (multiple) sclerosis by ultraviolet microscopy; she was also given advice by workers at the National Institute for Medical Research. She presently claimed to have discovered a virus as the causative agent of disseminated sclerosis; and from cultures she prepared a vaccine which was used, without scientific justification, by certain practising clinicians in the treatment of this intractable disease. When others found themselves unable to repeat her findings, suspicions were aroused; she was eventually given an opportunity of repeating her work under close supervision, but after negative results had followed her first essay she withdrew from the scene. She had described her alleged infective agent in terms closely similar to an account of the virus of bovine pleuropneumonia (one of the larger viruses, and not pathogenic for man) published from the National Institute; and it was later discovered that she had used cultures of that organism obtained from there. The whole episode had wasted a substantial amount of money from various sources and also a great deal of the time and energy of many people engaged in important work.

Again, in 1952, the Council sent to Italy two members of the staff of the National Institute, a virologist and a biophysicist, to see a new invention in ultramicroscopy for which extraordinary claims were being made, including magnifications of several million diameters. While the technician who had invented the machine was demonstrating an image to the virologist, the sceptical biophysicist unobtrusively displaced the object plate by several millimetres to one side; but the image on the screen remained perfectly still! When no satisfactory explanation was forthcoming for this, and for various other strange features to which the visitors drew attention, the deception stood completely exposed.)

Canine distemper

As already noted, the distemper of dogs had been given a high place among the virus diseases most likely to repay intensive study. An animal disease would clearly be preferable to a human one as a subject of experimental research; and there was obvious advantage in being able to study it in the species in which it naturally occurred. Work with dogs would be more expensive than with the usual smaller laboratory animals, but none of these was known to be susceptible to the infection. This question of cost was solved by a confluence of the special interests of dog-owners with the more general interest of medical research. It was, however, not feasible to keep a large number of dogs at the Hampstead site of the National Institute, in an established residential area (where earlier there had been complaints of disturbance by the Council's dogs before any had arrived!); here the answer was provided by the Council's acquisition of a site for farm laboratories at Mill Hill, a then relatively rural area in the north-western suburbs of London.

It was in October 1923, following some tentative indirect soundings, that Sir Theodore Cook, Editor of *The Field*, formally approached the Council with proposals for cooperation. Agreement was quickly reached, and a *Field* Distemper Council was formed to take charge of fund-raising and disbursing activities; the Duke of Portland was chairman. In February 1924 the Medical Research Council appointed a small Distemper Research Committee of scientists to take full charge of the research side; Sir William Leishman was the first chairman, but was shortly succeeded by Professor C. H. (later Sir Charles) Martin of the Lister Institute, while the present writer was secretary throughout.

At half-yearly intervals during the period of the research, these two bodies—or representatives of each—met at the Duke of Portland's London house so that the Committee might report progress to the Distemper Council. The task of conveying the inevitably highly technical considerations to minds attuned to very different lines of thought was no light one. Sometimes it seemed that what was not understood was suspected of being evasive; and here it was that Lord Mildmay of Flete, with a footing in both camps, played a valuable part in, as it were, vouching for the expert statements of men whom he had elsewhere learnt to trust.

The research work itself was at first in the hands of Dr W. E. Gye of the Council's staff at the National Institute, with the collaboration of Mr J. B. Buxton, veterinary superintendent of the farm laboratories. Dr Gye, owing to pressure of other interests, shortly handed over the responsibility to Dr P. P. (later Sir Patrick) Laidlaw; and when Mr Buxton left to take up an academic post he was succeeded by Mr G. W. Dunkin.

The first requirement was to build up, as subjects of experiment, a stock of susceptible dogs—that is, of dogs which could have no acquired immunity as a result of an earlier natural attack of the disease. In those days the infection was so rife that this could be achieved only by breeding dogs under the most stringent precautions of isolation, guarding against not only the transmission of the infection by other dogs but its transportation by human beings.

To this end kennels were built, and also a bungalow for two resident kennel-maids, within a compound surrounded by a dog-proof palisade. The only way in and out was through a small building forming part of this perimeter, with one door to the outside and another into the compound. Two internal doors divided this into three compartments, of which the middle one was a bathroom. A kennel-maid leaving the compound for her time off had to strip completely in the inner compartment, pass through the bathroom, and dress in the outer compartment into the other clothes which she kept there; on returning, the procedure was reversed but taking a bath was obligatory. Members of the scientific staff entered the compound only when enveloped in rubber clothing which had just been washed down with disinfectant fluid. Another small building had a door to the outside and a hatch to the inside, through which sterilised food was passed with all possible precautions. Only once in the years of the work did this barrier system break down; a fresh start had then to be made, with new stock, after everything inside the compound had been rigorously disinfected.

The first tangible result of the investigations was ample confirmation of Carré's view that canine distemper was caused by a virus, and that any bacteria involved were no more than secondary invaders possibly responsible for complications; this was announced in the Report for 1925–26. A finding of great practical importance at this stage was that ferrets are susceptible to canine distemper. It was Captain S. R. Douglas, Director of the Department of Bacteriology and Pathology in the National Institute, who suggested this line of investigation; from his sporting contacts he was aware that gamekeepers found that their ferrets died when distemper broke out in the kennels. Scientific proof was soon forthcoming that the disease was one and the same, transmissible from one species to the other at will; and this meant that a susceptible animal which could be readily handled under ordinary laboratory conditions was available for some of the experiments. Moreover, infection in ferrets usually had fatal results and there would thus be nothing equivocal about any success in producing prevention or cure. In fact, it was soon found possible to produce immunity in ferrets by administering a killed preparation of the virus; making a vaccine was at this stage precluded by inability to grow the virus outside the animal body. At first, however, the attempt to do the same thing with dogs met with only partial success, and a result capable of practical application was still not plainly in sight.

In the following year, with the use of improved methods, it was possible to report effective prevention in dogs and ferrets under experimental conditions and also in dogs leading normal lives.

Some of the young entry in a number of packs of foxhounds were inoculated, and where distemper broke out in the kennels almost all these animals escaped infection, whereas a majority of the others contracted the disease and many of them died. Good results were also obtained with many other kinds of dog, although accurate figures were less easy to secure. A commercial laboratory was by this stage actively working towards large-scale production of the vaccine, so that the benefits of the research work could be made widely available.

In the Report for 1927–28, where the foregoing facts were recorded, it was pointed out that the private fund had provided facilities and equipment of a kind and on a scale which the Council of those days could not have found from its ordinary resources. On the other hand, the supporters of the voluntary fund had gained advantages in the availability of a trained and organised staff in suitable laboratories, which they could not have provided independently without serious delay and much greater expense.

The work on distemper was also helping studies of other virus diseases, including the deadly yellow fever of tropical countries. Dr Edward Hindle, holding a Beit Memorial Research Fellowship in London and working with material brought from West Africa by American investigators, was greatly helped by the experience of the distemper team in finding a means of protecting monkeys, and presumptively men, against yellow fever. That, and trials already made in Brazil, held promise of means of controlling this highly dangerous disease; as the Report said, "if the slightest contribution has been made towards those means by these studies of dog's distemper, then the whole cost of this work has been fully justified, morally and financially, even if all the practical benefits gained for the dog are cancelled or forgotten".

Before long, Messrs Burroughs Wellcome & Co. in Britain and two firms in the United States were manufacturing the distemper prophylactic, and the method had become a routine of veterinary practice. The method, as first used, was described in the Report for 1928–29 as follows:

> Two inoculations are given to the dog. The first consists of a vaccine of the killed or inactivated virus of the disease. This produces a temporary state of resistance, of which advantage is taken a week or two later to administer a dose of fresh living virus; this second inoculation, consisting of infective material much more than sufficient to give an unvaccinated animal a severe and possibly fatal attack of distemper, has no untoward effects. As a result of the double process a solid and lasting immunity is produced, similar to that resulting from a natural attack of the disease.

A subsidiary problem was the occurrence of severe reactions to inoculation in a small minority of instances, and this was the subject of further research. Laidlaw and Dunkin also proceeded to develop an alternative method of protection which could have advantages in some circumstances; it involved the production of immune and hyperimmune sera, which conferred passive instead of active immunity.

The Council reviewed a very successful decade of work in its Report for 1931–32. This mentioned, incidentally, that the methods might prove to be of high economic value to the fur-farming industry in Canada. Dunkin visited that country by request of the Dominion Government, and thereafter Laidlaw and he showed that distemper in the silver fox was the same as in the dog. Meanwhile, however, the Medical Research Council was looking forward to valuable applications of the knowledge and experience to the study of virus diseases in human beings.

Influenza

The historic pandemic of influenza in the autumn of 1918 led the Medical Research Committee to plan a comprehensive attack on the problems presented by this disease. Various workers were invited to investigate different facets of the subject, grant-aid being provided where needed; the investigations are listed in the Report for 1918–19. A report on influenza in Army hospitals in France in 1918 was published in the Committee's series.

The experimental approach was handicapped by the lack of a susceptible animal—the so-called 'influenzas' of some species were in fact different diseases; and there remained for some time a division of opinion as to whether the causative agent of the human disease was bacterial or viral. In 1922 the Council included in its series a report adducing evidence incriminating the *Bacillus influenzae* of Pfeiffer, an organism frequently present; but that the conclusion was far from being generally accepted was made clear in the official preface.

In its Report for 1932–33 the Council recorded the frustrations of the past decade in the following terms:

> The direct attack upon the problem of influenza has for some time been almost at a standstill. The importance of the matter has been fully recognized, and lack of material resources has not been the limiting factor. The difficulty has lain simply in the absence of any means of approach that would yield a starting-point for research. Experimental methods were inapplicable so long as no species of animal was known to be susceptible to the disease, because the difficulties in the way of keeping human beings under adequately controlled conditions were practically insuperable. Mere observational study of the disease as naturally occurring in man was unlikely to lead farther, especially considering the frequent ambiguity of its clinical identification and the possibility that the causative organism was a virus invisible with the microscope.

This statement was followed by a cautious announcement of an apparent breakthrough, achieved by members of the Council's staff at the National Institute for Medical Research, building on their success with dog distemper. Laidlaw, Andrewes and Wilson Smith had, as was amply confirmed later, "succeeded in conveying human influenza to ferrets, and thus in bringing it within the scope of research by the exact methods of experimental science". Again the ferret! Filtered nasal washings from human cases were instilled into the nostrils of the animals, which with some regularity then developed the characteristic feverish and catarrhal condition; the latter could be transmitted in like manner to other ferrets. After recovery the animals were found to be immune, for the time being at least, to further attacks. An attempt to transmit the infection from ferrets to human volunteers was unsuccessful; but it was known that the blood of practically all of these, so soon after the widespread epidemic of 1933, contained an antibody to the virus. The next, and dramatic, step is recorded in the Report for 1935–36:

> During the past year an accident has effected the transmission which deliberate attempts had earlier failed to produce. Virus originally obtained from a human case, but since passed through 196 ferrets in series, was used to infect a small batch of ferrets. One of these, when heavily infected, sneezed violently at close range while it was being examined by Dr Stuart-Harris. After forty-five hours he experienced the abrupt onset of a sharp and typical attack of influenza, reaching its climax on the third day with a temperature of 102°F. Dr Wilson Smith was able to follow this attack from its onset and to obtain successive samples for investigation during and after the illness. Washings obtained from the nasopharynx up to the fourth day were directly infective not only for ferrets but also for mice, this being the first instance in which the latter had been successfully infected with material directly from a human case. Fortunately, a sample of Dr Stuart-Harris's blood serum, taken before the attack, was available for examination; and this was found to contain no demonstrable antibody for the virus of human influenza.

(Incidentally, this contemporary record must be preferred to an unofficial account, published more than thirty years afterwards, in in which Wilson Smith figures as a patient, instead of his colleague Stuart-Harris; the strain, still maintained, is designated as 'WS' in the literature, a possible source of ambiguity.)

Laidlaw and his colleagues had thus, in 1933, clearly identified a virus as the infecting organism. The next step was to prepare a vaccine, but clinical trials of this in the epidemic of 1936–37 gave inconclusive results; a report by Dr C. H. (later Sir Charles) Stuart-Harris and others was published in the Council's series. This disappointing outcome became explicable when American investigators showed that there were two or more strains of influenza virus, and that these produced rather limited immunity against each other.

The future of vaccine prophylaxis against influenza thus lay with early identification of the strain responsible for an incipient epidemic, in whatever part of the world this might arise, and with rapid production of adequate quantities of the appropriate vaccine—a matter of some difficulty if a new strain of virus was involved, as did happen with the epidemic of 'Asian 'flu' originating in 1957. To meet this situation, the World Health Organisation set up a World Influenza Centre in 1947; it was placed in the National Institute for Medical Research and under the general direction of Andrewes.

With this help it was found possible to reduce the attack rate of influenza, in vaccinated groups, although not to the extent that had been hoped. In view of the multiplicity of influenza viruses and of different strains, progress with vaccination was slow, but further progress was reviewed in the Report for 1954–55. By this date the Public Health Laboratory Service was playing an important part on the epidemiological side; and among its members Dr L. Hoyle at Northampton had for long been engaged in more fundamental studies.

The common cold

After the Second World War, Dr C. H. (later Sir Christopher) Andrewes was the senior remaining member of the former influenza team at the National Institute for Medical Research. He was anxious to attack the problem of the common cold, and the Council agreed to make this a major project. As there was no susceptible animal species, experimental work would be possible only by using human volunteers as guinea-pigs; fortunately there was a building that might have been designed for the purpose—a small hospital at Salisbury, Wiltshire, which the Harvard Medical School had built and staffed as a centre of research on medical problems arising from the war. At the end of the war this had been handed over to the British Government.

The wards were converted into self-contained six-room flats, each for two people; and volunteers were accepted only in pairs, including married (sometimes honeymoon) couples. Each member of a pair was subjected to the same procedure; neither had contact with anyone else except masked and gowned members of the medical staff; and meals were left on the doorsteps in special containers. Country walks were permitted on condition that the volunteers did not come within less than thirty feet of other persons, a restriction not too difficult to observe on the surrounding Plain. Each batch of volunteers remained for twelve days, and after an interval of two days was succeeded by another.

The object, as with the stock of non-immune dogs in the distemper investigation described above, was to provide a group of subjects free from infections other than those administered by design. The doses to be inoculated, including inert preparations used as controls, were labelled only with arbitrary letters to which neither the volunteers nor the medical staff dealing with them had the key. The volunteers of the first group were inoculated with nasal washings from cold sufferers, treated in various ways, in July 1946.

So the Common Cold Research Unit came into being as an outstation of the National Institute (later, of the Clinical Research Centre). Dr Andrewes was the general director, but there was a resident medical officer in charge.

For 14 years the work, disappointingly, yielded little more information than that the common cold was caused by a filter-passing virus, and that the infection could be transmitted from person to person by inoculation, remaining true to type. Then in 1960 it was at last found possible to grow the common cold virus in tissue culture. This opened up various new possibilities, but it also led to the disconcerting realisation that common colds may be caused by any one of a large number of 'rhinoviruses' and other viruses, capable of conferring little or no cross-immunity—and indeed no very lasting immunity at all.

Nevertheless, there was much to be learnt about these viruses, the modes of their spread, and such degrees of immunity as they confer. This work was generally reviewed in the Reports for 1948–50 and 1963–65. And in 1968 Sir Macfarlane Burnet expressed the view that the Unit would never lack problems of interest; and that the work should continue even if no 'cure' were in sight: "unless a steady surveillance on what is causing respiratory infections is maintained, important new viruses may fail to be recognised in time to do something effective about them".

(A mildly bizarre extramural activity of the Unit may be recorded. Twelve volunteers were marooned on a small uninhabited island, Eilean nan Ron (isle of the seals), off the north of Scotland, with only wireless communication with the mainland. At the end of ten weeks, when the party might have been expected to have acquired an enhanced susceptibility to colds, six new volunteers were added to it, all of them in process of developing colds artificially induced by inoculation at Salisbury; the two groups were then mixed in a variety of ways calculated to ensure that the spread of infection could be accurately traced. Unfortunately no members of the original party developed colds.)

Clinical trials of possible or alleged remedies for colds are mentioned elsewhere (Chapter 11).

Poliomyelitis
Poliomyelitis, with its common sequel of paralysis, had not until 1947 had any major manifestation in Great Britain, although the disease had for long been widespread in continental Europe, the United States of America, Australia and elsewhere. In that year it flared up in the largest outbreak that the country had known; this was followed by a second in 1949 and by others later. These events led the Council to institute virological inquiries to determine the distribution of the causative agent in the country during epidemic and inter-epidemic periods and to explain the method of infection and mode of spread; and also epidemiological inquiries to ascertain the part played by various factors, including injury to the tissues, in the activation of latent infections. In this work a large part was naturally played by the Public Health Laboratory Service, at that time under the Council's general control.

The Council's Report for 1951–52 reviewed progress in the research programme on the epidemiology, pathology and treatment of the disease. Laboratory investigations had been greatly facilitated by the American discovery of methods whereby this virus could be grown in tissue culture, and later in eggs, thereby dispensing with the need to use living animals for the purpose. The American work also held promise of a protective vaccine.

By the date of the Report for 1954–55 the position had been radically altered by the introduction of formolised vaccine devised by Salk and his colleagues in the United States; the successful result of a large-scale controlled trial in that country had been announced. Limited supplies of the American product were available for import, and manufacture in Great Britain was under way. Safety testing was a major problem, which directly concerned the Council in view of the special responsibilities for biological control. The Division of Biological Standards under Dr W. L. M. (later Sir Walter) Perry at the National Institute for Medical Research was allotted additional accommodation, equipment and staff to enable it to cope with a task of exceptional dimensions, but these new resources could not all be instantly deployed. As in vaccine prepared by the Salk method there was only a narrow margin between dangerous infectivity and protective inefficacy, it was essential that every batch should, before issue to the public, be stringently tested for both safety and potency.

The point was emphasised by a disaster in America, when certain batches of vaccine, although they had passed the prescribed test, proved to be infective and caused an outbreak of the disease instead of protecting against it. Inoculations were temporarily suspended in the United States and Canada until the safety tests could be suitably revised; after that, many millions of children were vaccinated in these and other countries without report of further accidents. Meanwhile, limited inoculations were being made in the United Kingdom with a modified formolised vaccine of British manufacture. At the same time, as the Report said: "For still further progress towards the solution of the problem of preventing poliomyelitis, one school of thought looks to the development of an avirulent live virus which can be administered by mouth, thus simulating the natural method of gaining immunity." The Report for 1955–56 describes developments on these latter lines, pioneered by Sabin and colleagues in America, and followed up by Professor G. W. A. Dick and others at the Queen's University, Belfast, with support from the Council. Financial help for the British programme was given by the National Fund for Poliomyelitis Research (now National Fund for Research into Crippling Diseases (Action for the Crippled Child)).

In July 1957 the Council was asked to advise HM Government, through the Lord President, on the position regarding the use of American Salk-type vaccine, imports of which had been banned. The opinion was given that the British-made vaccine was safer and apparently at least as effective. The Council therefore recommended that the policy should be to meet the home demand as soon as possible entirely from British production; but that if there was any substantial gap in supplies the desirability of importing Salk vaccine as a temporary measure, and subject to the same rigorous tests as were applied to British vaccine, should be considered. On purely medical grounds it would be difficult, in such circumstances, to continue to refuse to import Salk vaccine, having regard to the substantial protection which it conferred and the smallness of the risk now associated with its use; but it was considered that the medical profession and the public should be warned that a slight risk still remained even if the vaccine had passed the usual safety tests. Field trials for assessing the effect of the prophylactic on a large scale are mentioned elsewhere (Chapter 11). Salk-type vaccine, however, was soon replaced by the live attenuated oral vaccine developed in America by Sabin, and this is now exclusively used.

Viruses and cancer

In 1911 Dr Peyton Rous of the Rockefeller Institute in New York had shown that a virus might be a cause of malignant tumours. The crucial finding was that a naturally occurring tumour ('Rous sarcoma') of fowls could be transmitted to other fowls by the injection of a cell-free filtrate of the growth, and thus presumably by an infective agent of the nature of a virus. Subsequently, in 1933, he showed that the action of a chemical carcinogen in producing a tumour in an experimental animal could be accelerated and enhanced if a tumour virus was also present, the two factors apparently acting synergistically. The importance of this work was not recognised at the time, and it was not until 1966 that Rous, at the age of 87, was awarded a Nobel Prize; he had worked for much of his life on other subjects.

Meanwhile, in or about 1922, Dr W. E. Gye, of the Council's staff at the National Institute for Medical Research, turned his attention to following up the clue provided by Rous (and with the cooperation of the latter in supplying the initial tumour material for further experiments). In this undertaking, Gye had as collaborator J. E. Barnard, the distinguished amateur microscopist. They were quickly able to confirm the early finding of Rous, and were soon able to add further points. The filter-passing agent was corpuscular in nature, as shown by centrifugation of fluids containing it; and it could be cultivated artificially and thus used in isolation for experimental work. The cultivated and isolated organism, however, could not alone produce a new tumour but was active only in the presence of a second agent ('specific factor'), which could be extracted from the original tumour; this was found to be non-corpuscular and therefore non-living, in fact a soluble chemical substance.

Gye and Barnard published their preliminary results in a medical journal in 1925, and there was immediately a great burst of newspaper publicity, hailing the discovery of the cause of cancer; this in fact broke a few days prematurely as the result of a 'leak' while the companion papers were in the press. There was a great public interest; and among other happenings Gye and Barnard were received in private audience by HM King George V.

Although the Council was not responsible for this excessive publicity, it was subsequently—as one can see in retrospect—not guiltless of making over-optimistic claims. In its Report for 1924–25 the Council appeared to endorse Gye's hypothesis. The Report for 1925–26, however, sounded a note of caution about too ready acceptance of the interpretation placed upon the preliminary findings. There had, predictably and properly, been much technical criticism of the evidence upon which these findings were based—particularly that for the simultaneous existence of two different kinds of agent, which was the keystone of Gye's hypothesis. The Report concluded its reference to Gye by saying: "Whatever be the final outcome of his work it has at least drawn many other workers already to face this outstanding problem which has been left disregarded too long."

Later, Gye himself began to get discordant results in his attempts to perfect his evidence by variations in his methods. At one point he accepted an invitation from the Harvard Cancer Commission to visit America and perform experiments jointly with Dr H. J. Mueller, who afterwards paid a return visit for like purpose. It was agreed that they should publish a combined account of their findings, each adding his own statement of interpretation.

Dr Gye, joined by Dr W. J. Purdy and working at the Farm Laboratories at Mill Hill, later turned to the immunology of these tumour-producing agents, in an endeavour to elucidate their remarkable specificity. Some parallel experiments were made by Dr C. H. Andrewes at the main building of the National Institute at Hampstead. The work continued for some years; but little further progress was made in resolving the intractable dilemma. Gye left the Council's staff in 1935 on appointment as Director of the Imperial Cancer Research Fund. His surname was originally Bullock, but in 1919 (soon after joining the Council's staff) he changed it by deed poll to Gye, the maiden name of his first wife. The son of a railway employee, he had had a hard struggle to acquire his education and helped to pay for his medical course at Edinburgh by playing cricket as a professional.

In more recent years there has been renewed interest in viruses as a possible cause of cancer, and experimental work has been in progress in laboratories all over the world. Contributions to the understanding of the process and mechanisms of cell transformation by tumour viruses have come from the work of the Council's Experimental Virus Research Unit, and its successor the Virology Unit, and elsewhere; experimental studies on viral carcinogenesis were reviewed in the Report for 1966–67. Mention may also be made of work overseas by a member of the Council's external staff, Mr D. P. Burkitt, on what is now known as the Burkitt lymphoma found in African children.

The case for the occurrence of viral tumours in man, however, is as yet based on analogy and circumstantial evidence. The situation was summed up thus by Sir Christopher Andrewes (1970):

> For several years there has been increasing interest in the role of viruses in causing tumours in some birds and mammals and in their possible importance in human cancers. Whether or not they are concerned in human cancer, their study has led to important extension in our knowledge about the disease: of how viruses can lead to malignant changes in cells, and especially of the role of immunity in protection against cancer.

Although there has been some further evidence, the position is still much the same.

Fungal infections
The Council has from time to time made grants for research in medical mycology, which has applications in dermatology and to some diseases of the respiratory tract. The infections range from the common 'ring-worm' to different forms of aspergillosis, and to diseases more often found in tropical than in temperate climates. Some are associated with occupation—as for instance 'farmers' lung' due to *Aspergillus fumigatus*—and are mentioned elsewhere (Chapter 9). Dr Dagny Erikson, working at the National Collection of Type Cultures, made systematic reviews of, respectively, the aerobic and anaerobic pathogenic organisms of the *Actinomyces* group for publication in the Council's series of Special Reports (1935, 1940).

From 1943 to 1969 the Council was advised by a Medical Mycology Committee under the successive chairmanship of Dr J. T. Duncan, Sir Archibald Gray, and Professor J. T. Ingram. The Committee framed recommendations for names to be used in Great Britain for fungi pathogenic to man and animals, published in the Council's series of Memoranda. More specialised was a committee on Industrial Epidermophytosis, particularly concerned with a common infection of miners' feet.

The subject has been a difficult one in which to promote research helpful to the Council's purposes. There is no dearth of botanists interested in fungi as such, but the range of fungal infections in Great Britain is so limited that few investigators have been attracted to this field. From an early stage, and originally under the honorary direction of Dr Duncan, a small Mycology Reference Laboratory at the London School of Hygiene and Tropical Medicine formed part of the Public Health Laboratory Service.

Protozoology
The Council has assisted many investigations into diseases due to infection by parasitic protozoa—unicellular animals, as contrasted with the bacteria, usually assigned to the Vegetable Kingdom. These parasites include the plasmodia of malaria, the trypanosomes of

sleeping sickness, and the amoebae of one form of dysentery—
mainly tropical diseases (Chapter 10).

For many years the Council had on its staff, at the National
Institute for Medical Research, "one of the outstanding protistolo-
gists of all time". This was C. C. Dobell, who worked for the Medical
Research Committee during the First World War while holding an
academic post, but entered its permanent service in 1919 (when he
had already been elected a Fellow of the Royal Society at the age
of 32); he remained with the Council until his sudden death in 1949.
An obituary by Hoare and Mackinnon, already quoted, described
him thus: "A man of generous habits, fastidious tastes and wide
culture, he was an intellectual aristocrat and an erudite scholar".
His wartime work was related to the causative organism of amoebic
dysentery, prevalent among forces in the Mediterranean and tropical
areas; afterwards he principally studied the protozoa inhabiting
the human intestine, pathogenic and otherwise. In addition to
purely scientific publications, he was the author of a scholarly historical work (he had learnt old Dutch) on Leeuwenhoek, the pioneer
microscopist of the 17th century.

One recalls Clifford Dobell as rather short, dapper in appearance,
with fair hair brushed back and a trim moustache. He was a reserved
man, but with a warm humanity; in his personal parlance, he and
his friends were "animalcules" but certain heroes were "elephants".
He was almost obsessively dedicated to his work, resisting attempts
to divert his activity. In the 1920s he allowed himself an annual
holiday of only a fortnight, spent rock-climbing on the Cornish
cliffs; he constantly read far into the night, doing with four or five
hours of sleep. One thought of him in those days as a confirmed
bachelor, but he married at the age of 51. He was essentially a lone
worker, and a perfectionist; he preferred to do everything for himself. At one stage his work required monkeys and these he insisted
on keeping in his own laboratory, rather than in the animal house;
they were much appreciated by privileged visitors, because being
tended by Dobell himself the monkeys had the status and behaviour
of personal friends.

Metazoan parasites and vectors

Above the unicellular or protozoan level, there are many kinds of
animals that have an impact on human health, particularly in
tropical countries, acting either as predators, parasites, vectors
conveying infection, or intermediate hosts in the life-cycles of parasitic organisms. Leaving aside attack by carnivorous vertebrates,
(presenting problems of security rather than of medicine), direct
predation on human beings mainly takes the form of blood-sucking;
this implicates chiefly insects of various orders and certain arachnids
(ticks and mites), but also some annelid worms (leeches) and others.
Apart from the high 'nuisance value' of biting insects, they can when
sufficiently numerous have an adverse effect on health; and where

a bite is highly poisonous—as with certain insects, arachnids (scorpions), and snakes—there is very definitely a medical problem.

Some of the blood-sucking forms may be not merely occasional predators, but permanent ectoparasites. Of the metazoan endoparasites, worms (helminths) belonging to several groups are the most important. Vectors conveying infections are notably some of the blood-sucking arthropods (insects and arachnids). Certain molluscs, such as fresh-water snails, play an important part as the essential intermediate hosts of particular helminth parasites.

The foregoing indicates the scope of what may be termed medical zoology, a field in which the Council has supported many investigations. The two main sectors are medical helminthology and medical entomology (with acarology), but medical malacology is also important. The Council's role in each of these, in turn, may be briefly considered.

The Council's support of research in helminthology centred for many years upon Professor R. T. Leiper, at first in the old London School of Tropical Medicine and later in the London School of Hygiene and Tropical Medicine. He was the Council's principal adviser in this field, the leading British worker in it, and the head of a department with all the requisite facilities. Work on bilharziasis (schistosomiasis) done for the Council during the First World War, and later work by others, receives mention elsewhere (Chapter 14). The investigations otherwise undertaken by him covered a wide range of parasitic worms, responsible for different conditions found in temperate and tropical climates.

The Council's help to Leiper mostly took the form of grants for special expenses (sometimes including travel) and additional assistance in particular studies. It was not always easy for him, in a restricted field, to find or retain the skilled manpower necessary for his researches; on one occasion, when he had just lost a man from his staff on promotion and a woman grant-holder on marriage, he complained that the purpose of his department appeared to be "to find chairs for men and beds for women".

Similarly, much of the Council's help for work on arachnids was centred on the Quick Laboratory (later Molteno Institute), University of Cambridge, under the direction of Professor G. H. F. Nuttall and later of Professor D. Keilin. As regards entomology, a role analogous to that of Professor Leiper was played by Professor P. A. Buxton of the London School of Hygiene and Tropical Medicine. In this field the greatest medical interest lay in the role of mosquitoes and various flies as vectors of infections, but this was mainly a tropical problem. Others, such as the louse-borne fevers and those conveyed by arachnids (mites), were predominantly of wartime concern (Chapter 15).

Nearer home (in every sense) was the problem of the bed-bug. The infestation of human dwellings, and not only in slums, by this blood-sucking insect was a matter of concern to authorities responsible

for housing and public health. "At the least", as the Council said
in its Report for 1934–35, "the bed-bug is a source of discomfort, unpleasantness and mental distress". In 1934 the Ministry of
Health had issued a report by a special committee which it had set
up to review the practical aspects of the question. To quote the
Council from the source already cited:

> In their report, the committee stated that they had been struck by the lack
> of accurate information on which recommendations could be based. As so
> often proves to be the case in practical problems of this kind, the important
> deficiency was in fundamental knowledge of the natural history of the creature
> against which measures had to be taken. The matter thus becomes a question
> of further research in the field of medical entomology and the Council were
> accordingly approached by the Ministry of Health with a request that they
> would undertake the promotion of new investigations in this direction.

The Council accepted this suggestion and appointed a special committee to advise and assist it in promoting research on the subject.
The kind of information required had to do with such matters as
the effect of climatic conditions and food-supply on the bed-bug,
at all seasons and in every stage of its development and reproduction; also the conditions which attracted the insects, the distances
that they would travel, and so forth. Further experiments were
likewise necessary to determine the efficiency of different countermeasures. This Committee's report was published in the Council's
series in 1942. It may be added that, in spite of the general loathing
with which the bed-bug is regarded, it has never yet been shown to
convey infection.

Immunology
The Council was early very conscious of the great field for research
offered by the phenomena of naturally acquired immunity to
infectious diseases and by the possibilities of imitating these by
artificial means for prophylaxis or treatment. In its Report for
1924–25 the field of immunity and infectivity was specially reviewed,
and among other things it was said:

> Here is studied the intricate interplay on a chemical battleground between
> minute parasitic guest and the resources of its host. It is a contest between the
> infectivity or virulence of the attacking parasite and the resistance or immunity
> possessed, or acquired during the struggle, by the defending animal body.
> 'Normality' or health is not the absence of attack and struggle: the body is
> never, under ordinary environment, free from the incessant contest. Disease is
> the sign of temporary or progressive failure in defence. It is not surprising that
> on the whole the chief efforts of the pathologist have been drawn to the study
> of the resistance of the body to bacterial attack, to its 'immunity reactions'.
> No phenomena are more obvious and striking than those of the immunity won
> by the body after a first successful defence against a given infective organism,
> and no triumphs of medical science are greater in terms of humanitarian
> utility than those successful empirical imitations of this natural process which
> have given us the means of a broadcast anticipatory defence against small-pox,

cholera, typhoid fever, and the like. This study of immunology has naturally
attracted the eager efforts of workers in all countries, and immense accumula-
tions of data have been collected. The scientific analysis of immunity reactions,
however, offers extraordinary difficulties.

The use of prophylactics conferring passive protection had already
been introduced into medical practice after the discovery of antibodies to the organisms of diphtheria and tetanus. Since then
vaccines conferring active protection have been developed against
typhoid fever, diphtheria, tetanus, tuberculosis, yellow fever, whoop-
ing cough, poliomyelitis, measles, and rubella. The routine use of
these vaccines has led in Great Britain to the virtual eradication of
some of these diseases, including diphtheria (see below) and poliomyelitis. Similar success has attended the use of tetanus vaccine in
the Army, and of yellow fever vaccine among Europeans in the
tropics. The degree of protection conferred by some of the vaccines
mentioned is still under investigation, but there is reason to believe
that all of them are beneficial. In still other cases success so far has
been limited or negligible, as already mentioned with regard to
influenza and the common cold. Problems of special difficulty are
presented by diseases that confer natural immunity only after
repeated attacks, such as malaria.

Immunological preparations include vaccines, sera, antitoxins,
toxoids, and the like; all of them are derived directly or indirectly
from infective microorganisms, and their properties are related to
the reactions between such organisms and the human or animal
body. Some of them are used in diagnosis or therapy, but as a class
their greatest role today is in prophylaxis. There is a wider sense,
however, in which immunology has ceased to be the concern almost
solely of bacteriologists and pathologists, but has become an aspect
of many branches of biological research (Chapter 8).

As in some other fields, particularly of preventive medicine, the
Council had occasion to deplore the tardiness with which discoveries
in immunology were applied to practical human needs. In its
Report for 1937–38 it said:

> One of the most striking instances of the delay in the application of new know-
> ledge is the relative lack of public recognition, in Great Britain at the present
> time, of the existence of a method of proven value for the prevention of diph-
> theria. Diphtheria is the commonest single cause of death among school
> children. In 1937, there were 61 339 cases of this disease in England and Wales,
> causing 2963 deaths, nearly all in children between the ages of 1 and 15 years.
> This is pure tragedy, in view of the needlessness of such deaths, for since 1929
> prophylactic inoculation against diphtheria has proved increasingly successful
> wherever it has been properly used. In parts of the United States and of Canada
> (notably in the Province of Ontario), diphtheria as a clinical entity has prac-
> tically disappeared, as the result of preventive inoculation with diphtheria toxoid.

The responsibility lay with local public health authorities, but
these needed guidance from the centre and also financial help
towards the high cost of large-scale inoculations. It was Sir Wilson

Jameson who rectified this situation on becoming Chief Medical Officer of the Ministry of Health in 1940; he knew exactly what was required and he forcefully stimulated both the local authorities and the central administration to get it done, wartime though it was. The Council was able to give great help to the campaign for inoculating children with diphtheria vaccine (toxoid) through the Emergency Public Health Laboratory Service. The latter took much of the work off the shoulders of the medical officers of health; and Sir Percival Hartley's Department of Biological Standards at the National Institute for Medical Research also had an important role. The campaign was an immediate success, and the incidence of the disease in Britain—as earlier elsewhere—was dramatically reduced. In the decade 1930–39 notified cases of diphtheria in England and Wales had averaged about 60 000 a year, with deaths averaging over 3000; by 1950 the number of cases had dropped to under 1000 and the deaths to just under 50; and in 1969 there were 13 cases and no deaths.

In general, it must be admitted that British science has not played a leading part in the introduction of new immunological prophylactics—unless one goes back to Jennerian vaccination against smallpox, or to Almroth Wright's antityphoid vaccine at the end of the last century. The new agents have tended to come from abroad, especially from America and from Germany. Where Britain has taken a principal part is in the evaluation of prophylactics in large-scale controlled trials, and in the accurate standardisation of serological products; the Council's activities in both these directions are discussed elsewhere (Chapters 11, 12).

In 1966 the Council joined with the Health Departments and the Public Health Laboratory Service in setting up a small standing committee to advise on policy in the use and development of agents for active immunisation. It was thought that such a body would fill a gap in an essential manner without overlapping the existing formal machinery of the parent bodies. It was intended that it should be free to consult the industry as necessary, and that it should recommend appropriate action to the Health Departments with regard to industry, and to the Council with regard to research. In addition there have been numerous other committees and working parties concerned with particular aspects of immunisation.

Drug resistance

A serious and growing problem associated with the increasing use of antibiotics and other antimicrobial drugs is the emergence of strains of organisms resistant to them. A partial answer is to use such drugs more sparingly, especially those that are valuable in serious infections. This applies also to animals, since drug resistance originating from the use of antibiotics in animal feeding may be passed on to man; this was the subject of a report produced by a joint MRC/Agricultural Research Council committee in 1962.

A more basic approach to the problem is to investigate the mechanisms by which drug resistance develops and spreads in organisms, and the Council has supported a number of lines of work in this area; the Molecular Genetics Unit, already mentioned, has contributed to fundamental knowledge here. The Report for 1967–68 includes an article on 'Bacterial sexuality and infectious drug resistance', which describes the complex basis for the dramatic spread of resistance (now often to several drugs simultaneously) through bacterial populations.

Cross-infection and air hygiene

As the Council said in its Report for 1938–39, "To enter a hospital for relief of one disease and to die of another contracted there constitutes a tragedy which has for long troubled civilised man." The situation in this respect in the earlier part of the nineteenth century was indeed often appalling; but the introduction first of antiseptic and then aseptic surgical techniques, resulting from advances in bacteriology, had brought about a vast improvement. Nevertheless, the problem was by no means solved; maternity wards, paediatric wards, and surgical wards for diseases of the ears, nose and throat presented particular difficulties. Several investigations into cross-infection in hospital wards were promoted by the Council; some of these were interrupted by the Second World War, but work on the subject was resumed later.

A problem of key importance in obstetric medicine, up to the late 1930s, was the prevention and treatment of puerperal infection. In 1928 the Minister of Health appointed a departmental Committee on Maternal Mortality and Morbidity and among its members was Dr Leonard Colebrook of the Council's staff, then engaged in bacteriological studies of 'childbed fever' at Queen Charlotte's Hospital, London. At that time the Hospital was in process of moving to a new site at Hammersmith, and late in 1930 wards in a special isolation block were opened, followed a few months later by the inauguration of the Bernhard Baron Memorial Research Laboratories. Dr Colebrook, remaining in the Council's service, was made director of these laboratories and additional staff for them was provided from a grant made by the Rockefeller Foundation. Notable contributions to the findings of the Committee, which presented its final report in 1932, were made by Dr Colebrook and his colleagues. They continued their bacteriological work until their success with chemotherapy in puerperal fever transformed the whole picture, as recounted earlier (Chapter 3).

Research on air hygiene from other than the bacteriological point of view has been mentioned elsewhere. After the Second World War the Council promoted work on bacteriological contamination of the air, especially in schools and hospitals, and on methods for its prevention. Members of the Council's own staff and of the Public Health Laboratory Service cooperated in the investigations, with a jointly maintained Air Hygiene Laboratory at the Central Public Health Laboratory as their focal point. A report by Dr R. B. Bourdillon and others was published in the Council's series in 1948, dealing with the effects of different methods of aerial disinfection. The Air Hygiene Committee, appointed by the Council, itself reported in 1954 on an experiment in disinfecting the atmosphere of school classrooms by ultraviolet irradiation. The field of aerial disinfection, however, has proved disappointing; no method yet introduced has been shown to be of practical value in the control of infectious disease. This committee was followed by a Committee on the Control of Cross-infection, later reconstituted as the Hospital Infection Committee. Cross-infection has also been the concern of the Industrial Injuries and Burns Unit, directed by Dr J. P. Bull, and more recently the Division of Hospital Infection (under Dr R. Blowers) at the Clinical Research Centre.

Chapter 8
Basic Biomedical Researches

General policy—Extrinsic and intrinsic causes of disease—The place of
physiology—Natural chemical stimuli—Experimental biology—The chemistry
of steroid compounds—The biochemistry of microorganisms—The immune
response—The role of inheritance—Further work on human genetics—
Molecular biology—The significance of proteins—Human behaviour

General policy

In the original programme of research schemes prepared by the
Medical Research Committee in 1913, and quoted in the First
Annual Report, the general objective was defined as follows:

> The object of the research is the extension of medical knowledge with the view
> of increasing our powers of preserving health and preventing or combating
> disease. But otherwise than that this is to be the guiding aim, the actual field
> of research is not limited and is to be wide enough to include, so far as may
> from time to time be found desirable, all researches bearing on health and
> disease, whether or not such researches have any direct or immediate bearing
> on any particular disease or class of diseases provided that they are judged to be
> useful in the attainment of the above object.

This statement, which received ministerial approval, has continued
ever since to be the policy of the Council.

This policy has always stressed that medical science is ultimately
based on knowledge of the normal structure and functions of the
human body, and that advances in it depend largely upon increases
of that knowledge. The quest goes far beyond the scope of con-
ventional anatomy and physiology; the biochemist studies the processes of life in their most subtle reactions and the biophysicist these
processes in their smallest dimensions, while genetics is concerned
with the mode of inheritance and psychology with the functioning
of the mind.

Some of these branches of biology are subjects in their own right,
and may also have applications in other practical fields than medicine; one might therefore question how far such studies should
form part of a programme of medical research. The answer is
sufficiently obvious whenever the work relates, even distantly, to
human biology; it also seems reasonably clear when the problems
are of a more general kind, provided that adequate assistance for
the subject is not available through some different channel that
may be thought more appropriate. The important consideration is
that fundamental work should not fail of support simply because,

at the moment, it seems to have no stronger claim on one specialised research agency than on another.

Extrinsic and intrinsic causes of disease

The Council's Report for 1967–68 was the last to be issued before the retirement of the third holder of the office of Secretary. It includes a valedictory memorandum by Sir Harold Himsworth on 'Future trends in biomedical research', prepared originally at the request of the Council for Scientific Policy. This document may be cited here, being relevant to the need for basic research.

Himsworth's initial thesis was that, viewing the progress of medicine since the beginning of the century, the conditions for which more or less completely successful prevention or cure have been achieved are those primarily due to external influences. The extrinsic factor may be positive, as in the invasion of the body by microbial agents (Chapter 7); or it may be negative, as in malnutrition due to defective diet (Chapter 5).

In contrast, there are conditions which cannot yet be either prevented or wholly cured, but in which alleviation is now possible— ranging from restoration of near-normal health, for example replacement therapy with insulin in diabetes mellitus, to some lesser degree of mitigation. There is still, however, a large group of conditions of which understanding lags. Achievement has been least in respect of those in which the basic feature is degeneration or alteration of the body tissues—genetic and developmental defects, chronic diseases, cancer and ageing. With increasing control of acute illness, and the consequent change in the age structure of society, this group continues to increase in importance for research.

With regard to diseases of extrinsic origin, the essential aim of research has been to identify the external threat and to devise means of dealing with it; here the traditional disciplines of clinical medicine, pathology, microbiology, biochemistry and pharmacology play their parts. Despite its success, however, this line of attack has by no means reached an end; there remains a hard core of problems that require more subtle or sophisticated methods for their solution, calling for increased basic knowledge in such fields as microbial genetics, virology and immunology.

In respect of diseases of intrinsic origin, the need for fundamental biomedical research is even greater. To deal with apparently selfsustaining pathological processes within the body tissues, research must reach back into the cell itself; the relative failure hitherto may be ascribed to ignorance of cellular function and the mechanism of its control. For research on cancer, for instance, the whole range of methods of study is required, and a lack of knowledge at any point can hold up progress everywhere. There has thus been a rapid intensification of interest in biological studies that might earlier have seemed remote from the purposes of medicine. Himsworth summed up, in broad terms, as follows:

The continued progress of research concerned with the understanding of normal function is certain. The newest horizon relates, however, to the degenerative and chronic diseases. Now we can entertain the hope of understanding their nature and of investigating trains of events that reach right back into the normal cell. In this context the development of biology at the cellular level is not only desirable, it is mandatory.

The place of physiology

In its Report for 1917–18 the Medical Research Committee said:

It has been specially noticeable during the past year that physiology, the science of the healthy living organism and of its reaction to disturbance, has been more and more brought into practical service by special needs revealed by the war. The violences offered to the human body in warfare—whether through exertion and exposure, by terror or excitement, in physical damage by lead or steel or in chemical attacks upon it by poison, and not least through the incredible stresses of flying high and fighting in the air—all these have brought many new and urgent calls for precise physiological knowledge and for new studies by the physiologist. . . . If in a hospital in time of peace the most obvious call has seemed in the past to come from the side of infective disease and morbid process for the help of the pathologist, in war the stress laid upon the individual machinery of man has made the physiologist and his methods indispensable. The results of pain and fear, of haemorrhage, of 'shock' by wound and operation, all these have needed further analysis before sound treatment could be devised and improved. New studies have been needed of the changes in blood-pressure and blood-volume and in the qualities of the blood itself, new inquiries into the finer vessels of blood circulation and their relation to the nervous and other systems, and new analyses of the chemical mechanisms of the body, and of the modes by which want of oxygen is met by adaptation, or leads to final damage.

This is followed by a plea for the continuation, in time of peace, of close cooperation between physiologist and clinician. True though the claims were, one may detect in the insistence upon them a certain anxiety to convince those who controlled the public purse that the support of 'highbrow' researches had practical utility— a defensive attitude which the Council was later able to abandon.

In the following sections of this chapter a few examples are given of lines of research that have been strongly supported by the Council in the field of physiology and related laboratory sciences, including particularly biochemistry and biophysics. They are chosen from a wide spectrum, for—with particular reference to the National Institute for Medical Research—the Council was able to say in its Report for 1966–67 that "work during the past year has ranged from a physiological study of the impaired performance of Olympic athletes at high altitudes to the secondary structure of ribosomal RNA—the nucleic acid immediately concerned with the assembly of protein molecules according to their genetic specification".

Natural chemical stimuli

An early example of an apparently academic line of investigation, which continued for many years to figure prominently in the programme of the National Institute for Medical Research, concerned the nature of the mechanism whereby motor nerve impulses are transmitted to the voluntary muscles and other structures where the effect becomes manifest. The work led ultimately to one of the great generalisations of physiology. Also, although it had been primarily undertaken for the advancement of basic knowledge of bodily function, it resulted—sooner rather than later—in a number of important practical applications in medical treatment.

The programme originated in work by Dr H. H. (later Sir Henry) Dale and Dr G. Barger at the Wellcome Physiological Research Laboratories, before they had joined the staff of the then new Medical Research Committee close on the outbreak of the First World War. This was a pharmacological study of compounds isolated from an extract of ergot, of which acetylcholine and histamine proved to be of special interest for the effects which they could produce. Later, at the National Institute, Dr H. W. Dudley was able to demonstrate biochemically the presence of acetylcholine in the animal body, and this gave reality to the concept of a natural physiological role for the substance. A similar function of adrenaline in respect of impulses in the sympathetic nervous system had been known for some years.

At the National Institute, Dale himself reverted to the subject with a succession of colleagues—Dr J. H. Gaddum, Dr G. L. (later Sir Lindor) Brown, Dr W. S. Feldberg, Dr F. C. MacIntosh, Dr W. D. M. Paton, and others—some of whom continued in this field after his own retirement in 1942. It was soon shown that nervous impulses reaching the synaptic endings of preganglionic fibres, and the motor nerve-endings on voluntary muscle end-plates, caused a local release of acetylcholine; and also that artificial local applications of acetylcholine to ganglion cells and motor end-plates produced postganglionic impulses and contractions of voluntary muscle fibres. Thus came the generalisation that the physicochemical change that constitutes a nerve impulse causes the discharge of acetylcholine (or noradrenaline) at the nerve endings, and that the substance then activates the muscle or gland which the nerve controls. For his major part in this discovery, Dale was awarded a Nobel Prize jointly with Dr Otto Loewi, of Graz, who had reached similar conclusions by another route.

In particular, Dale showed that acetylcholine acted differently, in one of two ways, at different synapses; and that the two types of effect could be independently antagonised by appropriate pharmacological agents. Mention has been made earlier of some clinical applications of this knowledge, such as the development of muscle relaxants in surgery and of drugs for the control of hypertension (Chapter 3).

Dale likewise returned to the study of histamine, mentioned above, and in this his chief collaborator at the National Institute was Dr P. P. (later Sir Patrick) Laidlaw. Dale had had an earlier interest in the phenomenon of anaphylaxis, but this further work opened up a whole new field of inquiry. Here again is a case of effects produced by the relatively massive release, within the body, of a chemical substance naturally occurring there. In this instance the causative factors are traumatic in nature, histamine playing a part in the production not only of anaphylactic reactions but also of the wound and surgical shock that had great wartime importance (Chapters 14, 15). The central feature of the group of conditions concerned is the loss of the normal tone of the capillary vessels and the consequent tendency to peripheral stagnation of the blood. Sir Thomas Lewis, on the Council's staff in the Department of Clinical Research at University College Hospital, London, also paid much attention to the responses of the tissues to injury, particularly of the skin.

As the outcome of work in the 1950s in Italy, America and Australia, a substance known as 'HT' (5-hydroxytryptamine) was added to acetylcholine, noradrenaline and histamine, forming a group of natural chemical agents regulating the actions of the tissues locally. This was followed up by workers for the Council at the National Institute and at Oxford.

Experimental biology
The above heading would be appropriate to many things in this chapter, and indeed in others, but it was the chosen title of a sub-department headed by Dr A. S. (later Sir Alan) Parkes at the National Institute and is here used primarily to refer to his work. The original interest of Parkes and his colleagues was in sex hormones, as noticed earlier (Chapter 3); it later developed in various directions, of which two may be briefly mentioned.

It was a short step from the study of sex hormones and their actions to the complex physiological process of fertilisation, the efficiency of which is the prime determinant of fertility. Considerable additions were made by Dr C. R. Austin and others to knowledge of the particular process, in mammals, by which the spermatozoon penetrates the ovum, and also of the chemical changes that accompany the whole process of fertilisation.

An entirely new avenue of work—'cryobiology'—had earlier been opened up on the preservation of living cells at low temperatures. It was already known that certain lower forms of life, mainly unicellular organisms, could survive freezing at very low temperatures and be preserved in the frozen state for revival after a long interval. Little work of this kind had been done with cells or tissues of vertebrate animals, until in 1949 the discovery was made at the National Institute that, by using special procedures to prevent destruction of the cell during freezing, fowl spermatozoa could be kept at the temperature of liquid air ($-$ 192°C) for several months and still retain its fertilising power. (A pullet was successfully inseminated with spermatozoa from the same frozen batch as that originally used to fertilise the egg from which she developed.) The work was later extended to ovarian tissue and to red blood cells. There have been further developments since then in many laboratories, and the method has had important practical applications, as in the storage of living material for subsequent clinical use; the principle also underlies the use of hypothermia during certain surgical procedures. There is a Cryobiology Division at the Clinical Research Centre.

Workers in the Human Physiology Division of the National Institute have contributed to world-wide studies of another biological phenomenon. This is the existence in animals, including man, of certain physiological rhythms which are generally in phase with regular environmental changes but are to some extent inherent. Of special significance in human affairs is the diurnal (or circadian) rhythm which, when inherent, constitutes the so-called 'biological clock'. This has important practical applications—in relation, for instance, to changes in hours of activity or to changes in length of daylight—apart from variations due to long-distance travel at high speeds. The subject was reviewed in the Council's Report for 1963–65.

The chemistry of steroid compounds

A passage in the Council's Report for 1925–26 gives the following account of work on the chemistry of steroid hormones:

> The study of the structure and distribution of the sterols might at any time until quite lately have been taken as a good example of a highly academic investigation, giving little promise of contact with any practical problems of life and health. These substances, members of a group of complex solid alcohols, had been found to occur as constituents of almost all living tissues, animals or vegetable. The most familiar is cholesterol, which occurs in gallstones, in the natural grease of the skin, in the sheaths of nerve-fibres, and is widely distributed elsewhere in the animal body. What was known as the result of long and laborious investigations, of its origin and fate in the body, suggested that it was a relatively inert substance. Meanwhile chemical studies of great ingenuity and elegance had revealed the complex architecture of the cholesterol molecule, and its relation to that of other sterols occurring in animals and plants.

The biological importance of sterols and related compounds was at that time only beginning to become evident. The subject was destined to occupy many research workers throughout the world for years to come; many notable advances were made under the aegis of the Council, several of them by members of the staff at the National Institute.

One of the studies there yielded a better understanding of the structural formula of the sterol molecule. Dr Harold King devised a rearrangement of the traditional interpretation and tested it in collaboration with Dr Otto Rosenheim; the results were satisfactory, and when these were published the view won general acceptance. Of this Sir Henry Dale wrote (notes personally communicated): "I doubt whether there has been another instance of a change in the structural conception of a molecular pattern, common to a series of natural substances, starting from purely theoretical considerations and having an influence of so far-reaching importance for the progress of biochemistry, pharmacology, endocrinology and medical therapeutics." This group of substances was of particular interest to the National Institute in a number of ways; it was there that vitamin D was identified as a product of the ultraviolet irradiation of ergosterol, to which the name calciferol was given (Chapter 3).

Again, as already noted, the National Institute has been the scene of much research in endocrinology, particularly on sex hormones, by Parkes and his colleagues. The hormones of the adrenal glands and of the gonads are steroid substances, and of these the Report for 1933–34 said:

The advance in understanding of the physiological actions of sex hormones has been accompanied by a growth in knowledge of their chemical nature. Gradually, various substances that were at first identified only by their activity are yielding also the secrets of their chemical constitution. Here again a picture of a related system is being built up; for some of these sex hormones, with various other substances produced in the body, are found to be members of a series of compounds having much in common in their chemical structure, and making a strong suggestion that one may be formed from the other. This knowledge must reflect light upon the physiological aspect of the problem; it is also a necessary preliminary to any artificial synthesis of these compounds for use as therapeutic preparations.

In 1951, Professor Sir Robert Robinson at Oxford and Dr J. W. Cornforth of the National Institute were able to announce the total synthesis, for the first time, of an androgenic steroid hormone. In its Report for 1961–62 the Council reviewed the progress of work on the natural biosynthesis of sterols, to which members of its staff had contributed.

Steroid substances are important in various other ways. In the body cholesterol plays a part in fat metabolism and is important in arterial disease. Some powerful drugs such as cortisone are steroids. Certain steroid substances induce cancerous growth, others inhibit it. In 1958 the Council instituted a Chemical Pathology of Steroids Research Unit at the Jessop Hospital for Women in Sheffield. This establishment, during the five years of its existence, was concerned with problems arising from the metabolic transformations of steroids in health and disease; and particularly with methods for the detection and measurement of steroids in biological material, and their isolation from it.

The Council had already, from 1954, given financial support (supplemented by the US National Institutes of Health) to a Steroid Reference Collection, maintained at Westfield College, London, with Professor W. Klyne as honorary curator. The object was to provide reference samples of steroids for use as standards in chromatography, spectrography and other techniques, particularly for work related to the metabolism of steroid hormones. Some 600 different compounds came to be included; and the service thus made available is a measure of the extent of research work in this field.

The biochemistry of microorganisms

In its Report for 1933–34 the Council expressed the dual motivation underlying its special endeavours to promote research in the field of bacterial chemistry:

> Great knowledge of the conditions which govern the growth and multiplication of bacteria is a fundamental necessity for the better understanding and control of infectious diseases and of all morbid states involving sepsis. These conditions, respectively favouring and inhibiting bacterial growth, should be largely definable in chemical or physico-chemical terms, and the importance of the study of bacterial chemistry, by a suitable blending of bacteriological and chemical methods of investigation, is therefore apparent. The chemical study of the factors necessary for the growth of relatively very simple organisms also gives opportunities of investigating the nature of nutritional factors where their modes of action are exhibited in the least complicated form. From either point of view —and the two are complementary—the subject offers a rich field for research work likely to yield results both of theoretical interest and of practical value.

Attention was then particularly directed to the food requirements of bacteria, for the provision both of energy and of growth. It was of interest that different species of bacteria varied widely in their capacity to utilise particular chemical sources: for some, as in higher forms of life, there are certain essential compounds (compare vitamins) that the organisms cannot synthesise for themselves but must receive ready made. There are in fact different, presumably evolutionary, levels ranging from organisms that make relatively simple demands to those that have adapted themselves to the use of more complex nutrients; the former can satisfy their needs through a wide range of conditions, while the latter need a more specialised environment—in some cases one that can be found only in a particular form of parasitism. There were here matters for interesting speculation and also possible clues to the practical problem of infection.

The Council was already supporting work on the subject by various members of its staff, notably Dr H. W. Dudley and others at the National Institute for Medical Research and Dr Marjory Stephenson in the School of Biochemistry at Cambridge; it was also making grants for work by Professor J. W. McLeod and others in the University of Leeds, and by Professor F. W. Twort at the Brown Institution, London. The curious history of the last named centre—an animal dispensary and research laboratory in Wandsworth Road, endowed by a benefaction to the University of London for the investigation, study and treatment of "maladies, distempers and injuries" of "Quadrupeds or Birds useful to man"—has been recounted by Bulloch (1925).

The Council had also been making grants for research on the subject by Dr P. G. (later Sir Paul) Fildes and Mr B. C. J. G. Knight at the London Hospital. It now announced new arrangements whereby what later became known as the Bacterial Chemistry Research Unit was set up in 1934 at the Middlesex Hospital (in the Bland-Sutton Institute of Pathology and the adjoining Courtauld Institute of Biochemistry). Fildes joined the Council's staff as director of the team; Knight received a Halley Stewart Research Fellowship; and Leverhulme Research Fellowships were made available for another bacteriologist and another chemist. It was thus very much a cooperative effort; and it was the first of the Council's research units outside the clinical field (Volume One).

Among the important additions to knowledge made in the Unit was the finding of Dr D. D. Woods which suggested a rational explanation for the effect of chemotherapy with sulphonamide compounds. This was formulated in the 'Woods–Fildes hypothesis' to the effect that p-aminobenzoic acid is an essential metabolite of certain bacteria; that sulphonamides are antagonistic to it, because by reason of structural similarity they compete for a particular enzyme system essential for the growth of the organism; and that when the drug is successful the result is bacteriostasis. Work on these lines was rapidly taken up in other laboratories and the generalised form of the hypothesis that resulted has had a valuable influence on the search for new chemotherapeutic agents.

On the outbreak of the Second World War the Unit was moved to the Lister Institute. Shortly afterwards, however, most of its members were seconded to the Ministry of Supply for special duty at the Experimental Establishment at Porton, Wiltshire. After the war the Unit returned for a time to the Lister Institute; but on the retirement of the Director most of the staff were absorbed by the National Institute for Medical Research, where they formed a special section for continuing work on other aspects of the chemistry and physiology of bacteria under Dr M. R. Pollock.

Two other establishments for work in this field were formed by the Council. One was the Chemical Microbiology Research Unit attached to the School of Biochemistry at Cambridge. This was directed at first by Dr Marjory Stephenson, mentioned above, and later by Dr E. F. Gale; the former was one of the first two women to be elected a Fellow of the Royal Society, in 1945. It was taken over by the University of Cambridge in 1962.

The other establishment was the Cell Metabolism Research Unit under the part-time direction of Professor H. A. (later Sir Hans) Krebs in the University of Sheffield; in 1954 it was moved with him to the University of Oxford. The whole subject was reviewed in the Report for 1952–53 on the occasion of the award of a Nobel Prize to Professor Krebs (jointly with Professor F. Lipmann of Harvard) for his work on the series of metabolic reactions known as the citric acid cycle.

Later work, some of it supported by the Council, was directed to the chemistry of the bacterial cell wall and had relevance to the mode of action of penicillin on growing bacteria; the field was reviewed in the Report for 1960–61. More recently the Council has made long-term grants for the support of research work in or near this field: on the mechanism of microbial pathogenicity under Professor H. Smith in the University of Birmingham; on bacterial enzyme variation under Professor M. R. Pollock in the University of Edinburgh; on molecular biophysics under Professor D. C. Phillips in the University of Oxford; on the biosynthesis of macromolecules under Professor K. Burton in the University of Newcastle upon Tyne; on the genetics and biochemistry of bacteria and bacterial viruses under Professor N. D. Symonds in the University of Sussex; and on the structure and functions (mainly metabolic) of microorganisms under Professor D. E. Hughes in University College, Cardiff.

The immune response

The history of immunology goes back empirically to Jennerian vaccination in the eighteenth century, and more definitely to Pasteur in the middle of the nineteenth. Until the 1940s, however, it was almost solely concerned with the defence of the body against infectious disease; the Council's activities in this field, including the large-scale trial of immunological agents and their quantitative standardisation, are discussed elsewhere. Here something may be said about other branches of the subject, more recently developed, the main basis being an article contributed to the Report for 1968–69 by Dr J. H. Humphrey, Deputy Director of the National Institute for Medical Research. Immunology has ceased to be the concern almost solely of bacteriologists and pathologists, and has become an aspect of many branches of biological research.

The basic principle is that the body, in all vertebrate animals, responds in certain ways to the introduction (otherwise than by ingestion into the alimentary tract) of alien molecules, even of substances that are 'bland' in the sense of not having any pharmacological or toxicological effects. These substances, known as 'antigens', are highly specific in the reactions that they evoke. The reactions are of two kinds: first, the proliferation of lymphocytes, cells in the blood and lymphoid tissue that are adapted to interact with the particular antigen; second, the secretion into the circulation by some of the lymphocytes of antibodies, which are proteins (of a kind called immunoglobulins) likewise able to interact specifically with the antigens that evoke them. Such interaction activates a chain of ancillary factors present in the blood plasma, collectively known as 'complement', which augment the effect of the antibodies in various ways such as by causing inflammation. The effect of the lymphocytes and antibodies is to destroy or to neutralise the corresponding antigens; and the capacity to do this may endure, so that the body is readier to deal with further invasions of the same kind. This necessarily over-simplified statement may be helpful for an understanding of what follows.

In 1934 the Council included in its series of publications a review by Professor J. R. Marrack, of the London Hospital, summarising the then existing knowledge of the chemical reactions between antigens and antibodies; since that time these reactions have been further elucidated by research methods of great refinement. For instance, in 1958, Dr R. R. Porter at the National Institute for Medical Research was able to show that antibody molecules could be split by enzymes into two separate parts, one with the specific activity and the other without it. He was later, after an intervening step had been taken in America, able to propose a general model for the structure of antibody molecules. Further analysis has shown that one part of the molecule is extremely variable, in parallel with the wide range of immunological specificity; the other is relatively constant. Five main classes of the constant part can be distinguished, each associated with some biological activity of a more general kind. Professor Porter is continuing his work on the structure of antibodies as Honorary Director of the MRC Immunochemistry Unit in Oxford. In 1972 he was awarded a Nobel Prize, jointly with Professor G. M. Edelman of New York.

Again, an American discovery concerning the nature of the reaction with lymphocytes has been followed up in recent years in various countries, among others by workers at the National Institute and in the Council's Rheumatism and Cellular Immunology Units. A mechanism has been disclosed which can destroy not only recognisably foreign cells but also the body's own cells that have been altered (e.g. by virus infection or malignant change). Lymphocytes specifically responsive to an antigen do not themselves secrete antibody but are responsible for a defence process known as 'cell-mediated immunity'. A now well known example of such reactions is the rejection of a tissue graft from another individual, which is the main obstacle to success in the surgical transplantation of organs. The subject of organ transplantation was reviewed in the Council's Report for 1962–63, and more recently in Dr Humphrey's article in the 1968–69 Report; much of the pioneer work on the reaction to grafts of foreign tissue was done by Professor (later Sir) Peter Medawar, before he joined the Council's staff, and he was awarded a Nobel Prize in 1960.

In 1968 the Council entered into an agreement with the Wellcome Foundation and the National Research Development Corporation for the production of quantities of antilymphocytic serum (ALS) sufficient for clinical trial. This preparation is called in the 1966–67 Report "the most powerful and least toxic agent hitherto used for suppressing the otherwise virtually ineradicable resistance of adult

animals to grafts from other members of their own species".
However, its production is difficult and clinical evaluation is still
continuing.

The Council's workers have also contributed to an understanding
of certain immune responses that are not beneficial but produce
hypersensitivity. This opened an experimental approach to the
study of various allergy diseases, in which the Council's former
Clinical Immunology Research Group played a part. The same
applies—the Radiobiology, Rheumatism and Blood Group Units
as well as the National Institute being involved—to studies of the
body's immunological tolerance of its own constituents; and of conditions in which this natural tolerance breaks down, with the
formation of 'autoantibodies' that may be concerned in various
diseases of previously obscure aetiology. Thus, evidence has been
found that the local lesions of rheumatoid arthritis are mediated by
autoantibodies against immunoglobulins, with or without the aid
of associated sensitised cells. The progress of research on this disease,
in which the Council's Rheumatism Unit has notably participated,
was reviewed in the Report for 1967–68.

Still another area of study is on the occurrence of immunological
deficiency diseases, in which some part of the capacity to make
immune responses is lacking in the individual; many of these conditions are genetically controlled, sometimes sex-linked. There is a
practical application in that it is sometimes possible to alleviate
the deficiency by regular injections of normal immunoglobulin; and
the Council has been responsible for an extensive trial and long-
term follow-up study of this treatment in children suffering from
'hypogammaglobulinaemia'. A monograph on this work was published in the Special Report Series in 1971. A further problem arises
when there are immunological reactions between the pregnant
mother and her foetus, notably the sensitisation of a Rhesus-negative
mother by a Rhesus-positive foetus; a working party organised by
the Council has supervised a clinical trial aimed at the quantitative
assessment of anti-Rh antibodies required for treatment.

Of obvious importance is the development in recent years of an
immunological approach to the study of cancer. Various reasons
have been suggested to explain the inadequacy of the immunological response where this fails to control the growth of tumour
cells, but before any practical applications can be expected more
information is required on such fundamental problems as the
aetiology of cancerous growths and the control of immunological
responses. Workers at the National Institute for Medical Research,
the Clinical Research Centre and the Institute of Cancer Research
among others have made notable contributions in this field.

The role of inheritance
In the classical antithesis of 'nature and nurture', the Council's
programme was at first very heavily weighted on the latter side; the

extent of its interest in nutrition has already been noted (Chapter 5). The relative lack of attention paid to hereditary factors may have been due in part to pessimism about the possibility of putting further knowledge to practical use in the medical sphere; the motivation of scientific inquiry is so strong, however, that the chief reason was probably the absence of appropriate techniques for following various lines of investigation. The position has greatly altered in recent years, as will presently be noted, and affords a good example of advance by outflanking movements, so to speak, where frontal attack has met with strong resistance.

In the Report for 1933–34 the situation was assessed in these terms:

> In spite, however, of the great advances which have been made in the biological study of heredity, and in the application of its results to agriculture, the subject of human genetics has been relatively neglected. Two practical difficulties have stood in the way of the fuller investigation of inheritance in man. In the first place, the method of experiment—with its deliberate matings of individuals showing the characters under study—is clearly inapplicable. In the second place, observational methods are handicapped by the small size of human families and by the length of the interval between generations. There remain certain statistical methods of approaching the problem, although these are themselves subject to the disadvantage that they require the collection of very large masses of data of a kind not always easy to obtain.

It was for this purpose that the Council had in 1932 appointed a Human Genetics Committee, under the chairmanship of Professor J. B. S. Haldane. The other members were also distinguished geneticists—Dr Julia Bell, Dr E. A. Cockayne, Professor R. A. (later Sir Ronald) Fisher, Professor Lancelot Hogben, Dr L. S. Penrose, and Dr J. A. Fraser Roberts—presenting a formidable array of scientific talent; the present writer was privileged to be secretary of this body.

Dr Bell had been in the service of the Council since 1933, latterly as a member of the external scientific staff but earlier with a grant for assistance to Professor Karl Pearson. Her personal research work, in the Galton Laboratory of University College London, was mainly concerned with the inheritance of anomalies and diseases of the eye; and she continued for many years to make important contributions in this field. Dr Penrose was also working for the Council, and later became a member of its external staff. He was engaged in a study, begun in 1931, of the inheritance of mental defect. This was made in the Royal Eastern Counties Institution at Colchester, Essex, and was promoted jointly by the Council, the Darwin Trust and the Institution. A review of 1280 cases was published in the Council's Special Report Series in 1938.

Some impetus to the programme had been given in 1934 by the Report of the Departmental Committee on Sterilisation; this included recommendations for research on the role of inheritance in mental defect and disorder, and these the Board of Control referred to the Council. One valuable line was seen to lie in the examination of the offspring of consanguineous marriages and a comparison with those of other marriages. Another line of inquiry was concerned with cases of mental defect in pairs of similar and dissimilar twins.

The Human Genetics Committee undertook the organisation of a large-scale statistical investigation of the question of consanguinity. It did not seem feasible, considering the large number of data required, to take consanguineous parentage as the starting point and to compare the incidence of various abnormalities in the off-spring with that in a control group. It was sufficiently difficult to follow the alternative course of beginning with large groups of patients with particular diseases or defects and to examine the inci-dence of consanguineous parentage among them. This was achieved with the cooperation of a large number of hospitals throughout the country which agreed to record, during a sufficient period, the con-sanguinity or otherwise of all their in-patients. To make the answer meaningful it was of course necessary to know the incidence of con-sanguineous parentage in the general population, and here the Council's Report already cited made the significant comment: "It is strange to find that our elaborate system of marriage registration and of vital statistics gives no aid towards establishing this essential 'base line'." The inquiry had accordingly to be so designed as to yield this information at the same time.

Another extensive investigation organised by the Committee was a search for rare congenital defects in the course of the routine medical examination of school-children; this was done in London and north Lancashire, by arrangement with the authorities con-cerned. The first analysis produced 44 records as the result of about 28 000 examinations.

With the aid of a grant from the Rockefeller Foundation in 1935, the Council fostered a scheme for the genetic study of blood groups in the Galton Laboratory at University College London. This was under the honorary direction of Professor Fisher, and Dr G. L. Taylor was appointed as Research Fellow in charge. When the Second World War came, the staff was moved to Cambridge and was maintained there as part of the scientific emergency services for which the Council then had responsibility (Chapter 16). In 1946 the Council reconstituted the team as a Blood Group Research Unit, under the direction of Dr R. R. Race, at the Lister Institute. It was stated in the Report for 1945–48 that "the Unit is investi-gating human blood groups not only as to their clinical significance in blood transfusion and, in the case of the Rh groups, the relation-ship of blood group differences in parents to the causation of haemolytic diseases in the offspring, but also because blood groups form the best material yet available for the study of human genetics". The establishment may indeed be regarded as one of those devoted mainly to the study of human genetics in a particular aspect. Later it was this unit that discovered the sex-linked blood group Xg; the fact that this is determined by a gene on the X chromosome has made possible a variety of genetic studies.

Further work on human genetics

In its Report for 1954–55 the Council reviewed the question of research in human genetics, with retrospective mention of the pioneer researches in which British scientists had played so large a part and with a brief account of more recent work, some of it within the Council's own programme. In the next Report the subject was again considered, this time from the point of view of research policy. After a further reference to past work, the current position was assessed as follows:

> During this early phase of development comparatively modest resources sufficed for the support of research in human genetics. This situation was radically altered, however, by the advent of nuclear energy. The fact that exposure to radiation could give rise to fundamental changes in the cells of the reproductive organs and thus affect hereditary characteristics had been known since H. J. Mueller's first observations of this phenomenon in 1927, but no one could then foresee that there might be a general increase in the amount of radiation to which individuals and whole communities were exposed. The new fear that man might, through ignorance, permanently endanger his hereditary constitution made it urgently necessary to re-examine the whole scale and tempo of research relating to genetics and to consider afresh how far the available resources were adequate to the needs. In the light of this new development, it was at once apparent that there existed not only serious gaps in fundamental knowledge but also a shortage of workers with the necessary training and interest. Although there was sufficient knowledge to make possible a planned policy of development in this field, it was clear that the existing deficiencies could only gradually be remedied, progress being dependent upon the extent to which promising young workers could be encouraged to enter the field, and upon the opportunities provided for specialized training and for subsequent careers in the various types of research now envisaged.

During a period of nine years from 1954 there was a remarkable efflorescence of new projects, some of them based on earlier grant-aided work but all now brought within the Council's staff organisation; these were units for the study of genetics in a variety of special contexts. The first of them was the Wernher Group (later Unit) for Research in Ophthalmological Genetics. This was set up by the Council, with the financial support of the Alexander Piggott Wernher Memorial Trust, under the honorary direction of Professor A. Sorsby at the Royal College of Surgeons of England; conditions of the eye had of course for long been of particular interest to geneticists, and this was the subject of a review article in the Council's Report for 1956–57.

What later became the Experimental Genetics Research Unit was initiated in 1955 as the Group for Research in Mouse Genetics under the honorary direction of Dr H. Grüneberg at University College London. Many mutant genes of mice have close counterparts in man and are of medical importance; to other workers in this specialised field the unit circulated a periodical document called *Mouse News*, and Grüneberg's annotated catalogue of mutant genes of the house mouse was published in the Council's series of Memoranda in 1956. The long-term planning of experiments is facilitated in a rapidly reproducing animal; and this is even more true of bacteria, very large populations of which can be grown with ease and speed and be manipulated under controlled conditions. Moreover, it had been recognised that microorganisms possess biochemical and genetic systems essentially similar to those of animal cells, and that they could accordingly be used as relatively simple models for the study of cellular organisation. The genetics of microorganisms had thus developed into a basic biological science, and in 1957 the Council established its Microbial Genetics Research Unit mentioned earlier (Chapter 7).

The same year saw the establishment of a Mutagenesis Research Unit under the honorary direction of Dr Charlotte Auerbach; this was in the Institute of Animal Genetics headed by Professor C. H. Waddington in the University of Edinburgh. The work was experimental, but spontaneously occurring mutations provided a natural yard-stick. The role of ionising radiations and chemical agents as factors inducing mutations is a question of great social importance. There are also significant parallels between mutagenic, carcinogenic and carcinostatic effects. Also in 1957, a Clinical Genetics Research Unit was set up under the direction of Dr J. A. Fraser Roberts in the Institute of Child Health, Hospital for Sick Children, Great Ormond Street, London. The main objects were to investigate the role of inheritance in common, and usually chronic, diseases; and to study congenital malformations and hereditary abnormalities and diseases. Dr C. O. Carter is now Director.

The Population Genetics Research Unit, under Dr A. C. Stevenson at Oxford, was founded by the Council in 1958. The aim was to study "variations in real people in real populations". The work was to be mainly in the field, with clinical cooperation, although the hypotheses to be tested might be derived from theoretical or laboratory researches. Background information on consanguinity, early mortality and other factors in the population was to be built up; gene frequencies and mutation rates were to be investigated; and reproductive wastage was to be assessed, especially that due to congenital malformations. The general subject was reviewed in the Council's Report for 1958–59.

In 1959 the Psychiatric Genetics Research Unit was set up, under the part-time direction of Dr E. T. O. Slater, in the Institute of Psychiatry at the Maudsley Hospital, London. Mental disorders had for long been an important field for the study of hereditary factors, but new biochemical methods of genetic investigation had become available. The working hypothesis was that not only a number of forms of mental deficiency but also such conditions as manic depressive and schizophrenic psychoses are primarily metabolic disorders; and that, if this be true, biochemical genetic investigation must go to the heart of the problems presented. The Unit would adopt any new biological methods likely to be useful and would establish liaison with research departments in various institutions.

The Council decided in 1968 to give long-term support to an interdisciplinary programme of work in psychogenetics. This was proposed by Professor P. L. Broadhurst and Professor J. L. Jinks of the Departments of Psychology and Genetics, respectively, in the University of Birmingham. The broad aim was a study of the inter-action of genetic and environmental determinants of behaviour in various species, including an attempt to apply to human subjects the methods that had been used in studies of rats and fruit-flies. The programme was in part a continuation of work that had received financial support from the National Institute of Mental Health of the United States Public Health Service and in the United Kingdom from the Science Research Council.

The Human Biochemical Genetics Research Unit, under the honorary direction of Professor H. Harris, was established in London in 1962, placed at first in King's College but later in the Galton Laboratory at University College London. It was concerned with exploring the extent and the character of inherited enzyme variation in man, with the broad aims of elucidating the genetic structure of human populations and the interrelationships between genetic con-stitution and inherited disease.

In 1962 a Cell Genetics Research Unit was set up under the honorary direction of Professor G. Pontecorvo in the Institute of Genetics, University of Glasgow, to undertake genetic analysis at the cellular level in human and other tissue. By this time, techniques for the cultivation of mammalian somatic cells had advanced to a point where these could be handled like unicellular organisms. This made possible a study of a multiplicity of processes of genetic recombination, which consists of bringing together and reassorting genetic material from different lines of descent. Earlier, genetic analysis of this type had been restricted to the field of sexual repro-duction and was thus handicapped, particularly in man, by the relatively enormous generation gap and the small number of progeny.

During the period when the various units mentioned above came into existence, there had been a progressive shift towards genetics in the interest of Professor W. M. Court Brown and his colleagues in the Council's Clinical Effects of Radiation Research Unit in Edinburgh, of which something has been said earlier (Chapter 6). This was recognised in 1967 when the title of the establishment was changed to Clinical and Population Cytogenetics Research Unit; meanwhile a specialised branch of the Unit had been established under Dr D. Rutovitz to develop automated methods of pattern recognition with the aim of evolving a system of chromosome analysis by computer.

Some of the foregoing projects have already run their course; others remain in being at the time of writing. This history is, how-ever, mainly concerned with beginnings; and in this regard it is of interest to note how the changes were rung, by natural development rather than deliberate policy, between the experimental and the clinical approaches. The mechanisms of genetics at the molecular level are considered in the next section.

Molecular biology

The study of living matter is now pursued to a level of minuteness that would have been inconceivable, as a practical proposition, during the earlier part of the Council's history; the starting points of the main lines of investigation in molecular biology were established, notably by workers in America, only about a quarter of a century ago. The subject is thus still young, although it has already made most impressive advances. To these, members of the Council's scientific staff have made a very important contribution, as testified by the galaxy of Nobel awards which they have received (Appendix D).

The Council, true to its policy of fostering the 'growing points of knowledge', has in fact made a major effort to promote research in this field. In 1947 it set up its Molecular Biology Research Unit, under Dr M. F. Perutz, in the Cavendish Laboratory at Cambridge; the initiative had come from Professor Sir Lawrence Bragg, who—with others at Cambridge—was anxious to secure more stable support for this very promising work hitherto precariously maintained by temporary grants and fellowships from various sources. The original small unit has since become a large establishment, separately housed as the Laboratory of Molecular Biology and with three divisions of staff and many attached workers. In the same year the Council established a Biophysics Research Unit at King's College, London, under the honorary direction of Professor J. T. (later Sir John) Randall; Dr M. H. F. Wilkins was senior member of the Council staff and worked in the molecular field. This was later split into a Neurobiology Unit under Professor Wilkins and a Muscle Biophysics Unit under Professor Jean Hanson (died 1973). The Council also maintained a small team of workers at the Royal Institution, London, under Sir Lawrence Bragg. Other projects have more recently been supported by grants, including a Research Group in Molecular Biophysics at Oxford under Professor D. C. Phillips. Progress in molecular biology, with special reference to the part played by the Council's workers, was reviewed in an article contributed by Perutz to the Report for 1968–69; this has provided the main basis of the present section.

Biochemistry—especially in the study of unicellular organisms as already noted—had approached this field; but it was mainly concerned with elucidating the chemical reactions involved in the utilisation of food in building up living matter and producing energy. Genetics, as also noted, was concerned with the modes rather than with the mechanism of inheritance and the nature of genes. It was the convergence of these two streams, as Perutz has pointed out, that gave rise to molecular biology as a special discipline, together with the application of physical methods such as the X-ray diffraction technique earlier used for determining the structure of crystals. As Perutz has said, the aim of molecular biology has been "to explain the inheritance, development and behaviour of living organisms in terms of the atomic structure and interactions of certain large molecules", notably those of enzymes and other proteins and of nucleic acids (DNA and RNA), and it is "a coherent subject of great conceptual beauty".

An outstanding achievement of the subject in Britain has been the development of methods for determining the molecular structure of enzymes, and the interpretation of their specific roles (that is, catalysing particular steps of particular chemical reactions) in precise atomic terms. To work out the three-dimensional structure of such large molecules as proteins is a laborious task, involving the use of both chemical methods such as partition chromatography and physical methods such as X-ray diffraction. Outstanding has been the work of Perutz and of Kendrew on haemoglobins and myoglobin respectively, that of Sanger on insulin, and that of Phillips and others (in Bragg's laboratory in London and later in Oxford) on the enzyme lysozyme which had been discovered by Fleming in 1922.

In terms of heredity, the production of each protein is determined by one gene; and it has been shown that the determining factor can be chemically isolated as a specific form of deoxyribonucleic acid (DNA). The great achievement of Watson and Crick, in the Laboratory of Molecular Biology, was to explain in molecular terms the nature of the genetic information and the way in which it can be transmitted unchanged from one generation of an organism to the next, and through successive divisions of somatic cells. This made it possible to decipher the genetic code containing the information laid down in the chromosomes for translation into protein structure.

The elucidation of the structure of nucleic acids was due largely to the work of Wilkins and Rosalind Franklin on the helical molecular pattern of DNA, combined with that of Watson and Crick. It was to fit the X-ray data of Wilkins and Franklin, as well as other available information, that in 1953 Watson and Crick took the bold step of building an atomic model of the molecule. Incidentally, Watson has since given, in his book *The Double Helix*, a strikingly uninhibited and subjective account of the personal elements in the collaboration.

Watson and Crick also proposed, in 1953, an explanation of the genetic control of enzyme function. In brief, the information to be conveyed is 'coded' in the permutations of the bases fitted into the chain of the nucleic acid molecule. It is now a fundamental postulate that the sequence of groups of these bases is colinear with the sequence of the amino acids in the corresponding protein chain. Further work was concerned with the form of this genetic code

(although the actual 'meanings' of the triplets of bases were elucidated by workers in the United States), and progress has also been
made in explaining how the genetic message embodied in the code
is translated into action in the synthesis of the proteins through the
mediation of messenger, transfer and ribosomal RNAs (ribonucleic
acids).

Other work in molecular biology—just to indicate the extent of
the programme supported by the Council in its own establishments
and elsewhere—deals with the effects of mutations on protein structure, with the mechanism of muscular contraction, and with the
structure of small viruses. Much new ground is being broken, and
Perutz in his article surmised "that the great unsolved problems of
medicine, such as cancer and cardiovascular and degenerative
disease, may have to be approached by seeking an understanding
of pathological events at the molecular level". Molecular biology
therefore needed to extend its frontiers towards medicine through a
study of higher organisms.

Closely involved in molecular biology, and lying in common
ground between genetics and embryology, is the branch of science
known as developmental biology or epigenetics. It is concerned
with the causal mechanisms of the changes whereby the fertilised
egg develops into the adult and finally senescent and moribund
organism. Its principles underlie both normal development and
ageing, and it is hoped that the subject will eventually throw light
on such deviations from normality as congenital defects, tumour
growth and perhaps even the so-called degenerative diseases. It
seeks a link between the fundamental elementary processes of biology
and the characteristics of living organisms as usually encountered.
Its problems include the mechanisms by which genes are organised
into batteries, and by which these are switched on or off. How does
an apparently uniform mass of cells differentiate into a patterned
aggregate of different organs, and how do unstructured masses of
material acquire definite shapes? For work on these and kindred
questions, the Council supported an Epigenetics Research Group
under Professor C. H. Waddington in the Institute of Genetics,
University of Edinburgh, and a Division of Developmental Biology
has been set up at the National Institute for Medical Research under
Dr R. M. Gaze; the Laboratory of Molecular Biology has also
entered this field.

The significance of proteins

The biomedical significance of the vast array of organic compounds
known as proteins is by no means restricted to the field of molecular
biology; this was expressed in the Council's Report for 1950–51:

> The amount of attention given in the Council's laboratories to chemical,
> physical and biological investigations on proteins reflects the enormous impor-
> tance of these substances to the body's economy, both in health and in disease.
> The enzymes which control almost all the chemical reactions within the cells

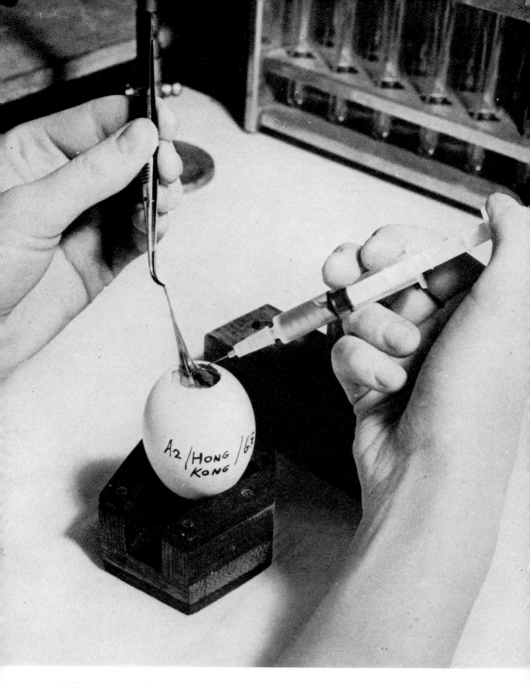

5 Influenza research at the World Influenza Centre (in the National Institute for Medical Research): inoculating an egg with influenza virus—a method of producing virus in quantity

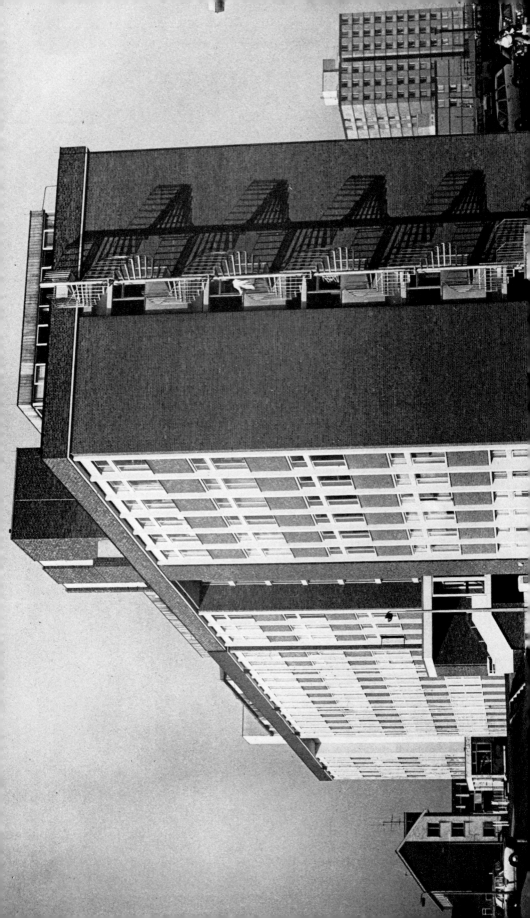

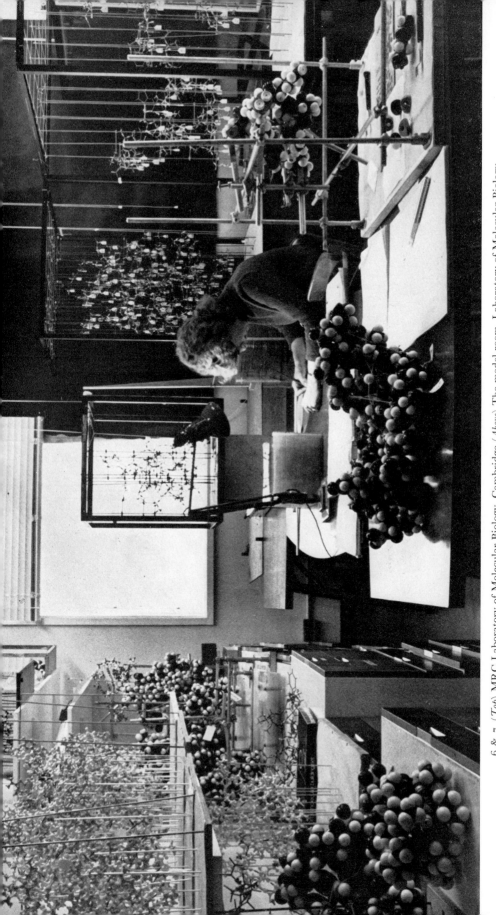

6 & 7 (*Top*) MRC Laboratory of Molecular Biology, Cambridge (*Above*) The model room, Laboratory of Molecular Biology

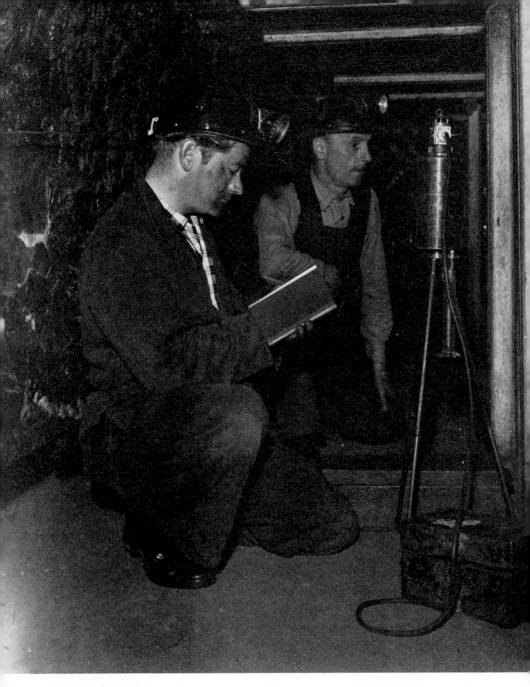

8 Dust sampling apparatus set up at a coal face by members of the MRC Pneumoconiosis Unit, South Wales

of the body or in the digestive tract are proteins; so are a great proportion of the hormones, such as ACTH and insulin; so are the toxins produced by micro-organisms and responsible for the damaging effects of infection. Each of these substances must possess specific structural characteristics which decide its special functions and which must be known in detail before its action can be fully understood.

All proteins break down into amino acids, of which there are twenty common kinds, and within the protein molecule these are linked in groups known as peptides, or polypeptides, which in various sequences form a chain or chains. The number of possible permutations is almost infinite. In 1945 Sanger, working at Cambridge on the Council's external staff, determined the structure of the insulin molecule, involving two kinds of peptide chain—a discovery which gained him a Nobel Prize.

Some proteins are relatively inert constituents of the tissues, notably muscle, but even these tend to be in a state of continuous breakdown and replacement. Many of the more soluble proteins have catalytic or enzymic properties essential to life. Each one is, in its molecular structure, specific for its particular function and commonly also, even if the function be the same, for the kind of animal.

Further major subjects could be mentioned in which proteins are of fundamental importance. For instance, in the 1950s new light was thrown on the classical problem of the contraction of muscle, largely made up of protein fibres, by the work of Dr H. E. Huxley of the Council's staff; this contributed to a new hypothesis concerning the physiological mechanism of the process. Again, members of the Council's Neuropsychiatric Research Unit at Carshalton were among the first to make a systematic study of the biosynthesis of water-soluble proteins in the brain; whereas this proved to be similar in mode to that prevailing in other tissues, the metabolism of the lipoproteins of the myelin sheath has features found to be specially characteristic of the central nervous system.

The study of proteins is of course one in which many laboratories in different countries take part. In the United Kingdom, as was said in the Council's Report for 1963–65, the National Institute for Medical Research "is a principal centre of research on protein synthesis—particularly on protein synthesis in subcellular particles derived from mammalian cells". Recent work there has been concerned with such matters as the synthesis of haemoglobin by small particles (ribosomes) from very young red blood corpuscles; the synthesis by a mouse virus of its characteristic coat of protein; and isolation of an agent (messenger RNA) which transcribes the genetic message contained in the molecule into a form in which it can be used to assemble the constituents of protein molecules in their proper order.

Human behaviour

Direct research both on diseases of the nervous system and on mental disorders falls within the general field of clinical science, and something about the peculiar difficulties of, in particular, research on mental disorders has been said under that head. There is not only a relation between the two subjects, but a certain analogy; clinical neurology was dependent on advances in nerve physiology, while progress in psychiatry was handicapped by inadequate knowledge of normal psychology.

In its Report for 1931–32 the Council took occasion to congratulate two of its members on the award of Nobel Prizes for advances in knowledge of neurophysiology. In discussing the bearing of such knowledge on the problems of disorders of the nervous system, the Report made this historical assessment:

> 'Half a century ago the foundations of our knowledge of nervous disease were being laid by Hughlings Jackson, Ferrier, Gowers, Horsley, and other members of a brilliant group at the National Hospital. By studies of central localization and by the use of new methods of disentangling and tracing the complex distributions of nerve cells and fibres, nervous diseases were given descriptions which expressed and interpreted their symptoms in terms of anatomical structure. Broadly speaking, that wave of progress, to which this country made such notable contribution, has in great measure spent iself. It could hardly have been carried farther forward by purely clinical methods. Steady advance, of course, has followed it, in the detailed working out and application of the knowledge gained, but it seems plain that further progress in the clinical field of any comparable vigour and novelty is now awaiting fresh stimulus and guidance from other directions of inquiry.

The obstacle had lain in lack of knowledge of the normal physiology underlying the anatomical complex of nerve cells, with their intercommunicating fibres and fibrils. This field was being opened as the result of Sir Charles Sherrington's work on the central integration (and summation) of the processes of nervous excitation and inhibition, quite distinct from the phenomenon of the conduction, and of Professor E. D. (later Lord) Adrian's work on the nature of the nervous impulse and of the excitation processes of nerve cells. Sherrington's work at Oxford had latterly had some aid from the Council; Adrian's at Cambridge was supported by the Royal Society. The Council was at the date of that Report forming its Neurological Research Unit, at the National Hospital, to apply this new knowledge to clinical problems.

Eight years later the Council was impressed by the potentialities of a more chemical approach, as witness the Report for 1938–39:

> It has been a common experience in medical research during the past fifty years that, when once investigation has been able to correlate chemical change with function, advance in knowledge has been rapid. Recently, this stage of investigation seems to have been reached in the case of the brain and nervous system generally, and there is ground for the hope that a new chapter concerning the chemical basis of nerve reaction, with all its peculiar manifestations, is

about to be opened up. It will be obvious that, in the case of the nervous system, the evidence of its activity is quite different from that of other systems of the body. In an organ such as the pancreas or kidney, activity can be measured by the amount and nature of its secretion; in a muscle, by its contraction; and in a ductless gland by its content of active principles or by the effect of these on other organs. When an indication of the activity of the brain is sought, however, only too often has reliance to be placed on unco-ordinated or peculiar movement, or on such intangible characteristics as consciousness, emotion, memory, judgement and other psychological qualities. Yet it is obvious that, if it were possible to correlate these functional activities of nervous tissue with specific chemical change, a new world of study would be at hand. Not only would such information be of great importance from the point of view of understanding brain activity, but it might well help towards the elucidation and control of many phenomena in the field of psychiatry, including abnormal thought, action and emotion, which form at present such an enormous social problem. It cannot be said that the newer knowledge has even approached this position, but there is now a distinct possibility of this stage being ultimately attained.

Some of the earliest work promoted by the Council in the field of mental disorders consisted of pathological studies in which a relation was sought between bodily abnormalities, especially of a chemical nature, and malfunctions of the mind. Little progress could be made, however, with the methods then available, and it is only in more recent years that the subject has developed more hopefully. Other early work was concerned with the inheritance of mental defect, and here also there have been recent developments.

It is therefore instructive to glance at the Council's effort, as shown by the number of relevant research units recorded in the Report for 1967–68—not to mention grant-aided work. There are in the first place, although they do not strictly belong to this chapter, the units making the direct psychiatric approach. The Clinical Psychiatry Unit under Dr P. Sainsbury at Graylingwell Hospital, Chichester, Sussex, is engaged in the type of work that its name implies. The Social Psychiatry Unit established in 1948 under Sir Aubrey Lewis (now under Professor J. K. Wing) at the Institute of Psychiatry at the Maudsley Hospital, London, studies the influence of social factors on the occurrence, continuance and outcome of mental illness and subnormality, and is concerned to evaluate social methods of treatment. The Unit for Research on the Epidemiology of Psychiatric Illness under Professor G. M. Carstairs (now the Unit for Epidemiological Studies in Psychiatry and under Dr N. B. Kreitman), in the University of Edinburgh, has studied sections of the population in which there is a high risk of particular psychiatric illnesses, and it examines clinical, social and psychological features in order to develop aetiological hypotheses and to pave the way for eventual preventive actions. The Developmental Psychology Unit under Dr N. O'Connor at Drayton House, London, is studying the psychopathology of cognitive development, and particularly the perceptual problems and physiological responses of psychotic children.

Secondly, there is a series of research units concerned with the underlying physiology and pathology of mental states. The Brain Metabolism Unit set up under Professor W. L. M. Perry (now under Dr G. W. Ashcroft) in the University of Edinburgh and associated hospitals, is studying the metabolism of amino acids and other substances in the brain and tissue fluids of animals and in the tissue fluids of normal volunteers and of patients with psychiatric and neurological disease. The Neuroendocrinology Unit under Professor G. W. Harris in the University of Oxford investigated the anatomical, physiological and behavioural relationship between the central nervous system and the endocrine glands. The Neuropharmacology Unit under Professor P. B. Bradley in the University of Birmingham is engaged in experimental work on the actions of drugs on the central nervous system, with particular reference to the correlation between electrophysiological and behavioural effects and to interactions with sensory stimuli. The Unit for Metabolic Studies in Psychiatry, under Professor F. A. Jenner in the University of Sheffield, and the Neuropsychiatric Research Unit, directed by Dr D. Richter at the Council's Laboratories, Carshalton, and the West Park Hospital, Epsom, Surrey, have been engaged largely in the study of patients with mental disorders.

Thirdly, the Psychiatric Genetics Unit, which was directed by Dr E. T. O. Slater in the Institute of Psychiatry at the Maudsley Hospital, but now disbanded, dealt with the effect of genetic factors in producing all types of mental ill-health, including mental deficiency, personality disorders, neurotic disturbances and the so-called organic and functional psychoses. The work included a follow-up study of twin pairs of which one member had been treated at the Maudsley Hospital during the past twenty years.

Fourthly, there is ethology—the descriptive and analytical study of normal behaviour. The other aspects mentioned above, it will be noted, relate to abnormal conditions—departures from the presumed norm of human behaviour. The definition of the norm itself lies within the province of the psychologist.

Psychology is a well established academic discipline, with methods of research that are generally not expensive. The pursuit of 'pure' knowledge within it has therefore been largely a matter for university departments; and although the Council has always made many grants in support of suitable projects it has had no major programme in this field. Its promotional efforts have been directed rather to applied psychology, particularly in relation to the performance of technical tasks in industry and the services as described elsewhere (Chapter 9). The Council's interest in ethology, however, has latterly been quickened by advances along other lines, such as those of neurophysiology and genetics; and various projects may be mentioned.

The Unit for Research on Neural Mechanisms of Behaviour, set up under Professor G. C. Drew at University College London, and now under Dr I. S. Russell, is primarily studying the role of the cerebral cortex in learning and memory. It is also concerned with cortical–subcortical interactions in such neural processes as the encoding, storage and retrieval of information during learning and memory processes, and it shows the endeavour of a psychological department to reach back into the underlying physiology—a characteristic trend in present-day research. The Speech and Communication (formerly Psycholinguistics) Unit under Professor R. C. Oldfield in the University of Edinburgh aimed at investigating psychological processes underlying language and other forms of communication in both normal and pathological conditions.

Experimental work assisted by the Council has included studies of animal behaviour undertaken primarily from the point of view of zoology and natural history. At a meeting early in 1969 the noted zoologist Professor N. Tinbergen, of Oxford, spoke to the Council on the case for including the investigation of animal behaviour in the field of medical research. He saw the principal contribution of such work as the development of a methodology that could be applied to research on man; but animal studies could also suggest clinical parallels and so indicate areas where further investigations were most likely to be profitable. A particular area, where methods found to be effective in animal studies might be applied to man, is the development of behaviour up to the adult stage. Thus, studies of the development of song and feeding skills in birds suggested that innate and learned behaviour should not be considered separately, but rather as two factors interacting to produce behaviour patterns. The experiments often involved modifying the environment in ways that would not be possible with human beings; but the parallels should not always be sought in primates, as both convergent and divergent forms of behaviour development could be fruitfully studied in a wider range of species possessing group organisation.

Also in early 1969, the Council decided to set up a research unit on the development and integration of behaviour under the honorary direction of Professor R. A. Hinde, holding a Royal Society chair in the Sub-department of Animal Behaviour of the Department of Zoology at Cambridge.

Such steps as these serve to illustrate recent and present trends in the direct study of behaviour; but there are other avenues of approach to which reference has been made. In 1962 Sir Peter Medawar, then Director of the National Institute for Medical Research, expressed the hope in a memorandum to the Council that neurophysiology and ethology would some day meet to explain the complexities of human behaviour.

Part II
Some Special Fields

Chapter 9
Industrial and Social Medicine

The special fields—Early interests in occupational health—The Industrial
Fatigue (Health) Research Board—Industrial physiology—Environmental
factors—Industrial psychology—Human factors in industrial productivity—
Accidents—Ageing—Occupational diseases—Dust hazards—Toxicology—
Epidemiology of non-infective diseases and genetic traits—Social medicine

The special fields
In certain fields the problems of medical research, although of
diverse nature, may be conveniently grouped together because they
arise in the same context. One such grouping is that of industrial
and social medicine; the former has to do with health in relation to
work—that is to say, occupation; the latter, in its narrower sense,
has to do with health in relation to community life, apart from
working conditions. Sometimes the term 'social medicine' is used
to include the whole; and this is logical enough, seeing that personal
health must be broadly related to the totality of the environmental
conditions under which an individual lives and works.

Industrial medicine has to take account both of the unusually high
incidence of some diseases in certain occupations and of the occurrence of disorders peculiar to those engaged in particular types of
work; it is also concerned with industrial injuries of all kinds. Both
curative and preventive aspects of medicine are involved. Further,
there is a wide range of problems that are not medical in the narrow
sense but lie in the realms of applied physiology and psychology:
these are related to the occupational efficiency of body and mind,
thus having a bearing on industrial productivity.

Early interests in occupational health
One of the earliest actions of the Medical Research Committee, in
1914, exemplified its particular concern with problems of tuberculosis. This was the appointment of a Special Investigation Committee upon the Incidence of Phthisis in relation to Occupations.
A report of this body, dealing with the boot and shoe trade, was in
fact the first publication (1915) in the Special Report Series. The
scheme then lapsed as the inquiries could not be prosecuted under
wartime conditions; but a study of the printing trade was completed
at a later date.

Investigations of dangerous dusts and gases were made for the
Factory Department, then the responsibility of the Home Office.
The Report for 1914–15 lists five grant-aided projects relating to

dusts. Dr J. S. Haldane of Oxford, provided with assistance by the Committee, was prominent in this field.

The First World War brought its own problems of industrial health. An example of a strictly medical subject was that of TNT (trinitrotoluene) poisoning among workers in factories manufacturing that explosive. Another category included investigations undertaken by the Committee's Department of Applied Physiology into working conditions in munition factories, such as ventilation, heating, lighting, general hygiene and canteen dietaries. Reports on these subjects were provided for the Health of Munition Workers Committee, advisory to the Ministry of Munitions of War. The Medical Research Committee also supported investigations by Dr H. M. Vernon into hours of work in munitions factories, and by Dr May Smith on fatigue among girls employed therein.

The Industrial Fatigue (Health) Research Board
The Health of Munition Workers Committee, mentioned above, was set up in September 1915 by Mr Lloyd George as Minister of Munitions, probably largely at the instigation of Dr Christopher Addison, his Parliamentary Secretary and eventual successor. Both Dr Walter Fletcher and Dr Leonard Hill were members. The Committee had an advisory function but soon found a need for better knowledge of some of the factors concerned; it accordingly turned to the Medical Research Committee with requests for the investigation of these.

This was the beginning of an expanding programme, long outlasting the war, for as described in the Report for 1917–18: "From many quarters the desire was expressed during last year that when the work of the Health of Munition Workers Committee had ended, arrangements should be made for maintaining on a more permanent footing an organisation for the systematic investigation of the natural laws of industrial fatigue."

So in 1918 the Industrial Fatigue Research Board was set up by the joint action of the Department of Scientific and Industrial Research and the Medical Research Committee, with the blessing of the Home Office. In practice the Board, beyond the limits of its autonomy, came to be administered by the Committee while the Department contributed a grant in aid. Sir Charles Sherrington was the first Chairman, and he had many distinguished successors in the post. Mr D. R. (later Sir Duncan) Wilson was seconded from the Factory Department to be Secretary of the Board, a position which he held until he returned to the Department in 1929 to become Deputy Chief Inspector and then Chief Inspector.

The Report for 1918–19 gives an account of the objects in view:

The terms of reference to the Board are to consider and investigate the relation of the hours of labour and of other conditions of employment, including methods of work, to the production of fatigue, having regard both to industrial efficiency and to the preservation of health among the workers. The functions of the

Board are to initiate, organize, and promote, by research grants or otherwise, investigations in different industries with a view to finding the hours of labour, spells of work, rest pauses, and conditions of other kinds best adapted to various industrial processes according to the nature of the work and its demands on the worker. It is plain that these objects are to be secured by researches which lie partly in the medical sphere and partly in that of industrial research, and are therefore fitly supported by joint action between the two appointing bodies. The primary studies in this subject must be physiological; they must gain further light upon the laws of the human body and brain, so that labour may be effectively and healthily applied to given tasks, and the undue onset of fatigue or any other industrial causes of ill-health prevented. These problems call for special study of muscular actions as well as of the neuro-muscular machinery and the psychological influences which play upon it. All the work on this side falls naturally in the province of medical research, in which will also be included hygienic studies of the effects on the body of attendant circumstances of work, like ventilation, temperature, unhealthy dusts, and the like. At the same time a very large part of the studies coming within the terms of reference must involve inquiries entailing detailed knowledge of industrial processes, reference to the effective use of engineering and other tools, while commonly the conditions of labour which may have medical importance can only be modified by the application of non-medical technical knowledge. On these sides the work is in the sphere of general scientific and industrial research.

In January 1921 the Council (as it had now become) was informed by HM Treasury that no special provision for the work of the Board could be contemplated for the coming financial year. This was tantamount to a death sentence; and as there was already less than three months left it was necessary to give members of the staff immediate formal notice of the termination of their engagements. Meanwhile, however, the Council appealed strongly against the decision.

The Treasury objection was clearly to the rather loose administrative control exercised under a condominium, and to the expansionist tendencies of the Board; as regards the importance of the work, it was suggested that industry should be asked to bear the cost of whatever investigations might be necessary. The Treasury eventually relented, in some measure, on condition that the Council would take sole and full responsibility for the Board's activities, and would integrate the administration with its own. On this basis a small addition was made to the Council's own grant in aid for the coming year; this made possible the retention of a reduced organisation— perhaps even improved in some ways by the enforced streamlining —and some of the letters of dismissal were withdrawn.

The Board itself was reconstituted as a body advising and assisting the Council; and on the scientific side it was reinforced by a group of specialist committees, appointed by the Council, on aspects of industrial physiology, on industrial psychology, and on statistics. This last committee came to have a much wider function in the Council's programme, as has been noted elsewhere (Volume One).

(In 1922 the opportunity of new premises was taken to integrate the Board's hitherto separate small office with that of the Council. In 1930 Mr Wilson was succeeded as Secretary of the Board by Air Vice-Marshal Sir David Munro, who had just completed his term as Director-General of Royal Air Force Medical Services; and on his retirement in 1942 his place was taken by Dr R. S. F. Schilling, formerly a Medical Inspector of Factories and later Professor of Occupational Health in the University of London. Finally, from 1946, the duty devolved on Dr Joan Faulkner, and from 1951 on Dr B. S. Lush, both of the Council's headquarters staff.)

In 1929 the word 'Fatigue' was replaced by 'Health' in the title of the Board. Not only was the former word too narrow in its connotation, but it had lost much of its significance. Originally, the big problem was in fact that of fatigue, owing to the excessively long hours worked in industry—especially under wartime conditions, when what was later shown to be a self-defeating attempt was made to increase production (over extended periods) by lengthening the working week. The introduction of shorter hours, the improvement of working conditions and the mechanisation of many laborious procedures greatly altered the perspective.

A later development was the growing number and importance of the scientific committees associated with the Board. The natural effect was that the advice of these committees tended, as a time-saving measure, to go direct to the Council as in the case of other committees; furthermore, the purely medical aspect of the programme had become predominant. The Board itself thus gradually became redundant, although the Council's work in the field of industrial health had increased. There followed a transitional stage during which the title was retained, for the good-will that attached to it, as a sort of bracket embracing the group of relevant committees; but in 1959 the Board was formally disbanded.

During the period of its existence, the Board had its own annual reports and its own series ('pink reports') of scientific publications.

Industrial physiology
Research in this subject has two main aspects. One is the study of the human body itself in relation to the tasks demanded of it. The other is the study of the worker's physical environment and its effects on his performance and well-being. Both aspects were from the beginning subjects of study in the programme of the Industrial Fatigue Research Board. In giving some examples of each, it is not intended to imply that psychological as well as physiological factors do not play some part.

The background of the modern study of optimum hours of work was delineated as follows in the *First Annual Report of the Industrial Fatigue Research Board* (1920):

The scientific study of the laws governing the healthy employment of the human mind and body in industry was strangely late in its development in this country, although it was in Great Britain that the industrial revolution had its first beginnings and industrial development was most rapid, and also that geographical, social and political conditions combined to intensify the evils arising from the neglect of scientific study. Even in the long parliamentary battles fought during the nineteenth century upon the specific question of the reduction of the daily hours of work, battles fought between the advocates of a *laissez faire* policy followed in the supposed interests of production and national wealth, on the one hand, and those pressing the claims of human charity upon the other, no appeal was made by either side to the laws of physiology or to the test of experiment, which might very rapidly have shown that a reduction of hours would have increased industrial output no less than human happiness and health. It was not until 1893 that Messrs Mather and Platt, of Manchester, conducted their well-known pioneer experiment on this subject. Mr Mather, later Sir William Mather, to whose initiative this work was due, primarily endeavoured to show that 'work before breakfast' was open to economic as well as to social objections. The working day, accordingly, during the two years' experimental period was shortened (permitting work to begin at 8 a.m. instead of 6 a.m.), and the breakfast interval was abolished. The experiment showed that the reduction in hours from 54 to 48 hours a week caused an increase in production and a decrease in lost time.

As an immediate result of the Manchester experiment, HM Government introduced the 48-hour week in its arsenals and shipyards. There was, nevertheless, no general adoption of this policy by industry. Nor did even the Government at that time promote any further organised scientific study of the subject, although at the beginning of the twentieth century industrial firms in Germany, Belgium and the United States of America were already undertaking analogous investigations.

At the end of the First World War, the Board took over from the Ministry of Munitions the responsibility for certain inquiries that had been initiated by the recently disbanded Health of Munition Workers Committee. At the same time it proceeded to draw up a plan for its future researches into problems of industry in normal times. In consultation with the Home Office, it decided that the following industries offered particularly favourable fields of study (for, among others, the reasons indicated):

Iron and steel (arduous and continuous character of work)
Cotton (work under hot and humid conditions)
Silk (fine nature of many processes)
Laundries (arduous work by women)
Boots and shoes (short normal hours; variety of processes and conditions)

Investigations were undertaken in all these industries, and in addition work was initiated on certain general problems without reference to the conditions of any particular industry.

As regards methods, the Board had recourse to (a) laboratory experiments; (b) statistical analysis of factory records, past and current; (c) observations in factories, including measurements of output under different conditions; and (d) large-scale factory experiments, involving trial alterations in hours of work or the introduction of rest pauses.

Use was also made of the methods of 'time and motion study'.

Here the object was to analyse the movements made by the worker in any given process, and to use the information to devise means of economising both his effort and the time taken. Trials were also made to determine the optimum height of the working bench for employees with different measurements. This is a simple example of the attempt to fit the machine to the man as well as to the job. It was a truism that when machines were designed for sale to the public great pains were taken to suit the convenience of the operator, but that when they were designed for use by factory employees this element was all too often lacking.

Study was also made of the physiology of muscular work, using laboratory methods, and of energy expenditure in different occupational groups. At a later stage, in 1958, investigations on the latter were facilitated by an important advance in technique, the development of an integrated motor pneumotachograph by Mr H. S. Wolff of the National Institute for Medical Research. This made possible the collection of samples of expired air from a subject over a period of hours, the measurement of the oxygen and carbon dioxide content of the integrated sample, and the determination of the total volume of air expired during the whole time. Yet the instrument, worn by the subject, did not interfere with ability to perform prescribed tasks. By this method, far more measurements of energy expenditure could be made in a given time than by the ordinary means of gas analyses, and basic data required by physiologists in many types of investigation of human beings could thus be readily provided.

Environmental factors

Essential to the worker's well-being and efficiency are appropriate ventilation, heating and lighting. These, together with avoidance of excessive noise and vibration, may be regarded as normal physiological requirements. In a different category, the subject of a later section, are measures for minimising the special hazards from harmful dusts, gases or radiations, from contact with toxic substances, and from infective microorganisms.

Ventilation and heating are closely linked and need to be studied, and indeed provided, together. The human requirements, and the means of meeting them, have been the subject of investigation from the earliest days of the Council. Work on the more general aspect, at the National Institute for Medical Research, has already been mentioned; studies in an industrial context came under the direction of the Council's Industrial Fatigue (Health) Research Board.

Following in the wake of Sir Leonard Hill's work at the National Institute, Dr H. M. Vernon made many investigations of factory ventilation on behalf of the Board. In 1926 a report by Vernon and others was published in the Council's series, dealing with the methods of studying ventilation and its effects; and in the official preface it was stated that "the ill-effects of bad ventilation do not result from the chemical impurity of the air, but from want of adequate cooling of the body and evaporation from it". On this basis it was concluded that "the successful ventilation of rooms, schools or factories thus depends primarily on both the temperature and the movement of the air (though the air should at the same time be kept free from dust and microbic infection)". Much effort went into inquiries directed to proving these propositions, to demonstrating their importance for industry, and to determining the precise conditions for putting them into practice. Many reports published in the Board's series gave the results of such investigations.

Further work for the Council in this field was largely in the hands of Dr T. Bedford. On the Council's staff as an investigator for the Board from 1920, he was recognised in 1947 as Director of a Group for Research in Industrial Physiology (No. 1); this later became the Environmental Hygiene Research Unit and was located in the London School of Hygiene and Tropical Medicine, and afterwards in part in the Medical Research Council Laboratories, Hampstead. Airborne dust was latterly included in its purview. After the Director's retirement in 1959 part of the Unit was absorbed by the National Institute for Medical Research. Other Council establishments concerned with climatology and air hygiene have already been mentioned in a more general context.

Much work on factory illumination and on other matters relating to the vision of workers was done for the Council by Mr H. C. Weston. He, also, was on the Council's staff as an investigator for the Board from 1920 and he was recognised in 1947 as Director of a Group for Research in Industrial Physiology (No. 2). This was subsequently renamed the Group for Research in Occupational Optics and was located in the London School of Hygiene and Tropical Medicine and later, until 1959, in the Institute of Ophthalmology, University of London.

Concern about industrial noise and its possible effects is of relatively recent origin. In 1962 the Ministry of Pensions and National Insurance commissioned an investigation into the subject that was undertaken jointly by the Council and the National Physical Laboratory, and the report, entitled *Hearing and Noise in Industry*, was published in 1970.

Some of the research was directed towards problems of work under exceptionally trying conditions. Vernon and other investigators for the Board, for instance, reported in 1927 on studies of coalmining in high temperatures. And in the Council's Report for 1957–58 some account is given of researches by the Council's Climate and Working Efficiency Research Unit at Oxford under the honorary direction of Sir Wilfrid Le Gros Clark. Some of the investigations were made at the request of the National Coal Board; they related not only to the normal working day, but also to the limiting conditions for short exposure of picked men to high temperatures in the course of mine rescue operations. Cognate work with a military objective is mentioned elsewhere.

The whole question of efficiency under unpleasant conditions is discussed in the Reports for 1963–65 and 1973–74. The point is made that, contrary to what might be supposed, uncomfortable conditions do not necessarily diminish efficiency; and that it is necessary to have recourse to objective experiment before deciding whether a particular stress is merely an unimportant annoyance or a true cause of inefficiency. The level at which some stresses appear to affect efficiency is indeed surprisingly high, although for others it may be quite low. Moreover, the effects of high-intensity noise, of excessive heat and of sleeplessness can sometimes be counteracted by altering the nature of the work in quite small ways. It is therefore necessary to ascertain, by research, the mechanisms on which different forms of stress produce their effects. Experiments on these lines have been made by Dr D. E. Broadbent and others in the Council's Applied Psychology Unit at Cambridge.

Another form of physiological stress due to abnormal environmental conditions is seen in the effects of high pressures encountered in the course of duty in submarines, in deep diving and during work in caissons. The problem, including that of preventing decompression sickness, is of importance for certain civil engineering and naval purposes; it is discussed in the Council's Report for 1965–66. Dr J. S. Haldane and his son, Professor J. B. S. Haldane, were both, in their generations, associated with the Council in this field of work.

Latterly the work of the Oxford unit mentioned earlier has been continued by the Council's Environmental Physiology Unit under Professor J. S. Weiner at the London School of Hygiene and Tropical Medicine.

Industrial psychology

The early investigations made for the Industrial Fatigue Research Board under this head were largely statistical and were aimed at assessing the effect of factors that were at least partly psychological in nature. They dealt with such problems as optimum hours of work and the value of rest pauses (partly physiological questions, as already noted), with the causes of absenteeism (only partly due to sickness), and with the influence of incentives and the part played by the monotony of repetitive work in producing boredom and fatigue. Studies were also made of methods of selecting and training workers for particular tasks, and of management–worker relationships and social life within the place of employment. Account had also to be taken of local or personal circumstances affecting the employee in non-working hours.

Most of this research was undertaken by teams of investigators working under the general direction of the Board. The senior members of staff were Dr S. Wyatt, for long attached to the University of Manchester; Mr E. Farmer, at first in London, but later in the University of Cambridge; and Dr May Smith, in London, who was especially concerned with women in industry. The collection of data, whether by direct observation or from the records, was done in factories, workshops, offices and the like.

At the beginning of the Second World War the Council found itself with a substantial concentration of workers in the Psychological Laboratory, University of Cambridge, headed by Professor F. C. (later Sir Frederic) Bartlett; some of these were members of the Council's staff, as in the case of Mr Farmer already mentioned, and others were in receipt of grants. Much of the work was for the time being directed towards work for the Services, but the problems were similar to those of industry. In 1945 it was decided, following a memorandum prepared by Professor Bartlett in 1943, to consolidate this group of workers as the Council's Applied Psychology Research Unit. Of this, Dr K. W. Craik was appointed Director at the early age of 28 but was unfortunately killed in a road accident in the following year. Professor Bartlett then took personal charge, with the status of Honorary Director, until Dr N. H. Mackworth was appointed Director in 1952; the latter was succeeded in 1958 by Dr Broadbent.

Bartlett retired from his chair in the University in 1952 and, as his successor there could be expected to have different interests, the main part of the Unit was transferred to a large private house which the Council acquired for the purpose. A residue of the members reverted to their former individual status within the University.

The Report for 1950–51 included an article reviewing the experimental study of human skill, a main theme in the programme of the Applied Psychology Research Unit. By that date heavy work in industry had largely been transferred to machines and what was required from the operative was not muscular exertion so much as mental effort—accurate and often extremely speedy—in controlling the machine. To facilitate this the design of machinery had to be adapted to human potentialities, raising problems for the physiologist and psychologist as well as for the mechanical engineer. The first stage to be considered was the identification and interpretation by the operator of certain information coming either from the environment (as in motor-driving) or more commonly from the machine itself in the form of signals provided by gauges and other 'display devices' or by the 'feel' of the manual control levers and the like. The second stage was that of making the appropriate controlling response to the information or stimulus received; this involved two factors, that of 'load' (the complexity of the sources of information) and 'speed' (the rate at which decisions must be made). There was also the question of the anticipation of signals. A related problem was that of the transferability of acquired skills from one situation to another, a matter of importance in designing methods of training in times of rapid technological change.

The advantages of laboratory work in this subject are expressed in the Report for 1954–55, again with special reference to the Applied Psychology Research Unit:

> Some problems are unsuitable for field investigation, since this may involve dislocation of production in many ways, for example by alterations to machinery in constant use; moreover the result of field studies are often open to criticism on the grounds of poor scientific control. In the laboratory, on the other hand, it is easy to keep irrelevant factors from interfering with a set problem, and it is possible to vary such important details as the sensitivity of the controls which are being compared; in addition, laboratory findings, besides providing useful guidance on a large number of practical issues, can at the same time furnish information of fundamental scientific interest.

The Report goes on to say that "Some laboratory experiments happily reinforce common-sense views of human performance; others produce unexpected results." Several popular fallacies have in fact been discredited by scientific studies in which the Unit has taken a large part—the fallacy that there is an inevitable steady decline in performance in the course of repetitive work; the fallacy that perceptual tasks are easy, for example that constant watch on an operation and inspection of its results is less tiring than more active participation; and the fallacy that there is an unchanging optimum in conditions of work (in fact repeated slight changes have for a time a beneficial effect on output). There have of course been parallel studies elsewhere, particularly in America.

Of the pioneer investigators for the Industrial Fatigue (Health) Research Board, mentioned earlier, Mr Farmer's small team was absorbed by the Applied Psychology Research Unit at the latter's inception. Mr Wyatt's Industrial Psychology Research Group (later Unit) continued to be centred on the University of Manchester until his retirement in 1952; thereafter its headquarters moved to London, where it came under the honorary direction of Professor G. C. Drew at University College until 1965, and then under that of Dr C. B. Frisby at the National Institute of Industrial Psychology for a final two years. Dr May Smith retired in 1944.

Special subjects of study have included problems of the resettlement of disabled workers (following a request by the Ministry of Labour in 1948), and problems of the employment of mentally subnormal people.

The prevalence of neurosis among industrial workers was investigated for the Council during the Second World War by Dr T. Russell Fraser and his assistants; the results were published as one of the Reports of the Board (1947). Disorders of this kind were further studied by the Unit for Research in Occupational Adaptation, under the honorary direction of Professor Sir Aubrey Lewis, as recounted in the Council's Report for 1953–54.

Early in 1967 the Council had presented to it, by Sir Austin Bradford Hill and Professor H. Kay, the report of a committee which it had set up to review the programme of research in industrial and applied psychology. Emphasis was laid on the importance of maintaining the Council's role in the provision, in particular, of a backing of medical expertise in this field; the vital need was for the collaboration of first-class investigators drawn from the medical and social sciences. The Council agreed in principle to expand its activities and to consult the Department of Education and Science, with other bodies as necessary, about committee structure and other administrative arrangements. The setting up of a Social and Applied Psychology Unit under Professor Kay in the University of Sheffield was a direct result, and also some expansion of the Applied Psychology Unit at Cambridge.

Human factors in industrial productivity
In 1948 the Council assumed, by official request, responsibility for a number of research projects recommended by the Panel on Human Factors of an official Committee on Industrial Productivity set up by the Advisory Council on Scientific Policy. These ranged in scope from an anthropological survey of a coalmining area in Fife to a study of the optimum size of batches of material issued to an operator for processing at one time, but most of them were concerned directly with human relations. Special financial provision was available for the productivity programme from Conditional Aid Funds (described as "counterpart funds derived from US economic aid").

The Committee on Industrial Productivity, before it dissolved, had recommended that the completion of these projects should be made the occasion of a review of the work of the Human Factors Panel, and this review became part of a wider survey undertaken jointly by the Council and the Department of Scientific and Industrial Research. The Council had gone into this venture with some misgivings because, although health and efficiency are obviously linked, it was less clear that productivity as such was properly a medical objective; strict conditions were stipulated, giving the Council full control in consultation with its own advisers. Moreover, it soon became evident that the difficulties in the way of scientific study of social behaviour had not yet been overcome; the Council accordingly appointed a new Committee on Methodology in the Study of Social Behaviour, under the chairmanship of Sir Frederic Bartlett, to consider the problems arising in this kind of inquiry.

In 1951 a joint report was made by the staffs of the Council and of the Department who were concerned with the project. This was followed by a joint memorandum by the Secretaries of the two organisations, making proposals about the division of responsibility for future work. As a result, it was proposed in the following year that a Joint Committee on Individual Efficiency in Industry should be set up to keep under review the progress of knowledge bearing on this aspect, to advise on general policy in the research, to call attention to gaps and make recommendations for filling them, and to report from time to time on requirements for training research workers and technicians in this field. It was further proposed to set up a Joint Committee on Human Relations in Industry to examine current activities in this line of study and to call attention to problems of special timeliness or promise on which applied or fundamental research might be undertaken or supported. These proposals were approved by the Lord President and HM Treasury in the following year, and the two Joint Committees, with Sir Frederic Bartlett and Mr A. B. (later Sir Bertram) Waring as the respective chairmen, came into being at the beginning of 1953.

These committees did useful service in reviewing the fields, and their reports were published in 1954 and 1958 under the joint authority of the two sponsoring bodies. It cannot be said, however, that they had much impact in originating research; little of value was done that would not have been done in any event. In negative fashion, the episode exemplifies the principle that successful research projects arise as natural developments of scientific thought and not from political motivation. Be that as it may, it was very soon found expedient to dismantle this rather ponderous machinery. The preface to the joint report of 1958 put it thus: "When the Conditional Aid scheme ended on 31st March, 1957, our two Councils reviewed the position in detail and agreed that they should work separately in future, each concentrating on problems within its own field of interest."

Accidents
From an early date the personal element in accidents was a subject of study by investigators of the Council's Industrial (Fatigue) Health Research Board; at first this work related only to ordinary industrial accidents, but its scope was later widened to include other types and particularly road accidents. The nature of 'accident proneness' was thus summarised in the Council's Report for 1933–34:

> It is now well established with regard to industrial risks that certain persons have a special liability to be the subjects of accidents. Thus, for instance, it may be found that if a large number of individuals are exposed to the same risks, seventy-five per cent of all the accidents occurring among them are sustained by a small minority of the group, possibly consisting of as few as ten per cent of its number. This is an entirely different result from that which would be found if the distribution of accidents among individuals were due to chance. The phenomenon, moreover, is independent of any question of responsibility or blameworthiness: the statistical result holds good even although the subject of numerous accidents may on some of the occasions appear to have been the victim of fortuitous circumstances or of the actions of others. The practical consideration is that the total number of accidents suffered by any group can be greatly reduced by detecting and eliminating the relatively small number of individuals who exhibit special liability.

In the special case of road accidents, and the possibility of reducing their number by eliminating a small minority of drivers shown by their insurance records to be accident prone, it was remarked that "The novelty of the method, as compared with judicial disqualification in isolated cases as at present, lies in the facts that it makes use of information provided by minor accidents, and that it is dissociated from any question of blame." The section concluded as follows:

> The question as to what practical steps it may be possible to take along these lines is not a matter coming within the purview of the Council. They believe, however, that a successful attack upon problems of road dangers will necessarily have to take into account, in one way or another, the existence of these phenomena of accident proneness which are being brought to light by scientific investigation.

Personal proneness is of course only one aspect of the problem of accidents, there being various specific causes against which measures can be taken. Faulty design of machinery—or of roads—is an obvious example; and also lack of adequate safeguards against mechanical risks. There are also factors in the environment that contribute to accidents, such as extremes of temperature, a high level of humidity, or poor illumination; and in evaluating these the Council's workers have played their part. There is also the psychological problem of lapses of attention on the part of even highly skilled operatives. This subject has been extensively studied in America and elsewhere, and has been one of the special concerns of the Council's Applied Psychology Unit at Cambridge. Its Director, Dr D. E. Broadbent, distinguished four different factors that could be shown by experiment to be causes of inattention—distraction, fatigue, expectancy (of particular signals), and arousal (a state of non-specific alerting activity). These concepts not only are of practical importance but, as the Council said in its Report for 1958–59, "contribute to our general understanding of the functioning of those mechanisms of the human nervous system which underlie behaviour".

In an article in its Report for 1954–55 the Council summed up the question of the causation of industrial accidents:

> Accidents are commonly due to multiple causes. Diverse personal factors, as well as defects of environment, equipment and materials, all combine in varying degree to produce them. Research into these different factors brings us into the fields of psychology, occupational hygiene, and engineering; and preventive measures, based on these separate approaches, can each be expected to affect a proportion of the accidents. The object of such researches should be to discover the most vulnerable links in the chain of causation, and these may well differ in different industries, factories and workshops.

A strictly medical aspect of the subject is the treatment of accidental injuries, from whatever cause, with the aim of securing an early return to health with the fullest function. Studies with this aim have been particularly the task of the Council's Industrial Injuries and Burns Research Unit, the origin of which is mentioned in a subsequent section. This is directed by Dr J. P. Bull in the Birmingham Accident Hospital.

In Great Britain, accidents have in recent years become the commonest single cause of death between the ages of one and forty. They may be divided into industrial accidents, transport accidents and domestic accidents; and the Council's investigators have been concerned with all three groups. Transport accidents occur mainly on the road; and the effects of alcohol on driving has been an important aspect of the study, as noted in an earlier chapter. Accidents in the home chiefly involve children, among whom burns are particularly common and severe, and old people. The subject of accidents, including accident proneness, was discussed in the Report for 1963–65.

Ageing
The increase in the proportion of old people in the population of economically advanced countries has added to the importance of the disabilities associated with ageing. These present a social problem as well as a field of medical practice and research. In recent years various aspects of gerontology have engaged the Council's attention. In its Report for 1960–61 the Council reviewed the question of mental disorders in old age. Both the overall incidence of psychiatric disorders and the frequency with which they complicate physical illness rise steeply with age. The suicide rate also reaches a peak in old age. On the social side, the Council's Clinical Psychiatry Research Unit in Graylingwell Hospital at Chichester, Sussex, has examined the indications for community rather than hospital care for old people, including the effect on families of maintaining aged relatives in their homes.

In 1955 the Council set up a Group (later Unit) for Research on Occupational Aspects of Ageing, under the honorary direction of Professor L. S. Hearnshaw, in the University of Liverpool. The work has been concerned with the physiological changes in performance, capacity and attitude that occur during the second half of working life, between the ages of 40 and 65. Two factors gave the study special importance: the increasing proportion of the labour force in the upper age-groups, and the increasing rate of technological change calling for personal readjustment and retraining. The results of a survey carried out by the Unit in manufacturing industry on Merseyside was published in the Council's Memorandum Series in 1961.

More recently the Council has supported a Research Group on the Biology of Ageing under Dr Alex Comfort at University College London. The fundamental biological aspects of ageing were discussed in the Report for 1966–67. And in 1969, wishing to be advised on possible lines of research, the Council invited Professor W. F. (later Sir William) Anderson of the Chair of Geriatric Medicine, University of Glasgow, to address one of its meetings; his statement has since been published (1970).

Occupational diseases

The concern of the original Medical Research Committee with the occupational incidence of pulmonary tuberculosis was mentioned early in this chapter. Work on diseases associated with dust hazards and with the manufacture or use of toxic substances are discussed in subsequent sections; so also are certain statistical inquiries of an epidemiological nature.

Between the two world wars the Council organised research on a number of morbid conditions associated with particular occupations. Notable among these was the eye disorder known as miners' nystagmus. Following a request from the Home Office (on the recommendation of its Miners' Lamps Committee), the Council appointed a special committee on the subject, and in 1922 and 1923 it was able to include two reports of this body among its publications. Dr T. L. Llewellyn of Nottingham was secretary of the Miners' Nystagmus Committee and also received a grant from the Council to continue his personal researches in the subject. In 1924 another item in the Council's series was a report by Professor E. L. Collis and Dr Llewellyn on the conditions of miners and others known as 'beat knee', 'beat hand', and 'beat elbow', associated with forms of continuing trauma such as the effect of using vibrating tools; the investigation was promoted by the Council at the instance of the Mines Department.

In 1924, the attention of the Council was drawn by the Mines Department to the occurrence of what appeared to be spirochaetal jaundice (Weil's disease) among coalminers in East Lothian. In association with the University of Edinburgh the Council organised a special investigation; and an arrangement was made with the Edinburgh Royal Infirmary to release Dr G. Buchanan from his post there, for a year, to enable him to give his whole time to work on the subject. The causative organism, *Leptospira icterohaemorrhagiae*, was identified not only in human cases but also in field-mice and rats in the area, and in roof drippings from certain of the pit tunnels.

During and immediately after the Second World War there was a great intensification of the Council's effort to promote research in the strictly medical aspects of industrial health. In the Report for 1945–48 it was remarked that:

Research into occupational health has shown unprecedented expansion in the last three years, and now represents a very substantial part of the Council's programme. Indeed, it may be said that the development of research in this field, and the initiation of research projects into the medical and biological aspects of nuclear physics . . . have been the two outstanding features of the Council's work in this country since the end of the war.

In addition to committees on occupational physiology and psychology, the Council was now advised by new committees on occupational medicine, industrial pulmonary diseases and toxicology. The Industrial Health Research Board, which had been reconstituted in 1942, acted as a reviewing body and continued to advise the Council on the field as a whole—but this function was soon found to be otiose and formal, so that dissolution of the Board followed in 1959, as already mentioned.

In 1943 the Council had set up a Department for Research in Industrial Medicine at the London Hospital, with Dr Donald Hunter as part-time Physician-in-charge. The programme in the early years included an inquiry into the risks of lung and skin cancer in workers handling arsenic, and investigations of the dust hazard in the vitreous enamelling trade, in iron and steel foundries, and in tin mining in Cornwall. Work was also done on Raynaud's disease associated with vibrations from machinery, on the toxicology of organic mercury compounds and other substances used in industrial processes or as insecticides and weed-killers, and on pulmonary damage attributable to beryllium and its compounds.

The Department also made an intensive study of the fluorosis hazard in and around aluminium works in Invernesshire, groups of the local population as well as factory workers being examined. This was undertaken at the request of the Department of Health for Scotland, after an outbreak of fluorosis had been noted among cattle and sheep in the area. Although there was considerable morbidity from fluorosis amongst the local domestic stock, and widespread contamination of the soil and herbage with fluorine compounds, only a few cases of skeletal fluorosis (without symptoms) were found amongst the factory workers. A full report was published in the Council's series of Memoranda in 1949.

An Industrial Medicine Research Unit, under the direction of Dr J. R. Squire of the Council's staff, was set up in the Birmingham Accident Hospital in 1946. This was evolved from the Council's wartime Wound Infection Research Unit, under the direction of Dr A. A. (later Sir Ashley) Miles, in the same institution. In its new form it was concerned largely with occupational skin disease, including cancer. Eventually, in 1952, it was combined with the Burns Research Unit which had been established in the Royal Infirmary, Glasgow, in 1942 under the direction of Dr Leonard Colebrook and moved to the Birmingham Accident Hospital two years later.

Dust hazards

A principal subject in the Council's programme of research in industrial medicine has from the earliest stage been the hazard of pulmonary disease arising from, or aggravated by, the inhalation of dusts of various kinds incidental to different mining and manufacturing processes. Even before there was any deliberate programme of the kind, Dr W. E. Gye of the Council's staff at the National Institute for Medical Research was collaborating with Dr E. H. Kettle of St Mary's Hospital, London, in pathological studies of the effects of silica dust on the tissues, with special reference to problems of industrial tuberculosis; the results were published in joint papers in 1922.

In 1930 the Council appointed a Committee on Industrial Pulmonary Disease, and as recorded in the Report for 1934–35:

This step was taken in response to a request by the Home Office for further research into morbid conditions due to the inhalation of dust associated with occupation. The practical importance of the subject may be gauged by the fact that one of these conditions, silicosis, has been certified as the cause of over 300 deaths annually in England and Wales during the last three years, and has cost in compensation alone more than £100 000 in a single year. Silicosis is a disease arising directly from exposure to the inhalation of the siliceous dust which occurs in various important industries and occupations: these include mining, quarrying, and pottery manufacture, and the exposure is thus widespread. Preventive measures are hampered by lack of exact knowledge. Silicosis is insidious in its onset, but it is not known how much of the dangerous dust must be inhaled, and over what period, to produce disabling effects. Much also remains to be discovered as to the influence—as regards degree of danger—of the size-distribution and concentration of the dust particles at the time of inhalation, although the chemical and mineralogical characteristics of the dusts that are harmful, and the nature of their specific effects upon the body, have already been determined to some extent.

The investigation depended on the availability of a satisfactory instrument for sampling dust clouds and measuring the concentration and size-frequency of the particles. For this purpose a suitable apparatus was devised by staff lent to the Council from the Chemical Defence Experimental Station at Porton. Further refinements in method were much later the subject of research by Dr C. N. Davies in the Council's own Industrial Physiology Research Unit and by Mr H. S. Wolff and others at the National Institute for Medical Research. From the latter there emerged a new dust sampler, named the 'conicycle', of which some account was given in the Report for 1967–68.

Another basic need was more information about the chemical properties of the dusts concerned, including the composition of the particles and their solubility under different conditions. Grants were accordingly made (in 1935) for chemical studies under the general direction of Professor H. V. A. Briscoe at the Imperial College of Science and Technology, London, in close cooperation with those working on the physical and pathological sides. Various biological investigations were at the same time continued. These included both pathological studies of material from human cases and experimental work, the latter chiefly under the general direction of Dr J. S. Haldane of Oxford and of Professor E. H. Kettle in (by that time) the British Postgraduate Medical School at Hammersmith.

The Report for 1937–38 describes the origin of a notably extensive scheme of research on pneumoconiosis among workers in coal mines:

In recent years it has become apparent that coalminers are subject to chronic pulmonary disease of a disabling nature which does not come within the accepted definition of silicosis. A condition occurs which clinically resembles silicosis, but is radiologically different from it. Thus, while in silicosis the lungs, on radiological examination, show shadows indicating distinct nodulation, in the condition referred to this appearance is absent and there may be instead a variety of other shadows, the significance of which, in relation to the occurrence and progress of disability, is not clearly understood. Apart, however, from the disabling nature of the disease, the matter is one of economic importance to the workers for, whereas silicosis is a disease allowing compensation, no such claim is allowed ordinarily to those who develop other forms of chronic pulmonary disease.

This important problem of health was presented to the Medical Research Council by the Home Office and the Mines Department with the request that an investigation should be made on the matter. The Council's Committee on Industrial Pulmonary Disease after close study reported that "there is a sufficient amount of disablement due to pulmonary conditions occurring amongst workers in the coal industry to call for thorough scientific investigation from the aetiological, clinical and radiological points of view and they recommend that such investigations be undertaken by the Medical Research Council". The Council accepted the responsibility for investigating this problem of health, with the object of obtaining new knowledge on which methods of prevention and treatment could be based. The administrative problem raised by this disease, namely, whether it should be scheduled as an occupational disease under the Workmen's Compensation Act along with silicosis, was clearly outside the province of the Council.

The investigations began in 1936 on a carefully planned basis, involving the deployment of staff and associated workers on different aspects of the problem. Dr P. D'Arcy Hart was appointed to the Council's staff to lead the research; and with him on the clinical side was Dr E. A. Aslett of the Welsh National Memorial Association. The anthracite coalfield in South Wales was chosen as the scene of the investigation, and in the first instance a particular coalmine was designated for intensive study. All the workers at this pit were examined, whether or not they were known to have pulmonary disease; and as complete as possible an examination of the environmental conditions in the pit was made. In all this the mine-owners and mine-workers most willingly cooperated; and a contribution to the cost was made from the Miners' Welfare Fund.

The Mines Department supplied the services of mining engineers and inspectors to advise on environmental conditions, and special studies of these were also made by Dr T. Bedford of the Council's staff and other experts. Biochemical and histological studies of post-mortem material were undertaken by, respectively, Dr E. J. King and T. H. Belt at the British Postgraduate Medical School in London. As secretary of the Council's Industrial Pulmonary Disease Committee, Dr E. L. Middleton of the Factory Department, Home Office, coordinated the different lines of inquiry.

As an outcome, three reports entitled *Chronic Pulmonary Disease in South Wales Coalminers* were published in the Council's series in 1942–45. Much work nevertheless remained to be done, and the need for a permanent research organisation on the spot was clearly indicated. So in 1945, after consultation with the Ministry of Fuel and Power, the Council established a Pneumoconiosis Research Unit at Llandough Hospital, Cardiff, to continue the work on occupational lung disease among coalminers on a larger scale. The first Director of the Unit, which soon ranked as one of the largest of the Council's establishments, was Dr C. M. Fletcher; he was succeeded in 1952 by Dr J. C. Gilson. The subject was again reviewed by the Council in its Report for 1953–54.

Although silica dust was always the most important, various other dusts were studied in relation to particular diseases. Thus, Professor Matthew J. Stewart, University of Leeds, and Dr J. S. Faulds of Carlisle were aided by the Council in work on the effects of haematite dust on those mining that ore. Later, special attention became directed to asbestos dust, the health hazards of which were discussed in the Report for 1967–68. In 1955 Dr Richard Doll of the Council's staff had shown, statistically, that there was a greatly increased risk of bronchial cancer in workers in scheduled occupations in the asbestos textile industry—a risk which became much less when exposure was limited to improved working conditions after 1931. About the same time investigations were made in South Africa; Dr J. S. Wagner played a leading part in these, and in 1962 he joined the staff of the Council's Pneumoconiosis Research Unit in South Wales and continued his work there. The Council has now a contract with the International Agency for Research on Cancer to investigate those aspects of the problem in which an internationally coordinated study is likely to be most helpful.

Various organic dusts, mainly of vegetable origin, have also come under investigation. Outstanding among these was the dust found in card-rooms in the cotton industry, producing a lung condition (byssinosis) in some of the operatives. A Home Office committee on the subject, reporting in 1932, had been helped by studies arranged by the Council. The results included finding histamine in cotton dust, an important clue to an apparently allergic condition and one which the Council was anxious to follow up. Arrangements were accordingly made for a thorough study by Professor Carl Prausnitz, a distinguished refugee from Germany to whom the Council gave a grant for some years. The work was done in Professor H. B. Maitland's department in the University of Manchester and a report was published in the Council's series in 1936. In its own Report for 1935–36 the Council gave an account of the investigation, concluding with these words: "It is satisfactory to know that Professor Prausnitz has narrowed this problem of industrial health down to its essence, and although he has not been able to produce the cure out of a bottle which many hope for in such work, he has been able to indicate the lines of action necessary for preventing the disease."

This was by no means the end of the matter, and work continued to be promoted by the Council not only on cotton dust but on other dusts such as those of flax, sisal and sugar-cane—this last causing a condition (bagassosis) attributed to the presence of a fungus. The whole subject of pulmonary hypersensitivity disease due to organic dusts, industrial or otherwise, was reviewed by the Council in its Report for 1966–67. Mention is there made of work on aspergillosis by Dr J. Pepys and others in the Clinical Immunology Research Group supported by the Council at the Institute of Chest Diseases, Brompton Hospital, London; the results of work of this kind have made serological tests a matter of routine in the diagnosis of 'farmer's lung' and like conditions.

Toxicology

The Council's wider interest in toxicology, and its establishment of a Toxicology Research Unit in 1947, has been discussed elsewhere (Chapter 6). Certain hazards, however, arise chiefly in the course of manufacture and affect particular categories of industrial employees rather than the general public.

In the Report for 1934–35 it was stated that the Council had been asked by the Home Office to investigate the possibility that various volatile organic substances might be injurious to the health of workers using them under industrial conditions, chiefly as solvents and to an increasing extent. Such a substance, used on a large scale and within an enclosed space, might be inhaled in substantial amounts. The effects might be either acute, as the result of massive exposure, or might arise insidiously from exposure to relatively low concentrations over longer periods; and they might not be obviously referable to a particular cause.

The Council appointed a committee under Sir Joseph Barcroft, to advise it in this field. On the recommendation of this body certain immediate investigations were promoted; but to provide a basis for a future programme Dr Ethel Browning was commissioned to compile a summary of available information on such solvents as were then in general use. Although not intended to be exhaustive, the resulting volume gave sufficient detail to show the extent of the problem and to indicate the most suitable points of attack. Publication in 1937, as a report of the Industrial Health Research Board, led to a heavy demand, no comparable work being available at that time. In 1946, the original edition being out of print, Dr Browning was asked to prepare a revised version. This was a formidable task, owing to the much greater number of substances to be covered and the amount of new information that had accumulated; it was thus not until 1953 that the new edition was published under the aegis of the Council's Toxicology Committee.

From the dates of their inception, work in the field fell largely to the Council's Department of Industrial Medicine at the London Hospital and to the Toxicology Research Unit. In a related area, a Carcinogenic Action of Mineral Oils Committee was appointed by the Council in 1948 and reported on a chemical and biological study in 1968.

Epidemiology of non-infective diseases and genetic traits

The term 'epidemiology' is commonly associated with study of the spread of infectious diseases, outbreaks of which may develop into epidemics on a large scale; that aspect is considered elsewhere. The word has nevertheless a wider meaning, embracing "study of the frequency with which disease occurs in different populations"; this definition was used in an article by Doll in the Council's Report for 1968–69, from which much of this section is derived; in it he discussed the epidemiological approach to the understanding of diseases that are not infectious. Aetiological factors may be disclosed by studying the incidence of such a disease in relation to seasons and geography, to occupation and conditions of living, to diet and habits, or to age and sex. The method played a large part in the discovery of vitamin deficiencies, and also industrial poisons, as causes of disease; but it was not until after the Second World War that it came to be generally applied to such conditions as cancer, arteriosclerosis, malformations and psychiatric illness. Sir Richard Doll, while Director of the MRC Statistical Unit, was himself concerned in much work of this type on the Council's behalf. This is true also of his predecessor in that position, Dr A. (later Sir Austin) Bradford Hill, who made early investigations of this kind for the Industrial Health Research Board; a report by him on the incidence of sickness, especially gastric, among London busmen was published in the Board's series in 1937.

An outstanding example, cancer of the lung and its relation to smoking, has been mentioned earlier (Chapter 6). Coronary thrombosis, occurring especially in men, is another condition which has in recent years increased in importance as a cause of death in developed countries. In the United Kingdom, Professor J. N. Morris of the Council's Social Medicine Unit has paid special attention to this. He and his colleagues have found evidence that, at each age, coronary thrombosis—particularly in a severe form—is commonest among men whose work calls for the least physical activity: an effect that may, however, be reversed by vigorous leisure exercise.

Leukaemia is a third source of increased mortality in recent years. Dr W. M. Court Brown, with other members of the Council's staff, identified ionising radiations (in the amounts used for treating a non-malignant condition) as one of the causative factors in this disease. Work at Oxford under Dr Alice Stewart, grant-aided by the Council, likewise showed that even small dosages, as in the X-ray examination of pregnant women, could be responsible for an increased incidence of leukaemia and other malignant conditions in young children.

Air pollution is a factor in the exacerbation of chronic bronchitis and increased mortality therefrom; the Council's Air Pollution Unit has shown that chemical pollution of the atmosphere, rather than bad weather, is responsible for making the condition of patients more acute. The study eventually broadened out into a programme of research on all aspects of the causation of chronic bronchitis; in this the Council was advised by a Committee on the Aetiology of Chronic Bronchitis, which it set up in 1955. The subject was reviewed in the Reports for 1959–60 and 1967–68; and in 1965 the Council, with the help of a small group of experts, prepared a report on chronic bronchitis and occupation, which was sent to the Ministry of Pensions and National Insurance at the latter's request.

Dr A. L. Cochrane and his colleagues working in the Council's Pneumoconiosis Unit in South Wales used the method of cross-sectional surveys of populations living under different environmental conditions. In the face of various difficulties, they successfully applied the method to the study of chronic and degenerative disorders. In 1953 they were able to make a census of the entire population of a whole valley, the Rhondda Fach, obtaining the cooperation, for X-ray examination, of 90 per cent of those aged five years and over—in all nearly 25 000 persons. The prevalence of many diverse conditions has thus been compared with other characteristics of the different populations and their environments, and a much clearer picture of the natural history of certain disorders has emerged. The use of community surveys by Dr W. E. Miall in the study of rheumatoid arthritis is a case in point.

In 1960, the Epidemiological Research Unit (South Wales) was hived off from the Pneumoconiosis Research Unit and placed under the honorary direction of Professor Cochrane. Its primary concern is with the development of techniques for calculating the attack, progression and prevalence rates of various conditions in a defined population. Dr Miall was Director of a similarly named unit set up by the Council in Jamaica.

Epidemiological methods may also be used for assessing the results and possible side-effects of therapy, but the organisation of clinical and prophylactic trials is considered elsewhere. The Council's Statistical Research Unit collaborated with the Royal College of General Practitioners and the Committee on the Safety of Drugs in assessing the possible side-effects of oral contraceptives.

Since 1962 the Council has supported the National Survey of Health and Development under Dr J. W. B. Douglas, now Director of the MRC Unit for the Study of Environmental Factors in Mental and Physical Illness. The survey has consisted of a study of more than 5000 children born in Britain during a week in March 1946, contact having been successfully maintained with about 90 per cent of them. Much information has been published relating the social and economic circumstances of the families to the occurrence of infectious diseases, hospital admissions and accidents, and also to the educational and social progress of the young people. One of the subjects of special study has been the occurrence of delinquency among the boys in relation to their family backgrounds.

Mention may also be made here of certain lines of research that impinge on the field of anthropology, and that are sometimes concerned with the incidence of physiological traits rather than actual diseases; they are likewise of special interest from the standpoint of genetics. It has, for instance, long been known that the blood groups of the ABO system—the first to be recognised—differ widely in their frequency between races and nations. Information on this point, and about other systems, has greatly increased as the result of testing several millions of blood donors in many countries. The findings have made a considerable contribution to anthropology; but the chief medical interest is that the incidence of certain diseases, such as peptic ulcer, some forms of cancer, and pernicious anaemia, shows an association with the incidence of particular blood groups. The Council's workers have played a part in the investigation of this subject, which was reviewed in the Report for 1960–61.

A kindred problem is presented by the geographical incidence of certain atypical forms of haemoglobin in the blood. Much of the work on this subject has been done by the Council's Abnormal Haemoglobin Research Unit, under the honorary direction of Professor H. Lehmann. Around a hundred variants of the haemoglobin molecule are now known, and a few of these—affecting millions of the world's population—are associated with diseases that present a significant problem of public health. The most important is sickle-cell haemoglobin, which occurs simply as the sickle-cell trait if normal haemoglobin is also present, but in a proportion of individuals—those who are homozygous for the gene—produces sickle-cell anaemia, a disease highly lethal for children. The trait is found in a few parts of Europe and Asia, but widely in tropical Africa and Madagascar, and appears to be associated with a degree of immunity to malaria. The subject was reviewed in the Council's Report for 1965–66.

Also discussed in the same report was the question of enzyme diversity in human populations. It has for long been known that certain rare 'inborn errors of metabolism' are due to genetically determined deficiencies of particular enzymes among the very large number that contribute to the chemical processes of the body. These rare metabolic disorders represent extreme examples of a form of inherited enzyme variation which is widespread. The Council's chief contribution towards the elucidation of this fundamental matter has been by the Human Biochemical Genetics Unit directed by Professor H. Harris. As the Report says, "Each of the different enzyme polymorphisms and rare variants . . . poses a whole range of intriguing problems in biochemistry, medicine and genetics".

Social medicine
Epidemiological studies such as have just been described make up much of the content of 'social medicine'. It was in 1948 that the Council first used the term in designating one of its establishments, a new Social Medicine Research Unit. This has been successively located in the Central Middlesex Hospital, the London Hospital,

and the London School of Hygiene and Tropical Medicine. Dr J. N. Morris has been Director throughout, formerly as a member of the Council's staff but latterly, on his taking up a chair at the London School of Hygiene, in an honorary capacity; Dr R. M. Titmuss was his colleague in the initial stage.

The Unit started with investigations on biological and social factors in infant mortality (with the General Register Office); on social and psychological aspects of reproductive efficiency (with the Department of Midwifery, University of Aberdeen); on schizophrenia; and on the occupational incidence of heart disease in middle life (with medical officers and others in various industries and professions). Other subjects soon taken up included social factors in the incidence of duodenal ulcer and the value of group therapy; the occupational incidence of coronary disease (as mentioned in the preceding section); the functions of general practitioners in relation to the development of medical and social services; and problems of young people in the local community.

More generally, the purpose of the Unit can be described as being to investigate social factors influencing health and sickness, and their interaction with other factors. Throughout the years main interests have continued to be reproductive efficiency, duodenal ulcer and coronary disease, together with the critical appraisal of medical and social services.

It is part of the philosophy of the Unit that the so-called 'chronic diseases' especially merit study. These are the metabolic, malignant and mental diseases, particularly of the second half of life and having increasing impact on the practice of medicine with the growing number of older people in the population. They tend to be characterised by insidious onset, prolonged course, and profound familial repercussions. Better treatment is often not an answer, as the conditions may become apparent only through sudden death (coronary disease) or when it is too late for effective action (cancer). The aim has therefore to be control and prevention, which can be secured only by the aid of better knowledge of early subclinical signs, of precursor disturbances, and of high-risk groups that are particularly likely to show these disorders. The prevention of disability from chronic diseases that have reached the clinical stage is also an important aim. Rationalisation of the collection and collation of morbidity records, so that they may more readily yield the necessary information for epidemiological studies, is an intermediate requirement.

The Council has several more specialised establishments in this field, most of which have been mentioned elsewhere: the Social Psychiatry Research Unit in London; the Unit for Research on the Epidemiology of Psychiatric Illness in Edinburgh; the Unit for the Study of Environmental Factors in Mental and Physical Illness at the London School of Economics (work mentioned in the preceding section); and the Medical Sociology Research Unit in the University of Aberdeen under the honorary direction of Professor R. Illsley. Also relevant was the Population Genetics Research Unit. In 1944 the Council appointed a committee, under the chairmanship of Sir Joseph Barcroft, to consider problems of the physiological aspects of human fertility, on which the Royal Commission on Population sought advice, and a coordinated programme of experimental research was initiated.

Researches on the effects of smoking tobacco and of drinking alcohol have been mentioned earlier (Chapter 6). These present problems that have a social context, and this is even more emphatically true of drug addiction, preferably termed drug dependence. In 1968, in view of the widespread public concern at the increase in drug dependence, the Council convened a conference to advise on further profitable and feasible lines of investigation. On the recommendation of this meeting, the Council set up working parties on (a) the pharmacology and biochemistry of drug dependence, (b) clinical trials of therapeutic measures, and (c) the epidemiology of drug dependence. In the Report for 1971–72, in a section on the development of scientific policy, it was mentioned that special efforts were currently being made to expand appropriate research on drug misuse and dependence, particularly in relation to smoking and alcoholism. A programme grant was made for appropriate work by the Addiction Research Unit in the Institute of Psychiatry at Denmark Hill, London.

Chapter 10
Tropical Medical Research and Expeditions

The Council's interest—Historical setting—Tropical diseases in the First World
War—Origin of the London School of Hygiene and Tropical Medicine—
Colonial Office reviews (The Edgerton Committee; The Chalmers Committee;
The East Africa Commission)—Research in India—The first Colonial Medical
Research Committee—Stringent interlude—The Council's Tropical Medical
Research Committee—Nutritional problems in the Colonies—The second Colonial
Medical Research Committee—Liaison with India—Reassessment of the
Colonial situation—The Tropical Medicine Research Board—The Council's
tropical activities between the wars—The Council's Laboratories in the Gambia
—Other overseas establishments and staff of the Council—Home-based staff
working overseas—Restatement of policy—Expeditions

The Council's interest
The broadest ground for the Council's concern with research in
tropical medicine is that medical science is indivisible; no part of the
field can be neglected without detriment to knowledge of the whole.
This view was early emphasised by one of the Council's members
particularly concerned with the tropics, Lieut.-General Sir William
Leishman, and in an obituary tribute to him the Report for 1925–26
said that:

> While he gave all his influence to the promotion of specialised investigations
> in tropical medicine, in which he had himself played so distinguished a part,
> he urged increasingly that this study is no separate branch of medicine but
> touches all the fields of medicine and needs the services of all the medical
> sciences.

There are also special reasons, arising from the obligations and needs
that the United Kingdom has had, and still has, in respect of health
in tropical countries; as the official agency charged with the promotion of medical research, the Council clearly has a responsibility.
There are the further points that travellers can reach the United
Kingdom within a few hours of leaving countries where exotic
infections are rife; and that only relatively advanced countries are
as yet in a position to undertake major research in this field.

The cooperation of the Council, as a specialised agency, was
welcomed from the beginning by most government departments
with problems that called for advances in medical knowledge. The
War Office, notably, made the fullest use of the services of the
original Medical Research Committee from the earliest stages of the
First World War. By contrast, the Colonial Office was slow to avail
itself of the Council's help, although it lacked any expert technical-
administrative machinery of its own for promoting research; it made
a few grants to institutions at home, but otherwise its provision of a
190

medical service for the territories overseas was for long regarded as sufficient. There was certainly a marked official resistance to any intrusion, as was early shown by the attitude taken up in 1920 by the Colonial Office representative on a medical subcommittee of the Cabinet Committee on the Coordination of Research (Volume One).

There was moreover, in the 1920s, some sign of reluctance on the part of the Treasury to regard expenditure on work overseas as a desirable charge on the funds with which it supplied the Council. The view was expressed as late as 1935, although only in semi-official conversation, that such expenditure might constitute an indirect subsidy to the government of the particular territory. It was only later that full acceptance, by the Treasury, was won for the thesis that knowledge which may be universally applicable should be sought where the best opportunity is presented—sometimes even on foreign soil.

No objection was ever based on the ground that tropical medicine was outside the Council's unwritten terms of reference. On the other hand, it is difficult to accept as other than hindsight the suggestion that the Charter incorporating the Council in 1920 was deliberately worded to permit activities overseas. The Council was placed under a Committee of Privy Council for, in the main, quite different reasons.

The first overt authority given to the Council to support work in the tropics derives from the Order in Council of 26 July 1926 whereby the Secretary of State for the Colonies was, among others, added to the Committee of Privy Council for Medical Research (Volume One). Even so, the authority was little more than inferential; but in fact, as will be seen, some activities in the tropics had preceded this. It was also in 1926, as it happened, that the Council received a private benefaction to be used as an endowment for research in tropical medicine (Volume One).

Historical setting
In the period between the two World Wars, when the Council first seriously sought to enter the field, the general situation of British work in tropical medicine was different in several respects from that now existing. On the one hand, the overseas liabilities of the United Kingdom were more obvious. On the other hand, there were valuable assets for tropical research that have since largely disappeared. Of the latter, the most important was the Indian Medical Service, which was something of a *corps d'élite* and attracted many of the ablest medical graduates of British universities; its officers spent the best part of their lives working in the subcontinent, and there were institutes offering excellent opportunities for research to those posted to them. The numbers were increased by officers of the Royal Army Medical Corps, who often spent much of their service in India. There was thus a substantial body of British experience in tropical medicine and a research effort of high distinction. There

was also the more widely dispersed Colonial Medical Service, with generally less good opportunities for research work. Nor should one forget the British medical officers working in what was then the Anglo-Egyptian Sudan, and some others elsewhere.

What was lacking at that time was a sufficiently broad home base for tropical medicine in the United Kingdom itself. The chief institution at the beginning of the period was the Liverpool School of Tropical Medicine, which had an overseas station in Freetown, Sierra Leone; the London School was then a smaller affair—subsequent developments will be mentioned presently.

From 1897, the Treasury had included in the Colonial Services Vote a grant for "Tropical Diseases Investigation" (Tropical Diseases Research Fund). Before the First World War, the annual amount was £1000 and this was nearly quadrupled by contributions from India and the Colonies (a term which in those days included the self-governing Dominions). The total revenue was allocated, on the recommendation of an Advisory Committee appointed by the Secretary of State, in grants for work in London, Liverpool and Cambridge. Similar financial provision was made, and a Managing Committee appointed, for the Tropical Diseases Bureau; this was established in 1912 as a development of a Sleeping Sickness Bureau founded in 1908, and has now for long been called the Bureau of Hygiene and Tropical Medicine. Its principal function has been to compile and issue three (latterly two) abstracting bulletins. From 1920 the Council was represented on both the Committees mentioned—at first informally, but explicitly from 1924.

It is of interest that in 1919, when the future of the two projects was under consideration after a period of reduced activity during the war, the Treasury semi-officially asked Sir Robert Morant, at the Ministry of Health, whether he thought that either or both of these (and, by implication, perhaps also the Imperial Bureau of Entomology) should be brought under the Medical Research Committee. It was appreciated, however, that the Colonial Office and the Colonies would probably object to diversion of the administration from the existing committees with which they were familiar—described as "separate bodies specialising in tropical diseases". The probability was indeed a certainty.

In a letter to the Ministry of Health at that time Sir Walter Fletcher expressed the view that:

All research into tropical diseases should ultimately—and indeed as soon as possible—be brought under the Medical Research Committee, or at least into close organic connexion with their work. The chief practical reason for this of course, is that the technical methods used are the same in nature for all kinds of diseases, the same research worker may often be profitably transferred from one sphere of work to another, and it is of great importance that there should be the freest intercourse between workers in all fields.

Yet it took many years to bring about even the obviously desirable "close organic connexion". Even so there still remains the anomaly that official responsibility for research on trypanosomiasis is vested in a separate body on the ground that the major problems lie in the veterinary field.

Tropical diseases in the First World War
The Medical Research Committee in fact made an early entry into the field of tropical medicine; but this was under the impetus of war, in 1914, and so exemplified no principle and created no precedent. One of the Committee's first actions, in the autumn of that year, was to send Dr John Freeman of St Mary's Hospital to the Eastern Front, in Galicia (now a part of southern Poland), to study the different strains of cholera vibrio that were currently infective there; admittedly the area was far from the tropics, but the disease has its primary focus in tropical and subtropical Asia. There was considered to be a risk that movements of enemy troops might bring these infections to the Western Front. Dr Freeman was accompanied by an interpreter and temporarily enjoyed the rank of Lieut.-Colonel in the Russian Army. He was able to bring back cultures of the chief strains to the Inoculation Department at the Hospital, which was shortly able to supply large quantities of anti-cholera vaccine to the Serbian Government and to the British forces in the Mediterranean area.

A more ambitious expedition was undertaken at the end of the same year, in cooperation with the War Office and the London School of Tropical Medicine, when it was agreed to send Dr (temporary Lieut.-Colonel) R. T. Leiper and two assistants to Egypt to apply the results of recent discoveries regarding the life history of the worm *Schistosoma (Bilharzia) haematobium*, and to extend them by further investigations of the debilitating parasitisation endemic in the Nile Delta—a serious hazard to British forces in Egypt as well as to the local population. In short, the expedition confirmed beyond doubt that the parasite passes part of its life-cycle in an aquatic snail, and established that infection is always acquired from the water in which the mollusc lives and never directly from man to man. Many points in the natural history of the parasite and its intermediate host were determined, and this knowledge provided a basis for sounder hygienic measures. Prevention was all important, because no method of ridding the human body of the infestation was known. Some experimental work on this latter aspect was indeed undertaken in the Committee's Department of Biochemistry and Pharmacology, but without any immediate result of practical value.

The Medical Research Committee was also concerned during the war period with other diseases that occur mainly in tropical and subtropical countries, notably amoebic dysentery (Part III).

Origin of the London School of Hygiene and Tropical Medicine
A most important contribution to provision for the subject was made in the 1920s by the establishment of the London School of Hygiene

and Tropical Medicine. In this the Council took a substantial part through its Secretary, who was active behind the scenes and served on various committees concerned with the matter. Fletcher did this by virtue of his office, and although the innumerable questions that had to be settled did not figure as Council business, they took up a great deal of his time and energy. He was probably largely responsible for interesting the Rockefeller Foundation in the project, and he was certainly influential in shaping the plans so as to secure generous financial support from that quarter.

The action arose from a confluence of two originally independent streams of thought. The one was to create a more effective centre for the teaching and study of tropical medicine in the metropolis. The other, which had sources even before the First World War, was for concentrating the London postgraduate teaching in public health, hitherto wastefully diffuse. In the period 1909–14, the Board of Studies in Hygiene of the University of London had urged the need for "one well-equipped Centre for Hygiene in London to be provided in connection with the new University Buildings". It was stated that in London "140 candidates for the Diploma of Public Health work at 10 different centres and demand part-time service from 44 Lecturers and Demonstrators". Even at that stage the scheme was to include a 'Centre of Special Tropical Hygiene'.

After the war, in January 1921, the question was revived when, at the request of the University Grants Committee, the Ministry of Health appointed a committee under the chairmanship of the Earl of Athlone (and with Fletcher among its members) "to investigate the needs of medical practitioners and other graduates for further education in medicine in London and to submit proposals for a practicable scheme for meeting them". The report was published in May of the same year, and among other things recommended the establishment of an 'Institute of State Medicine' under the University of London. It said: "The formation of such an Institute would not only relieve the undergraduate schools of a certain section of work for which it is difficult to make satisfactory arrangements at present but would foster the development of an increasingly important branch of medicine throughout the Empire."

The new London School of Hygiene and Tropical Medicine was opened in stages during the period 1924–29, moving into its present building in the latter year. Meanwhile there had been other developments.

Colonial Office reviews
The Edgerton Committee—In 1919 the Secretary of State for the Colonies appointed a Committee to inquire into the Colonial Medical Services; this was under the chairmanship of Sir Walter Edgerton, and the six other members included such eminent medical men as Sir James Kingston Fowler, Sir William Leishman and Sir Humphrey Rolleston. The Committee's report was published in the

following year, and the keynote of its recommendations was that "the ideal is a unified service". Although it was seen that there were difficulties in the way of complete implementation at an early date, a scheme for a single Colonial Medical Service was propounded. Among other things, there were to be specialist appointments so that the highest ranks should be open to men who did not wish to turn to administrative duties. The opening paragraph of the section on promotion quaintly reads: "The prospect of promotion is a necessary incentive to good work for all except a chosen few who are imbued with the spirit of research and who live for that alone." The section directly concerned with research deserves quotation in full:

44. *Field for research work in Tropical Colonies*. Every witness who has been questioned on the subject has agreed that great opportunities in medical and the allied sciences exist in all the tropical Colonies, and owing to the absence of a Research Service they are being lost. There is no better investment for the money of any Colony than scientific research, both medical and economic, and the Committee recommend the creation of such a Department as part of the Colonial Medical Service.

Any medical officer who may show a capacity for research work should receive every possible encouragement, and such officers in charge of clinical laboratories as give evidence of such capacity should be promoted to the Research Service, but appointment by special selection should not be excluded.

The Committee venture to express the hope that in future it will not be necessary to go outside the Colonial Medical Service to find officers fit to undertake any medical or scientific work in any of the Colonies.

Research Institutes. The Committee recommend that a Medical Research Institute under a Director should be established in every important Colony or group of Colonies, and that wherever possible the Institute should be placed near to the largest and best equipped hospital, so that the two institutions may mutually influence each other's standard of work.

With regard to the penultimate paragraph of the section, it is not to be supposed that men such as Leishman were advocating a 'closed shop' policy in research, rather than just an adequate degree of self-sufficiency. With this proviso, the views expressed seem enlightened even today; unfortunately they were never given full effect.

The Colonies, however, already had the renowned Institute for Medical Research at Kuala Lumpur in the Malay Peninsula, established in 1901 at the suggestion of Sir Patrick Manson. Among other investigations, important work on beri-beri was done there by Dr A. T. (later Sir Thomas) Stanton and Dr H. Fraser, collaborating in 1907–16.

The Chalmers Committee—On 19 November 1920 the then Secretary of State, Lord Milner, appointed a Committee on Research in the Colonies "to consider and report what steps can be taken to secure the assistance of the Universities of this country in carrying out the research work which is essential to the protection of the inhabitants of the Colonies and Protectorates from disease and to the successful development of their veterinary, agricultural, and mineral resources". The Committee received evidence from the universities and on 6 April 1921 submitted a report to a new Secretary of State, Mr Winston Churchill, which was in due course presented to Parliament. The Chairman of the Committee was Lord Chalmers, late Joint Secretary to the Treasury and a former Governor of Ceylon; and among the members was the Council's Secretary, Sir Walter Fletcher, who signed the report with a reservation.

The Committee considered that the universities could help in two directions, first in a fuller training of students who might be recruited to scientific departments overseas, and second by building up a corps of advanced workers whose services could be utilised in emergencies or for investigating the more complex problems. To this end postgraduate study should be encouraged by increasing the number of research fellowships and studentships. It was also proposed that scientific posts in the Colonies should be filled on the nomination of universities and not by competitive examination. The universities would require more staff, and it was suggested that funds might be obtainable from industry.

Fletcher's reservation was with regard to the vagueness of the recommendation for the creation of a cadre of experts who could be appealed to for help. He argued that the proposal left untouched "the prime questions of practical interest: Who will make the appeal? What appeal? By what mechanism or in what modes? And on what occasions?" In his view, the scheme would be impracticable without coordination by small scientific committees in the respective main divisions of subject matter. These would be expected to advise all relevant government departments and research agencies, and to have powers of initiative in doing so: "They must be able, that is to say, to offer the Secretary of State the promptings of their scientific foresight without waiting for the specific appeal from him; they should be expected by him to be as forward with proposals for preventive measures as with advice invited on emergency."

In the subsequent letter from the Colonial Office, forwarding copies of the report to the heads of universities and other institutions, the main recommendations were endorsed; but Fletcher's point was brushed aside somewhat complacently with an expression of confidence in the adequacy of existing arrangements for advising the Secretary of State.

The East Africa Commission—In July 1924, the Secretary of State appointed an East Africa Commission to visit (using the names then current) Northern Rhodesia, Nyasaland, Tanganyika Territory, Uganda and Kenya; the aim was to obtain information on a wide range of matters bearing on acceleration of the general economic development of these British dependencies and on amelioration of the social conditions, including health, of the natives of East Africa. The Commission consisted of three Members of Parliament drawn from the several parties: The Hon. W. Ormsby-Gore (Conservative) as Chairman, Major A. G. Church (Labour), and Mr F. C. Linfield

(Liberal), with Mr J. A. Calder of the Colonial Office as secretary. The Commission spent four months in East Africa, and its report was published as a command paper early in 1925.

The East Africa Commission, although its remit was of a general kind, deserves a place in this history because of the eye-opening impact that it clearly made on the leader himself; in his ministerial capacity as Under-Secretary of State for the Colonies, Ormsby-Gore (later the 4th Lord Harlech) was able to exert considerable influence on policy for implementing the advice given by himself and his colleagues, including that pertaining to medical research. This resulted in the first real cooperation between the Colonial Office and the Council, as described later. There can also be little doubt that Major Church, a scientist by training and a parliamentary member of the Council, played a valuable part in bringing out these questions in the course of the Commission's inquiries.

The Commission's report was an important publication, but concerned only to a minor extent with medical services or scientific research. In these respects, as in others, it had a sorry tale to relate. Except in Uganda the medical services, originally concerned only with the health of the European population, were still covering only a small minority of the native inhabitants, for whom there was little hospital provision. The tsetse fly problem, as regards both human sleeping sickness and the diseases of domestic stock, bulked largely but was not being tackled consistently on any well founded plan. (In Northern Rhodesia an official handbook, published in 1922, had called the fly "one of the assets of the country" on the astonishing ground that the inability of the natives to raise cattle in some areas ensured a supply of labour for mining.) Scientific research in general, although badly needed for the solution of many problems, was not being promoted on an adequate scale—and notably in the two territories, Northern Rhodesia (now Zambia) and Nyasaland (now Malawi), under the direct financial control of HM Treasury. Even the fine agricultural research station built by the Germans at Amani, in Tanganyika, had been reduced (for the time being) to a 'care and maintenance' basis.

The picture as regards medical research was more favourable, as work of high standard was being done by the staffs of various laboratories—again, notably in Uganda; but the scale of the effort fell far short of the requirements. For instance, one reads that in Kenya "the retrenchments carried out in 1922 added greatly to the duties of the small research staff, who had thereafter to devote the greater part of their time to ordinary medical practice"; and, likewise, the pathetic plea that "there is a real need in Kenya for a medical entomologist".

To the research work that was being done due tribute was paid, together with a constructive proposal:

We were impressed by the number, complexity, and interest of the problems in connection with the investigation of disease in East Africa, and by the high standard of the workers and the exceptional quality of the research which is being carried out. We suggest for the consideration of the Colonial Office the possibilites of formulating a scheme whereby research workers from Great Britain would be encouraged to spend some time in original investigations in the laboratories in East Africa. We also suggest that the Medical Research Council should be approached with a view to its devoting to this purpose some of the funds put at their disposal. We need hardly emphasise the great advantage it would be to young research workers to spend a year or two attached to laboratories under the direction of men with great experience and knowledge of local conditions, in districts where cases for investigation are numerous and varied. We feel convinced, moreover, that the various faculties of medicine in the universities and the tropical research institutions would be only too glad to co-operate further in working any such scheme put forward.

As a gloss on the report, a semi-official comment made by Ormsby-Gore a few weeks after publication may be cited. It was contained in a letter written by him from the Colonial Office on 29 May 1925 to the Earl of Balfour, who then not only held ministerial office as Lord President but was also Chairman of the Medical Research Council. It read (almost in full):

> Apropos of Tse-tse fly and sleeping sickness . . . something more than the limited League of Nations' scheme wants doing, and . . . as the report of my Commission has shown up the degree of starvation of our scientific work in Africa and public opinion is keenly interested at last, something might usefully be done soon.
>
> I saw the Rockefeller people this morning—en route from New York to British Nigeria, where they are going to do our yellow fever research for us.
>
> I am really pained at the inadequacy of our own research work all along the line in the tropical empire.

Research in India

As related in its Report for 1927–28, the Council gave the Secretary five months' leave of absence in that period to allow him to accept an official invitation to visit India. Fletcher's task was to chair a small committee appointed to report on the organisation of medical research under the Government of India, with special reference to the establishment and location of a Central Research Institute and its relations to other research activities under the auspices of the Government of India, of the Provincial Governments, or of the Indian Research Fund Association. Some problems of recruitment, of training and of research into questions of nutrition were also referred to them. After an extensive tour, the four members were able to submit a unanimous report. Fletcher had incidental opportunities for making various useful contacts, notably with the Indian Research Fund Association. Of that body the Council's Report says:

> This Association supplies an organization well adapted to promote direct, rapid and flexible co-operation between India and Great Britain and any other part of the Empire in medical research work. It is interesting to note that it was founded by the Government of India as early as 1911, with a foresight remarkable at that time. It was designed to combine Government financial

resources with monetary aid derived from private sources and to provide an organization to hold and use these funds of double origin for the promotion of medical research. It was given a constitution which allows it to assist approved research work by approved persons upon independent scientific advice and by its own administrative machinery, while remaining in close co-operation with the established services of the Government.

The position of research in India after the Second World War is mentioned later.

The first Colonial Medical Research Committee

In 1926, Dr A. T. (later Sir Thomas) Stanton was appointed to a new post as Chief Medical Adviser to the Colonial Office as the result, it was said, of the keen interest taken by Mr L. S. Amery and Mr Ormsby-Gore—respectively Secretary of State and Under-Secretary of State—in the scientific work on which the better development of the colonial empire depended. Stanton and Fletcher had useful discussions, the outcome of which was that in April 1927 the Council had before it a memorandum on cooperation with the Colonial Office, proposing the appointment of a joint committee. In May the Colonial Office agreed to this, although in practice the formula was modified to appointment by the Secretary of State in consultation with the Council. In June the Committee was appointed, with the Rt Hon. William Ormsby-Gore as chairman (a personal appointment, not as Parliamentary Under-Secretary of State), and with an ex-colonial officer as deputy chairman. In addition there were six members appointed on scientific grounds, together with the Medical Adviser to the Secretary of State and the Secretary of the Council ex officiis. At the same time the Advisory Committee for the Tropical Diseases Research Fund was dissolved.

The terms of reference of the new body were: "To advise the Secretary of State for the Colonies and the Medical Research Council upon the initiation of schemes for medical research to be conducted either at home or overseas with a view to the preservation of health, the control of disease and the improvement of efficiency within the Colonial Empire; upon the recruitment of the necessary personnel; and upon the management and allocation of any funds made available for these purposes." These were encouraging words; but there were in fact no funds—at least none that were not already committed or firmly under the control of the separate Colonial Governments.

The Committee was to have a medical secretary, who was to spend half his time at the Colonial Office and half at the office of the Council. This seemed to be a good arrangement, and the post was held first by Dr William Fletcher, retired from Malaya, and afterwards by Dr H. H. (later Sir Harold) Scott, retired from Hong Kong. These were men well qualified for the task through their experience of pathological research in the tropics; and they were personally most acceptable as colleagues by the Council's staff. They had, however, been conditioned by their years of service to regard the Secretary of State as one whose views, as attributed by his various officials, must be treated as absolute. The degree of liaison which they were able to provide may be inferred from the apologetic statement of one of them that he was not allowed to pass on to the Council's staff any information which he acquired at the Colonial Office.

Nevertheless, there was at first an illusion of progress, although this was slightly marred by irritation caused by the unilateral action of the Colonial Office in appointing a purely administrative officer as Deputy Chairman of what the Council regarded as a scientific committee. (In 1929, with the Council's concurrence, the post of Deputy Chairman was abolished and two Members of Parliament were given seats on the Committee.) After describing the new machinery in its Report for 1926–27, the Council went on:

> If the Committee succeed in their task there can be no doubt that workers, whether at home or in the Colonial Empire overseas, will alike gain greatly by new opportunities for collaboration and new facilities for intercourse. It ought indeed now to be recognized that the time has gone by for usefully thinking of 'tropical diseases' as a separate subject of medical research. For many, if not most of the diseases peculiar to the tropics the preliminary observational studies of field and clinical inquiries have already been made, and the stage is set for intensive laboratory investigation wherever that can best be done, whether in bacteriology or in biochemistry or in the difficult studies of 'viruses'. The part played by errors of nutrition either in producing 'deficiency' diseases or in lowering resistance to specific infections is being more and more recognized, and this may point to places of experimental work far remote from the immediate site of the phenomena observed. On the other hand, there is probably, for instance, more tuberculosis, or again, measles, in the tropics than in England, and from some points of view those diseases may perhaps be better studied overseas than at home, just as the control of a purely tropical disease may spring from clues discovered in a northern laboratory. With every year of progress in science it becomes increasingly clear that medical science is one and indivisible, whether for temperate or tropical climates, and that nothing but gain can come from ignoring all geographical considerations as such. The work should be done wherever the man best fitted for it can most easily find his opportunities for progress, whether in laboratory work or in a field inquiry, and whether at home or far overseas. As the Committee proceed with their programme it is not unlikely that they will find that the organized research service is imperceptibly shaping itself, as right provision is made for needs as they arise. In this way may come about a veritable 'Imperial Research Service', to use a phrase lately much in use, not through the invention of paper schemes, logically contrived and brought by artifice into being, but through a gradual and perhaps unconscious process of development along the natural lines of growth.

These high hopes, however, were doomed to disappointment. That the Committee had been brought into existence at all, and functioned for three years in a limited way, was mainly due to the personal friendship between Ormsby-Gore and Walter Fletcher. When the former left the Colonial Office in 1929 the previous attitude quickly reasserted itself. (Ormsby-Gore returned as Secretary of State in 1936, but that was after Fletcher's death.) In the spring of 1930 Fletcher described himself as "heavily depressed" by a meeting of the Committee; and soon afterwards the Colonial Office decided that Scott's post should be combined with that of Assistant Director of the Bureau of Hygiene and Tropical Medicine (with a view to succeeding as Director, which in due course he did). A few months later the Colonial Office proposed that the functions of the Committee, on the Colonial Office side, should be transferred to the existing Colonial Advisory Medical and Sanitary Committee, giving the unconvincing reason that it was inconvenient to have two committees. To this the Council was in no position to raise effective objection; and in any event the joint arrangement had clearly failed of its purpose. The first Colonial Medical Research Committee was accordingly dissolved by agreement on 31 December 1930.

Stringent interlude
On 4 November 1930 a letter from the Colonial Office about the proposed dissolution of the CMRC had said that "The Secretary of State fully appreciates the importance to the overseas medical services of association with the work of the Medical Research Council in this country and he is satisfied that the new arrangements will involve no interruption in this valuable cooperation in the field of medical research". Early in 1931, however, it was realised that there was no effective liaison at all; and on 14 April Fletcher wrote to Stanton, the Medical Adviser:

> The actual result in fact has been that the improved intercourse you foreshadowed has not taken place, and the association to which the Secretary of State referred has been abruptly and completely discontinued. A soundproof curtain was lowered somewhere about November, and nothing has passed it from your side ever since.

This protest, however, was unavailing; in fact the question seemed to die away in somewhat desultory correspondence and verbal exchanges. During the next four years there was occasional consultation of the Council by the Colonial Office on specific questions, but cooperation in research was for all practical purposes in abeyance.

One reason why the Council did not press the issue at this time was the exceptionally severe financial crisis in the latter part of 1931, which among other things led to a reduction in the Council's resources, with attendant administrative difficulties. Another was Fletcher's illness during part of the period, and eventually his death and the subsequent interregnum. It was not until 1934 that his successor, Edward Mellanby, was able to revert to the problem.

Meanwhile, however, the Council had been independently able to initiate one important new project in the field of tropical medicine, consisting of laboratory studies in the United Kingdom. This was concerned with malaria, and the Council's view of that problem at the particular time is worth quoting from its Report for 1931–1932:

> The common and erroneous belief that the Manson–Ross discovery has freed the world from malaria has had some disastrous results in checking the development of further research work. That discovery had all the merit, and deserves all the credit, rightly belonging to a first step. We are still waiting, however, for many further advances in knowledge, and no general success in the fight against malaria can come till these have been attained.
>
> After Manson had propounded the hypothesis of the mosquito carriage of malaria and Ross had demonstrated its truth, it was hoped by many that the practical conquest of malaria was close at hand. Nearly forty years have passed, and yet the best available evidence indicates that the total number of sufferers from malaria has increased rather than diminished. The financial losses due to the disease are quite incalculable. Their magnitude is indicated only in small part by the fact that in the world as a whole the annual expenditure upon quinine alone amounts to about £2 500 000, of which about £450 000 is incurred within the British Empire. The number of cases of malaria which could be effectively treated by the quinine purchased in those amounts is 47 000 000 and 7 000 000 respectively.
>
> Experience has long shown that the frontal attack upon malaria in terms o direct war upon the mosquito is too costly for general use, and that it gives a provisional and purely local result, only lasting so long as expenditure in labour and money is maintained.
>
> The campaign against malaria cannot be generally effective until we can design co-ordinated plans of attack upon it at every assailable point, and by means that are practicable and cheap under various conditions of place and time. For this we need better knowledge in many different directions. In spite of our immense annual bill for quinine, for instance, it is not known even yet how quinine acts or how to avoid relapses after its use. Valuable new synthetic compounds, such as 'plasmochin' and 'atebrin', have been produced in Germany, and have their effects upon other points in the life-history of the parasite; this country has done almost nothing to aid on this side of the work. Innumerable problems in the life-histories and habits of the many different species of mosquito that carry malaria have still to be worked out. The chemical and physical properties of the parasite itself that may give it vulnerability at particular points now unsuspected are still waiting study. Yet the two centres of research which we owe to the vision of Joseph Chamberlain, the Liverpool School of Tropical Medicine, and Manson's own school, now the London School of Hygiene and Tropical Medicine, have never had funds sufficient to enable them to make any adequate and combined attack upon the problems in sight.

The Report goes on to mention that the Council had for some years been maintaining, in the Molteno Institute at Cambridge under Professor D. Keilin, a study of the effects of quinine and various synthetic drugs on bird malaria; and that "the Council have for long been reluctant to leave work in this field to be developed on so small a scale when such vital and financial issues are at stake". It then records that an opportunity had been seized to aid the formation of a team for malaria research within the London School of Hygiene and Tropical Medicine and to secure for its direction the services of Sir Samuel Rickard Christophers, a distinguished worker in this field who had recently retired from the Indian Medical Service, in which he had for many years been Director of the Malaria Survey. This was made possible by financial help from the Trustees of the late Lord Leverhulme and provision in kind by the School. The enterprise became known as the Malaria Research Unit.

The Council's Tropical Medical Research Committee
In May 1935 Sir Edward Mellanby saw Sir Thomas Stanton, the Medical Adviser at the Colonial Office, about the possibility that the Council might take over the Trypanosomiasis Institute at Entebbe, Uganda, which it was proposed to close. Stanton appeared to welcome this idea, but a few days later he wrote regretfully to say he had found that there was no immediate prospect of the laboratory's becoming available for the Council; the Colonial Office would, however, have laboratories at Entebbe and Nairobi with ample accommodation for research workers from this country if the Council decided to embark on a policy of expansion overseas. He added that "any such development would be most welcome to the Colonial Office".

With this encouragement, conversations between Mellanby and Stanton continued, until on 29 October there emerged a proposal that the Council should have a committee of its own on tropical medical research. On the 8 November 1935 Stanton sent Mellanby a letter, with a covering note saying that this had received official approval in draft; the important passage, seeking both to explain past failure and to be constructive for the future, read as follows:

> The Colonial Medical Research Committee which Fletcher and I caused to be set up in 1927 was ineffective, in my opinion for the following reasons: it had too many members (13) and too many of these (5) were non-medical men; it was associated for administrative purposes with the Colonial Office instead of the Medical Research Council and in 1929 with a change of Government it assumed a political complexion; it had very little money at its disposal and failed to get more. In 1930 this Committee was dissolved; it served no important purpose in the conditions then existing.
>
> A revival of the Committee under the Medical Research Council would I now think serve a useful purpose in the following conditions:
> (a) if the Medical Research Council is willing to interest itself more fully in research in the tropical Colonies; (b) if the cooperation of the Colonial Office and the Colonial Medical Service is assured; and (c) if the cooperation of the Schools of Tropical Medicine is similarly assured.

So, at the beginning of 1936, the Council's Tropical Medical Research Committee was appointed, under the chairmanship of Professor J. C. G. (later Sir John) Ledingham and with the present writer as secretary. There were ten members in addition to the chairman, all of them medical or other scientists and most of them closely concerned with tropical problems; they included representatives of the Liverpool and London Schools and Stanton from the Colonial Office. The project had indeed the full blessing of the

Colonial Office, which issued a despatch on the subject to Colonial Governments on 30 July 1936.

The terms of reference were "to advise and assist in the direction of such investigations as the Council may be able to promote, whether at home or abroad, into problems of health and disease in tropical climates, and to make suggestions generally as to research in this field". The work of the new Committee was to be closely coordinated with the other activities of the Council, and full use was to be made of the advice obtainable from the existing committees dealing with special subjects. It was contemplated that expenditure of the order of £5000 per annum, from the ordinary funds of the Council, might be incurred on work in the tropics on the advice of the Committee.

The Tropical Medical Research Committee met for the first time on 3 April 1936. Its inception was described in the Report for 1935–36 in terms which recapitulated some of the past history already described in this chapter. After referring to the demise of the earlier committee, it said:

> The Council had meanwhile not lost sight of the desirability of instituting a wider programme of work in the tropics, although the question was necessarily in abeyance during the period of financial stringency. They have now proceeded, accordingly, to appoint a new Tropical Medical Research Committee and are prepared to make grants for work in the tropics on the recommendation of this body. This step was taken during the past year with the full concurrence of the Colonial Office.

The report goes on to describe the first policy recommendation of the Committee, which was to build up a cadre of trained investigators to undertake research in the tropics:

> The new Tropical Medical Research Committee have already made farreaching recommendations, on which the Council have begun to take action. The Committee have advised that the most effective means open to the Council of promoting investigations in this subject is the establishment of a small staff of highly-qualified workers giving their whole time to research under the best possible conditions. This involves the selection of men with special aptitude for research, their training in the appropriate methods of investigation, and the provision of facilities for work unembarrassed by routine or administrative duties. Arrangements will have to be made in due course as to the centres in the tropics to which these men can be attached: it is proposed, however, that they should spend a greater proportion of their time in this country than is allowed in the case of ordinary tropical appointments, in order to carry out in the most favourable circumstances such part of their investigations as can be done in Europe.
>
> The Council fully accept the view that an important service which they can render by their entry into this field will be the recruitment of able young investigators willing to work in the tropics under a scheme of the kind indicated. It is appreciated, however, that the chances of success in recruitment will depend very largely on the prospects that are held out as open to promising workers: they have therefore thought it important to announce at once their definite intention of eventually establishing some permanent posts for research in

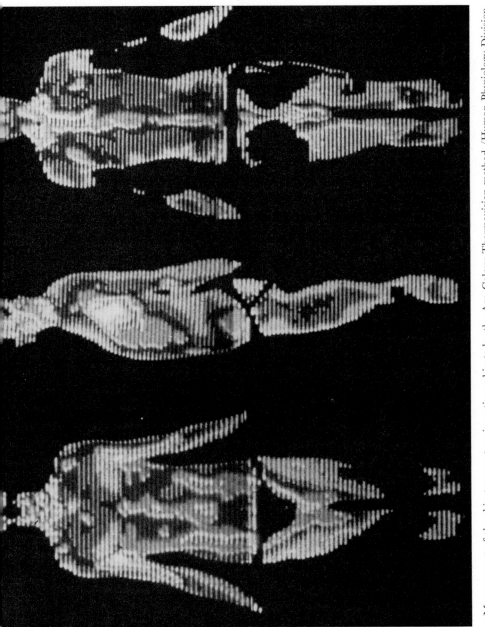

9 Measurement of the skin temperature in active subjects by the Aga Colour Thermovision method (Human Physiology Division, National Institute for Medical Research, Hampstead)

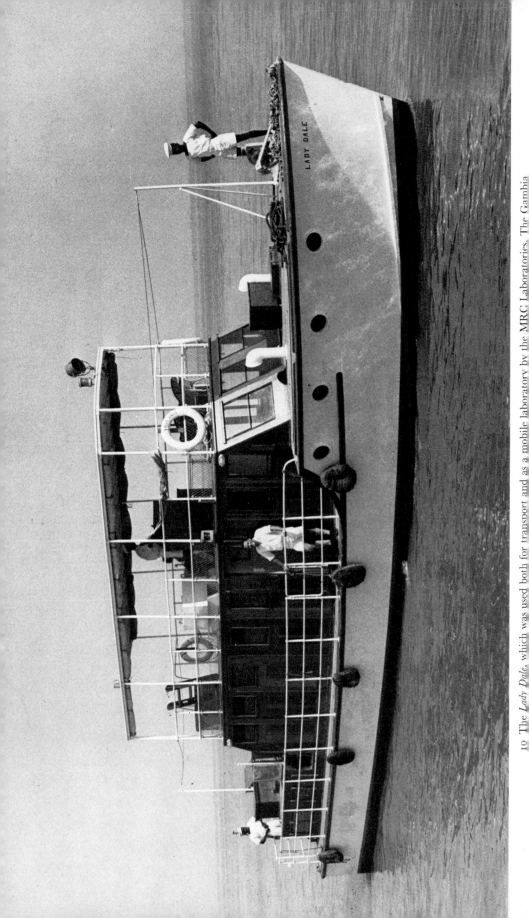

10 The *Lady Dale*, which was used both for transport and as a mobile laboratory by the MRC Laboratories, The Gambia

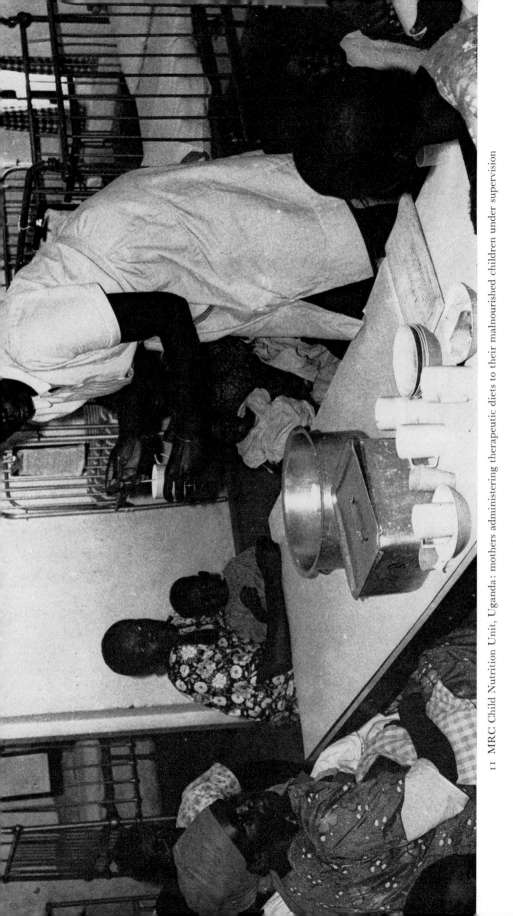

11 MRC Child Nutrition Unit, Uganda: mothers administering therapeutic diets to their malnourished children under supervision

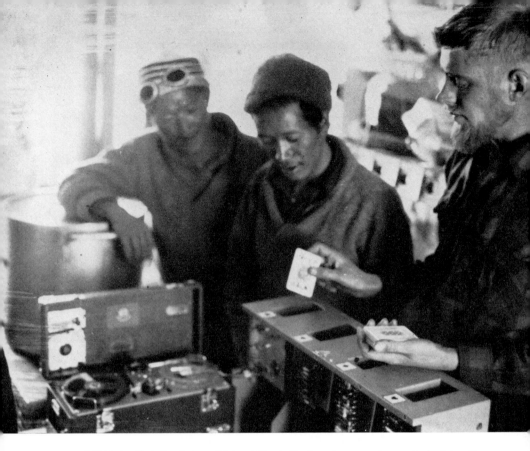

12 MRC Applied Psychology Unit: (*Above*) Card-sorting experiment devised by the Unit to test the effects of altitude and fatigue on performance, being demonstrated to two Sherpas on the Himalayan Scientific and Mountaineering ('Silver Hut') Expedition of 1960–61, which wintered in a portable hut at 19 000 ft, under the scientific leadership of Dr L. G. C. E. Pugh of the National Institute for Medical Research (*Below*) Tracking and signal detection apparatus used to measure effects of stress (sleep loss, alcohol, noise etc.) on attentional selectivity; the subject is guiding a model Concorde aircraft along a wavy line

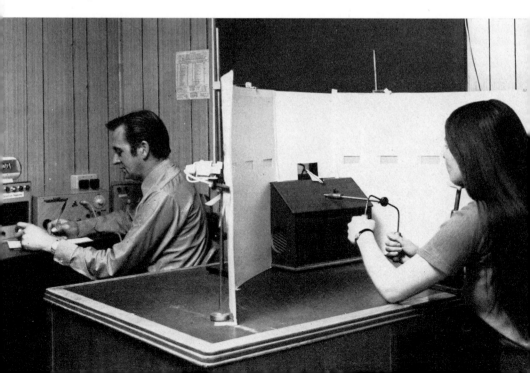

tropical medicine, to which workers engaged at first on a temporary basis may reasonably aspire. Even with this inducement, it will necessarily take time to secure and train the required workers, and the first step has therefore been the award of a few research fellowships.

Under this scheme, two junior fellowships have already been awarded to qualified men wishing to receive training with a view to careers in research work in tropical medicine. Subject to satisfactory reports, the fellowships will be tenable for three years. The first year will be spent at a school of tropical medicine; the second in doing research in the same or some other institution at home; and the third largely in work under direction at some centre in the tropics. The Council believe that men who undergo this training will be well qualified for other appointments, apart from the prospects of further employment under the scheme.

It has been intimated that, in due course, senior fellowships will be available for candidates who have shewn promise while holding the junior fellowships just mentioned. These will be awarded for a further period of three years, and the time will be spent mainly in research work in the tropics. Two such fellowships have been immediately awarded to candidates who have already had adequate experience.

The Council's further intention is to establish, as suitable investigators become available as the result of the fellowships scheme, permanent and pensionable appointments for research work in tropical medicine, including senior posts. Members of this research staff will work partly in the tropics, and partly in institutions at home to which they will be severally attached. The terms of service will be not less favourable than those which apply to other Government appointments at home or overseas for men of similar professional standing.

In addition to launching this main scheme of fellowships and appointments, the Council are prepared to assist research in tropical medicine in other ways as opportunity may offer. In particular, grants will be available in suitable cases to enable workers in established positions at home, particularly those not having the facilities already possessed by the staffs of schools of tropical medicine, to make short visits to the tropics for the purposes of research or the collection of material.

Two years later the Report for 1937–38 recorded that in the three years since the scheme was initiated, eight junior and three senior fellowships had been awarded. Fully trained investigators had been sent to The Gambia, Uganda, Tanganyika and Sierra Leone to study various problems. In 1939, however, the advent of the Second World War began to erode this promising development so that it eventually came to an end; it was not afterwards revived in this form.

Nutritional problems in the Colonies

Also at about this time a new opportunity of assisting the Colonial Office arose from the world-wide interest in nutritional problems. The Economic Advisory Council had set up a committee on problems of nutrition in the colonies, using the machinery mentioned in Volume One. Subsequent action is described as follows in the Report for 1937–38:

In 1936 the Secretary of State for the Colonies sent out a circular despatch drawing the attention of Governors of colonial territories within the Empire to modern aspects of nutrition and their relation to health, and asking for their comments and advice on such matters as they affected each territory. The response was surprisingly great and resulted in the setting up of an Advisory Committee on Nutrition in the Colonial Empire upon which the Medical Research Council were represented. Many of the replies received from Governors of colonial territories, while showing the greatest interest in the subject and realisation of its importance, also made it clear that much more information of the actual dietetic and nutritional problems to be faced in each territory was needed, and that this information could be obtained only by further investigation. To meet this situation, the Advisory Committee on Nutrition set up a sub-committee, with Sir Edward Mellanby as Chairman, to prepare a coordinated plan of field surveys and research.

The sub-committee just mentioned recommended that the Council should be asked to appoint, for a period of five years in the first instance, a small staff whose duty would be to undertake the scientific coordination of a series of field surveys of diet in relation to health and physique in the colonial territories—the actual field surveys to be made by officers seconded from the colonial service in each territory concerned. These suggestions were approved by the Secretary of State, and the Council willingly agreed to accept the responsibility entrusted to them. It was arranged that the Council should pay the salaries of the staff appointed by it to coordinate the programme of work, while other expenses should be borne by the Colonial Development Fund.

Dr B. S. Platt, who had had great experience of nutrition and deficiency diseases in the Far East, was appointed to the Council's staff as head of the coordinating unit. Nyasaland was chosen for the first inquiry because of the interest already taken in that country by the International Institute of African Languages and Cultures, from the anthropological and social points of view. It was thought well to combine these investigations into one, and further to graft on related inquiries into the agriculture of the country. There was thus initiated a comprehensive investigation into the condition of Nyasaland, involving dietetic, nutritional, agricultural, anthropological and social studies. This particular investigation was expected to be more intensive and prolonged than those to be subsequently undertaken in other territories, as it was hoped to learn the best methods of inquiry and standards for adoption in further work of the same kind.

The section in the Report already quoted carried the following peroration:

The benefits that might accrue from such inquiries are unlimited. It will be possible not only to see in what way the diets of native populations are defective, and the conditions of malnutrition which are developed in consequence, but also to determine means of remedying these defects by native crops grown in best accord with the agricultural, economic and social conditions of each country. Probably one of the important developments of this scheme will be the greater encouragement of the production of food crops for improving the physical and mental condition of the population. At the same time, investigations of this nature cannot fail to bring to light many other agricultural and economic possibilities which will certainly benefit the trade of the colonial territories.

The Second World War interrupted these developments at an early stage; but much work on such lines, under various auspices, was subsequently undertaken in different territories.

The second Colonial Medical Research Committee

The Colonial Development Act 1940 provided for an annual grant of £500 000 for research, and in spite of wartime difficulties this took effect in 1943. The money was applicable to all kinds of scientific research, including medical research, and allocation among the different fields was to be made with the help of a new Colonial Research Committee (later Council) under the distinguished chairmanship of Lord Hailey; the Secretaries of the three Research Councils were members of this body.

The Council naturally welcomed this development; but it had serious misgivings about proposals that were being formulated for implementation of the scheme in the medical field. It was proposed that the controlling body for medical research should be set up within the Colonial Office and be there provided with an administrative staff. This would have created an organisation parallel to that of the Council, duplicating the latter administratively but providing nothing comparable with the resources of scientific advice that have contributed so much to its effectiveness. A further suggestion harked back to an earlier proposal for the establishment of a separate Colonial Medical Research and Laboratory Service; this, in view of experience of the ease with which government research institutions overseas could become predominantly routine service laboratories, did not command confidence.

Many discussions ensued, with much redrafting of memoranda, until early in 1944 agreement was reached between Sir Edward Mellanby on the Council's behalf and Sir George Gater, Permanent Under-Secretary of State for the Colonies. The amended scheme was then accepted by the Council and approved by the Secretary of State. A new Colonial Medical Research Committee was to be set up conjointly by the Colonial Office and the Council to advise both parties. Equal numbers of members of this body were to be appointed by the Colonial Office and by the Council, but all appointments were to be agreed between them before being made. These members were to be selected as scientific advisers on their individual merits, although in practice it would be desirable always to draw some of the members from the staffs of the two principal tropical schools. There were to be joint secretaries appointed by the respective parties; or if a single secretary were agreed upon between them he would have access to the Council's administrative staff and to its committees advising in relevant special fields (e.g. nutrition, bacteriology, chemotherapy and therapeutic trials).

Thus, early in 1945, the second Colonial Medical Research

Committee came into being under more favourable auspices than its predecessor. At the suggestion of the Colonial Office, Mellanby was appointed chairman—to be followed in due course by Himsworth, his successor in office with the Council. At first Dr F. Hawking of the Council's scientific staff was sole secretary; he was joined next year by Dr A. F. Mahaffy from the Colonial Office, and in the year after that Hawking was succeeded by Major-General Sir John Taylor (IMS, ret.) from the Council's side. Later, Mahaffy was succeeded by Dr R. Lewthwaite, who eventually became sole secretary. Changes in membership took place from time to time; and various subcommittees were set up to deal with special subjects not covered by existing committees of the Council. The Colonial Medical Research Committee first met on 29 May 1945.

In the Council's Report for 1945-48 it was stated that "the expansion in recent years of the Council's work in association with Government departments has been specially notable in the case of the Colonial Office". The history of the earliest steps taken to promote this particular cooperation, as described in the present chapter, was recalled; and the establishment of the second Colonial Medical Research Committee was rightly hailed as an advance: "Assisted by three active subcommittees, on malaria, helminthiasis and nutrition, respectively, the Committee has sponsored an extensive programme, though here again progress has been slowed by shortage of suitable investigators." Nevertheless, the Colonial Office did not feel able to accept the widely held view that it should remit to the Council the responsibility for recruiting research staff for work overseas and preferred to set up its own service. The Council's outlook on the means of solving the recruitment difficulty was expressed in the following paragraph:

To encourage further recruits to medical research in the Colonies, the Colonial Office, since the end of the war, have undertaken the formation of a new Service —the Colonial Medical Research Service. Even when this is in full activity, however, it is certain that the Council will still have a large part to play in promoting and developing such studies, and a close interweaving of the structure of the new Service with that of the Council's research organisation in this country is highly desirable. Many members of the Council's scientific staff have specialised knowledge and experience which could prove very useful in Colonial medical research, and the value of sending such workers to underake field investigations in particular Colonies has repeatedly been demonstrated. In certain cases, moreover, there will probably be advantages in making Research Units of the Council the home bases of investigators whose main work is in the tropics: after spending a period abroad, such workers would, on their return to this country, be brought again into contact with their colleagues in the Units, and thereby have the opportunity both of discussing recent developments in the fundamental problems of medical science and of becoming familiar with new technical methods. The practical value of close association with the Council's research establishments has, indeed, already shown itself in cases where a team of workers has been sent to the Colonies, or elsewhere in the tropics, in order to study a particular problem from a number of angles. Investigations of this kind often require research workers with widely differing qualifications and training, and the selection of these teams is by no means easy without a large home organisation to call upon.

Liaison with India

As association with research in India (still the whole subcontinent) was outside the scope of the Colonial Medical Research Committee separate arrangements were made for liaison with that country. In 1945 a Medical Research Liaison Committee was set up in London by arrangement between the Council and the Government of India, with representatives of each, for the exchange of information and the coordination of investigations in the two countries. The chairman was Sir Henry Dale, and there was a distinguished membership; it was hoped that two of the representatives of India would usually be investigators from that country temporarily working in the United Kingdom.

The Committee remained in being for some years, and at first some useful arrangements were made. Two members of the Council's scientific staff visited India—Mr P. Bruce White, on an invitation conveyed by the Indian Research Fund Association, to collaborate with Indian research workers at Kasauli in bacteriological studies of cholera; and Dr T. Bedford, at the request of the Government of India, to advise on the organisation of industrial health research. Conversely, an Indian research worker visited the United Kingdom at the invitation of the Council. The political climate, however, was not favourable to the smooth working of cooperative enterprises; and profound changes followed the achievement of independence by India and the separation of Pakistan. The Committee, despite attempts to revive it, gradually died of inanition.

Reassessment of the Colonial situation

After eight years' experience of the working of the second Colonial Medical Research Committee, and of the new financial resources first made available by the Colonial Development and Welfare Act 1945, the Council again reviewed the position in its Report for 1952–53. Some sentences will suffice to indicate the trend of thought:

> In practice tropical medicine demands a first-hand experience of actual conditions in the tropics and thus tends to segregate the practitioners as specialists, but in research the essential contacts are not geographically determined; they range over all relevant studies of the particular part of the subject. . . . Every advance in medical research reveals the fundamental unity of its problems wherever, and in whatever circumstances they occur . . . Knowledge on any medical subject obtained anywhere may, at any time, become relevant elsewhere. Medical research is indivisible. Any measure which tends to segregate it according to whether it is done in the tropics or in this country is not merely artificial; it is actively harmful. . . . Of necessity applied research must be carried out in the tropics; but basic research may be undertaken either at home or overseas. Some basic research can be carried out only in the home country, because it is only there that the necessary specialised facilities and research

personnel are available. Some, in which access to tropical conditions is necessary, can be carried out only overseas. Yet other basic research may need to be developed, at different stages, in both places.

In the tropics provision needs to be made for work requiring local knowledge and experience or access to the field, and also, in so far as it is possible, for basic work; in this country the greater need is for work which is predominantly basic. But these provisions should not remain separate; they must be integrated. Workers in this country, whether from the universities or the research organisation, must be free, and be encouraged, to work in the tropics when their work has reached the appropriate stage. Workers in the tropics should be able to come to this country, or to move to other territories, as and when their investigations require them to do so.

The Report was able to record some progress towards implementation of these ideals. New centres for medical research had been established in Tanganyika, Kenya, Uganda and Nigeria; and additional support had been given to the existing centre in Malaya. Recruitment of medical investigators to the new Colonial Research Service had been opened in 1949. On the advice of the Colonial Medical Research Committee, a policy had been adopted of decentralising work based in the Colonies and creating interterritorial research organisations (e.g., the West African Council for Medical Research) to supervise this, while retaining home-based research and recruitment of specialised personnel under central control. The terms of reference of the Colonial Medical Research Committee were revised in 1953 to accord with the newer concept of its duties and thereafter read:

> To advise the Secretary of State for the Colonies and the Medical Research Council on all matters of medical research in and for the benefit of the Colonies; and in particular regarding:
> (a) medical research in the Colonies financed from Colonial Development and Welfare Funds;
> (b) the promotion of such basic and long-term work as is required to be based on the United Kingdom and the supervision of workers engaged for this purpose;
> (c) the promotion of work in, and for, the Colonies by home universities and research organisations.

The fiftieth and final meeting of the second Colonial Medical Research Committee was held on 12 July 1960, with Sir Harold Himsworth in the chair, before the Committee's duty was taken over by the new body described in the next section. During the period of its activity the Committee had been able to promote many research projects by means of grants made from the substantial resources available for the purpose under successive Colonial Development and Welfare Acts.

Progress during the Committee's term was reviewed in the Council's Report for 1958–59:

> When this Committee began its work, only two universities existed in the [tropical] Colonies—those of Singapore and Hong Kong—and these had not yet recovered

from the effects of the Second World War. In tropical Africa and in the Caribbean there were no centres of higher medical education, although in Uganda and in Nigeria institutions existed which gave a limited licence to practise. In several of the Colonies there were medical research institutes; but in general these were so burdened with routine that their staff could devote little time to investigation. Even had these resources been entirely available for medical research, the vast distances and the small numbers of personnel would have made them insufficient. Within ten years, however, the picture was changed substantially.

The first step was to recruit workers and to set up bases. An Overseas Research Service was created under the Secretary of State for the Colonies. Bases were built at strategic points, and the Rockefeller Foundation, with characteristic understanding and generosity, transferred their Institutes at Lagos and Entebbe. In this period, universities began to develop, and soon full medical schools, of which any country might be proud, came into existence at the University Colleges in Uganda, Nigeria, and the West Indies. Parallel with these changes, the increasing interest in the basic medical problems related to the tropics developed in the universities and research institutes of the United Kingdom.

But, despite these encouraging developments, it was early evident that no single territory contained, or in the foreseeable future was likely to contain, sufficient resources for medical research to deal with more than a fraction of its problems and opportunities, and, further, that the division of effort between them was such as to render those resources that were available less effective than they might have been. It was therefore suggested that neighbouring territories might combine their efforts. In this way there came into being a West African Council for Medical Research, covering Nigeria, the Gold Coast (as it then was), Sierra Leone, and the Gambia; an East African Council covering Kenya, Uganda, Tanganyika and Zanzibar; and a Standing Advisory Committee for Medical Research in the British Caribbean. Each of these organisations contained two members from the United Kingdom, nominated by the Secretary of State for the Colonies, and was thus related to the Colonial Medical Research Committee. As a consequence of these developments the role of the latter Committee began to alter. It became less concerned with individual schemes of research overseas, and more concerned with co-ordinating policy (including the integration of home-based and overseas research programmes), initiating the opening up of promising new fields, and acting as a consulting organisation and clearing-house of knowledge. In discharge of these functions an important factor was its promotion of visits to tropical territories by relevant experts and by visitors to undertake research of some duration.

It may be added that two of these regional bodies still have useful relations with the Medical Research Council; but the West African Council was brought to an end in 1962 by the withdrawal of Ghana from its operations.

The Tropical Medicine Research Board

By this time, however, two new factors were changing the scene, as the same Report mentions; one was scientific and the other political. The scientific factor was a shift in emphasis from a dominant concern with the tropical diseases in Africa under relatively primitive conditions to an interest in diseases such as tuberculosis, and also hypertension and other cardiovascular conditions, which were being favoured by the adoption of urbanisation and other western social structures, and which in a tropical environment might pose new and unsuspected problems. This latter state of affairs was already strongly marked in the more sophisticated conditions of the Caribbean. The political factor was of course the rapid emergence of former colonial territories as independent countries within the Commonwealth. These passed from under the aegis of the Colonial Office, and like-wise ceased to be eligible for aid from Colonial Development and Welfare funds.

There was thus a necessity for new arrangements in the United Kingdom, as regards both scientific sponsorship and financial aid for medical research work in the tropics. It had at last become in-escapable that the main scientific responsibility ought to lie with the Council; and it was proposed that the latter should appoint a Tropical Medicine Research Board, including representatives of the Colonial Office, to advise it in this field. The formula was accepted, and made workable by the provision of funds, although only after prolonged interdepartmental argument. Valuable time was thereby lost, while the position of medical research work in the tropics, and not unnaturally the morale of workers in the one-time Colonial Research Service, continued to deteriorate.

On 24 November 1959 the Council's Secretary, Sir Harold Himsworth, reiterated the case strongly to the Overseas Research Council, which at that time had a general responsibility for advising on policy. There were non-medical considerations—military, politi-cal, commercial; the medical reasons were the familiar ones given in this chapter. There were diseases common to temperate and tropical climates but with illuminating variants in the latter; and there were purely tropical diseases—all of them infectious and there-fore relevant also to Europeans. The Council must remain concerned with these problems in the interests of the United Kingdom, if for no other reason. The important thing at the time was trying to maintain experienced research workers in the tropics under the new conditions, and approaching new countries in a spirit of collabora-tion rather than of paternalism.

At length, on 26 May 1960, the Secretary was able to report to the Chairman of the Committee of Privy Council that the Treasury had agreed to let the Council have £50 000 per annum, additional to the ordinary grant in aid, for a holding operation to prevent the crumbling away of the amount of research then being done in the tropics; at least at this stage, no expansion was envisaged. Three measures were urgently required to prevent further deterioration of the existing research structure:

(a) to underwrite the appointment of key personnel now overseas so as to en-courage them to stay in post and so to remain to us the linchpins upon which our effective action primarily depends.

(b) to maintain the flow of small project grants to tropical universities.

(c) to continue the necessary supporting services at home as and when support now derived from Colonial Development and Welfare funds is withdrawn or curtailed.

It was also considered urgent "to bring into being the proposed Tropical Medicine Research Board so that it can be widely known in the tropics that a home-based body like the Medical Research Council has made medical research for the tropics its permanent concern".

Three stages of action were envisaged: (i) in the immediate future, to halt the current deterioration; (ii) during the next two or three years to prevent any curtailment of research consequent on territories becoming independent; and (iii) to obtain a decision on the extent to which the United Kingdom was prepared to develop its own overseas research interests.

The new Board was set up by the Council on 15 July 1960. The Chairman and members were appointed by the Council in agreement with the Colonial Office, half of the ordinary members being nominated by the latter in the first place. A medical officer of the Council's staff was secretary, conducting the business from the Council's office; medical representatives of the Colonial Office and the Commonwealth Relations Office were assessors. Existing scientific subcommittees of the expiring Colonial Medical Research Committee were taken over as advisory committees of the Council in special relation with the Board. The terms of reference of the Board were:

To advise

(i) the Secretary of State for the Colonies, through the Medical Research Council, on all medical research in or for the Colonies financed from Colonial Development and Welfare funds;
(ii) the Council on all medical research in or for the Commonwealth financed from the United Kingdom Exchequer; and
(iii) the Council on all medical research in or for tropical or subtropical countries financed from their own budget.

The Board's terms of reference were amended in 1963, with the creation of the Department of Technical Cooperation, to read as follows:

To advise

(a) the Secretary for Technical Cooperation, through the Medical Research Council, on all medical research overseas or in the United Kingdom financed from the funds of the Department of Technical Cooperation;
(b) the Medical Research Council on all medical research in or for tropical or subtropical countries financed from their own budget.

Further governmental reorganisation necessitated another amendment in 1964, at which time clause (a) was changed to read:

the Minister of Overseas Development, through the Medical Research Council, on all medical research overseas or in the United Kingdom financed from the funds of the Ministry of Overseas Development.

The above-mentioned changes in the Board's terms of reference reflect the new arrangements made by the Government in the United Kingdom for aiding former colonial territories. A new Department of Technical Cooperation, succeeded by a Ministry of Overseas Development, became the important financial authority with which the Council had to concert its activities in this field. In 1965 a much diminished Colonial Office merged with the Commonwealth Relations Office, which in turn combined with the Foreign Office in 1968. The Council, for its part, was at last firmly established as the focal scientific agency for the promotion of research in tropical medicine by aid of United Kingdom funds. It remained for the future to show the extent to which it would be given the means to develop this opportunity.

The Council's tropical activities between the wars
What may be regarded as the 'political' history of the promotion of research in tropical medicine has been brought up to date in the preceding section. It is now necessary to go back to consider what actual projects in this field the Council itself was able to develop. Between the two World Wars the Council had maintained a substantial contribution to the subject in the form of laboratory work in the United Kingdom, and the main items may be briefly mentioned.

Work on malaria, particularly that of the Council's Malaria Research Unit in London, has been considered in an earlier section of this chapter. Mr Clifford Dobell's studies of amoebic dysentery, begun during the First World War, have been mentioned elsewhere (Chapter 7, 14). Also at the National Institute for Medical Research, there was work by Mr P. Bruce White on the serological diagnosis of cholera; and experimental investigations of leprosy by Mr S. E. B. Balfour Jones, and later by Sir Patrick Laidlaw, associated with work in the Hebrew University of Jerusalem assisted by a grant from the Council to Professor S. Adler. Grant-aided research on the virus of yellow fever was done by Dr G. Marshall Findlay and Dr F. O. MacCallum at the Wellcome Research Institute in London. In the sphere of medical entomology, Professor P. A. Buxton at the London School of Hygiene and Tropical Medicine was provided by the Council with the whole-time assistance of Dr Kenneth Mellanby for work on the effect of climate upon the functions and numbers of biting insects.

In 1926 the Council sponsored publication of a report by Sir Leonard Rogers on the relation between smallpox and climate in India, where he had had long experience, and on the consequent indications for forecasting epidemics. Likewise, in 1931, the Council sponsored a report by Dr J. B. Orr (later Lord Boyd Orr) and Dr J. L. Gilks, contrasting the physique and health of two African tribes, the Kikuyu and the Masai, of widely different dietetic habits; here again the investigations had been made under other auspices.

Much of the programme of work on chemotherapy, described elsewhere, was directed towards the treatment or prevention of tropical infections (Chapter 3). Field trials of some new compounds which showed promise in experimental work were arranged through existing services and institutions in the tropics. For instance, trials of the trypanocidal activity of compounds produced by Professor J. B. Cohen at Leeds, and tested by Professor C. H. Browning at Glasgow, were made in Tanganyika and South Africa; and different bismuth compounds supplied by the Association of British Chemical Manufacturers, at the request of the Colonial Medical Research Committee, were compared in the treatment of yaws in tropical Africa. In 1925 the Council issued the report of its Committee upon Cinchona Derivatives and Malaria, giving the results of clinical comparisons of quinine and quinidine therapy; these trials had been arranged with the cooperation of the Ministry of Pensions, the Colonial Office and the Sudan Government.

During the whole period the Council had scant footing actually in the tropics, and insufficient funds to employ a staff of its own to work there. One method of getting round this difficulty was tried in 1928, when an arrangement was made with the Government of Nigeria whereby the Council paid part of the salary of a medical officer from its private Tropical Medical Research Fund (Volume One). Under this scheme, Dr R. M. Burnie was released from much of his routine duty to undertake special research work on tropical ulcers of the skin, and later on relapsing fever. It did not, however, seem that a basis for any more extensive programme was likely to be found in borrowing personnel in this way from the Colonial Medical Service.

Also in Nigeria, Dr A. Clark—previously working at the London School of Hygiene and Tropical Medicine with a grant from the Council—made a survey of nutritional problems in the territory. This was at the request, and partly with the support, of the Nigerian Government, but financial help was also given from the Council's Tropical Medical Research Fund and the Colonial Office. This preceded the more general attack on colonial nutritional problems already described.

It has been mentioned elsewhere that the Council had the award of Dorothy Temple Cross Fellowships in tuberculosis (Volume One). In the first year, two senior fellows were assigned to the study of some aspects of tuberculosis as manifested among native populations in tropical climates. Dr R. J. Matthews, in the service of the Welsh National Memorial Association, worked in Zanzibar; and Lieut. S. M. Burrows, RAMC, attached Sudan Defence Force, worked in the Bahr el Ghazal Province of the Sudan. Under other auspices, Dr C. Wilcocks made a similar study in Tanganyika; and all three reports were combined in a special publication edited by Colonel S. L. Cummins.

Some of the Council's Tropical Medical Research Fellows,

appointed under the scheme mentioned in an earlier section, worked in the tropics. Just before the Second World War, Dr F. Hawking was in Tanganyika and elsewhere studying the trypanocidal activity of tryparsamide in the blood plasma, and Dr C. J. Hackett was studying the bone lesions of yaws in Uganda. These were experienced workers holding Senior Fellowships; some of the Junior Fellows also worked for a time in Africa.

Work on nutrition in colonial territories, by Dr B. S. Platt and other members of the Council's staff, began shortly before the Second World War, as mentioned earlier in this chapter. Work on scrub-typhus was a wartime activity (Chapter 15).

The Council's Laboratories in The Gambia

Immediately after the Second World War the prospects for bringing the Council's scientific resources to bear on tropical problems had greatly improved. A basis for satisfactory cooperation with the Colonial Office had at last been established; the Council had for the first time more than trifling sums for the purpose in its own budget; and additional finance could be obtained from the new Colonial Development and Welfare Fund. The question was how the Council could best utilise this opportunity.

The logic of the situation seemed to demand that the Council should do more than deploy members of its scientific staff for short visits to the tropics, or for longer periods of attachment to existing centres overseas—in fact that it should have one or more overseas establishments of its own. To these it could post staff specially recruited for regular work in the tropics; and it could also send there, by arrangements within its own control, visiting workers from its home staff or from other institutions in the United Kingdom. Nevertheless there was some hesitation about incurring commitments of this kind; and in the event the first steps towards the adoption of the idea as a matter of Council policy were almost fortuitous.

In accordance with a pre-war policy mentioned earlier, the Council's Human Nutrition Research Unit under Dr B. S. Platt had an explicit remit to make investigations overseas. Owing to the enterprise of Dr Platt, a suitable location for an out-station of his Unit was found in The Gambia in 1947. At Fajara, nine miles south-westwards along the coast from Bathurst, the hutted premises of a wartime military hospital were standing empty; there was also a strange all-steel, three-storeyed building which had before the war served as a rest-house for the Lufthansa. Leases to the Council were readily obtained from the Gambian Government, and the whole was adapted for use as a research station—a small hospital, laboratories, library, and living accommodation for staff and visitors. A small sub-station was also established at the up-river village of Keneba for use as an inland research centre in a rural community.

This project was financed partly from the Council's own funds, through the budget of the Unit, and partly from a special grant made to the Council from the Colonial Development and Welfare Fund. From the latter source there was also a grant to the Gambian Government for an experiment in agricultural development (Nutrition Field Working Party) at the up-country village of Geniere; Dr Platt had charge of this also, but separately from the matters in which he was responsible to the Council. The Nutrition Field Research Station at Fajara was not administered directly by the Council but through the Human Nutrition Research Unit, of which it was regarded as an integral part. Dr Platt divided his time between London and Africa, at appropriate seasons.

It did not in the event prove satisfactory that the Council should have responsibility for a distant establishment over which it had only indirect control. Misgivings also arose as to whether the cost was justified by the output of research limited to a particular subject. Early in 1952, accordingly, the Council sent out a subcommittee to examine the question on the spot; this consisted of Major-General Sir John Taylor, Brigadier J. S. K. (later Sir John) Boyd and the present writer. The subcommittee concluded that the existing arrangements should not be continued, but that the opportunity be taken to convert the station into a research establishment of wider scope, to be administered directly by the Council. The Council accepted the recommendations, and these were implemented within the next few months.

The station was renamed 'Medical Research Council Laboratories, Gambia' and Dr J. Newsome was appointed Director. He was succeeded in 1954 by Dr I. A. McGregor, who had been working there since 1949. The latter was thereafter responsible, under the Council, for the large development of the station, with new buildings, an increased staff and a broader programme of research.

Retrospectively reviewing this development of policy, in its Report for 1957–58, the Council said:

For these purposes the Gambia presents a number of advantages. It is the nearest of the British territories in Africa. It has an excellent climate during more than half the year, although the humidity is high during the rainy season; near the coast the weather is seldom excessively hot, and during the dry season the nights are cool with a breeze off the sea. The health record of Europeans nowadays—in strong contrast to earlier times—is good. The African population is cooperative, and the Government has warmly welcomed the presence of a research project which makes an important impact on the life of a small community. Relations on all sides are cordial, to the benefit of everyone concerned.

These considerations remained largely valid after the country was given independence in 1965. The small hospital not only provides beds for patients whom members of the staff wish to treat or keep under observation, but is also a 'bread-and-butter' undertaking which earns the goodwill and cooperation of the indigenous population.

The research programme of the resident staff under McGregor has been largely concerned with malaria and related problems, including entomological studies, this disease being hyperendemic in the territory and under local conditions intractable to prevention by mosquito control. Much of the work is done at the village of Keneba, where a relatively stable population of some seven hundred persons is little affected by the urban influences felt nearer the coast. This community has now been under close and almost continuous observation for over twenty years; and control studies are made in neighbouring villages.

At first, although the advantages of doing so much of the research work up-country were undoubted, poor communications imposed a serious practical difficulty. There is no railway or internal air-service in the territory, and the up-country roads were difficult—indeed often impassable in the rainy season—although of late greatly improved. The natural means of transportation was by river, but for this the Council had to depend on hired vessels, not always suitable even when available. The Council had thus good reason to be grateful to the Wellcome Trust for a generous grant to provide a vessel for its own use—a sixty-foot twin-diesel launch built specially for the purpose and with one of its cabins, usable also for sleeping, fitted as a small laboratory. This the Council named the *Lady Dale*, in honour of the wife of the then Chairman of the Trustees. It arrived in The Gambia at the end of 1958 and greatly added to the facilities for research; not only did it simplify journeys to and from Keneba, which is within easy reach of a navigable *bolon* (creek), but it opened up the possibility of work further up the river, where the conditions are different.

Special attention was naturally directed to the early stages in the development of disease, and in its Report for 1957–58 the Council gave an outline of this problem as presented in the population of the particular territory. The reason for concentrating investigation on malaria was then stated as follows:

Highly important in this complex picture is the protozoal infection, malaria, because of its very high incidence in the infant and child population. In the Gambia, mangrove swamps fringe the rivers and the creeks for over a hundred miles inland, and form innumerable and invulnerable breeding places for malaria-carrying mosquitoes. These breeding places are greatly increased with the onset of the rains by the formation of countless transient sites beyond the swamp margin. As a result infection is widespread, and so prevalent among children living in rural areas that malarial parasites can be demonstrated in their blood with a frequency that rises rapidly during the first year of life, and approaches a hundred per cent during the second year. Thus, during the highly vulnerable first two years of life, when innumerable other hazards to health and survival are also encountered, the Gambian child is almost continuously infected with malaria. Yet, despite the persistent presence of malarial parasites in the body, the overt clinical illness of malaria develops only intermittently.

In this situation, important and difficult questions arise concerning the role of the universal malaria infection in producing high mor-

tality at early ages, in permanently affecting the health of survivors, in producing and maintaining an effective immunity against
malaria, and in so doing perhaps placing an excessive burden on
the body economy.

These and subsequently emerging questions engaged the attention
of McGregor and a succession of collaborators, both on his own staff
and at the National Institute for Medical Research or elsewhere in
the United Kingdom—and indeed also in other countries, including
the adjacent Senegal (Dakar). Important publications have been
made, and knowledge of the epidemiology and immunology of
malaria has been greatly advanced. In the field of child health,
long-term investigations have led to the identification of factors
having an important influence on the growth and health of rural
African children. Reviews of work on immunity to malaria and on
the chemotherapy of malaria appeared in the Council's Reports for
1960–61 and 1967–68 respectively.

Other diseases have also been studied in The Gambia, either by
resident staff or by visiting workers; they have included filariasis and
schistosomiasis, and there have also been studies on aspects of social
and obstetric medicine. From 1958 a small section of the Council's
Trachoma Unit was attached to the Laboratories, but under scientific direction from the headquarters of the Unit at the Lister
Institute in London; the field work on this eye infection (the greatest
single cause of blindness in the world) was formerly done in Jordan,
until conditions there became unfavourable.

Other overseas establishments and staff of the Council
The station in The Gambia was the Council's first permanent
establishment overseas, and it remains both the largest and the most
self-contained. Several others have since been added, originating in
different ways; of these the first was the Child Nutrition Unit in
Uganda, set up at Kampala in 1953—under the title of Infantile
Malnutrition Research Unit—on the basis of a team working there
since 1950 under Dr R. F. A. Dean of the Council's staff. The Unit
was attached to Mulago Hospital but had its own building com-
prising a ward and a laboratory, its own staff and its own transport;
the expatriate members of the staff were allotted flats rented by the
Council. The main subject of study has been the condition known
as kwashiorkor, the manifestation of malnutrition associated particularly with a low protein intake, of which the first full description was published by Dr Cicely Williams of the Colonial Medical
Service. After the death of Professor Dean (he had received the title
from Makerere University) in 1964, Professor R. A. McCance took
charge of the Unit for a couple of years, after which Dr R. G.
Whitehead was made Director. The basic diet for malnourished
children worked out in this Unit was used to great advantage at the
end of the Nigerian Civil War in 1970.

The Council's creation of a third overseas establishment in 1955 extended the field of operation from Africa to the West Indies. This was the Tropical Metabolism Research Unit attached to the University College (now University) of the West Indies at Kingston, Jamaica. It was placed under the direction of Dr J. C. Waterlow, a member of the Council's staff who has since been appointed to a chair at the London School of Hygiene and Tropical Medicine. The Unit, which was taken over by the University in 1970, was concerned mainly with the effects of malnutrition in children and with adaptive processes in metabolism; it collaborated with the World Health Organisation and the Government of Jamaica in the study of practical nutritional problems.

In 1962 another establishment was set up at Kingston under similar arrangements. This, the Epidemiological Research Unit, was placed under the direction of Dr W. E. Miall, a member of the Council's staff from the similarly named establishment in South Wales. A capital grant was made by the Wellcome Trustees. The Unit has made long-term epidemiological studies of cardiovascular and pulmonary diseases, and also growth and development studies of children, in samples of the general population in the Caribbean.

Individual workers overseas hold positions as members of the Council's external scientific staff. They include Dr B. O. L. Duke, who is Director of the Helminthiasis Research Unit at Kumba in the Federal Republic of the Cameroon, an establishment which is largely supported from Overseas Development funds, with the help of the Wellcome Trustees, and which by arrangement with the Government of the Republic is administered by the Council and responsible to it scientifically.

At Tanga, Dr A. Davis of the Council's staff until recently directed a Bilharziasis Chemotherapy Centre maintained under a tripartite arrangement between the Council, the World Health Organisation and the Government of the country. Of the Leprosy Research Unit in Malaysia, which ranks as a field station of the National Institute for Medical Research in London, something is said later.

Various members of the Council's staff appointed for work overseas have been attached to institutions in different parts of Africa and the West Indies. They include a surgeon, Mr D. P. Burkitt, who was appointed to the staff in 1964 so that he might continue his pioneering studies of malignant lymphoma in African children and the geographical incidence of other forms of cancer. Cancer, like tuberculosis, is an example of a widespread disease that presents special aspects in the tropics and may thus provide clues for research. Such statistics as exist indicate that in at least some African populations cancer incidence does not rise steeply in later life as in European communities. There also appear to be gross differences from one tropical country to another in the incidence of cancer of particular bodily sites, and the possible relation to these of various environmental, nutritional and constitutional factors may be important for a better understanding of malignant disease as a whole. Cancer, however, has a low priority among the medical problems of the countries concerned; but as the information could be relevant to other communities it was advisable that the United Kingdom should take responsibility for collecting it. These considerations led the Council, in 1963, to appoint a Committee for Research on Cancer in the Tropics, including corresponding members overseas. An article on cancer in the tropics was included in the Report for 1961–62.

Home-based staff working overseas
In a different category from overseas establishments are a few in the United Kingdom which have had more or less permanent detachments in the tropics. The former Human Nutrition Research Unit has already been mentioned, and so also has the Trachoma Unit. Another case in point, for a number of years, was the Bilharzia Research Unit. This had its origin from the time, in the autumn of 1947, when by arrangement with the Egyptian Government the Council sent a small team to Cairo to collaborate with local investigators in studies of schistosomiasis (bilharziasis); of this Dr J. Newsome was the senior member. On return to the United Kingdom the team became the Council's Group for Research on Bilharzia Disease, as it was originally called, and was accommodated at the field laboratories of the London School of Hygiene and Tropical Medicine at St Albans, Hertfordshire. Experimental work was undertaken on the aetiology and treatment of this mollusc-borne helminth infection. Dr Newsome was absent in 1953–54 while acting as Director of the Council's Laboratories in The Gambia, as already mentioned; and in 1959 Dr A. Davis was detached from the Unit to work in East and Central Africa. In 1962 the Unit as such was disbanded.

Some of the Council's home establishments that are not particularly orientated towards tropical problems have nevertheless found useful ways of extending their investigations by sending staff overseas. This is true of the National Institute for Medical Research in several fields, including its work on leprosy in Malaysia. In laboratory studies at the Institute, Dr R. J. W. Rees succeeded in producing in mice a disease closely resembling leprosy in man and thus opened up possibilities of experimental leprosy research such as people had been seeking in vain for a century. In clinico–pathological work based on their studies, the Institute's field unit at Sungei Buloh, near Kuala Lumpur, was able to follow the course of the disease and assess the effects of chemotherapy by objective laboratory tests. This work was described in the Annual Reports for 1966–67 and 1970–71.

Another example was the Statistical Research Unit, members of which were sent to Fiji in 1964 and to East Africa in 1966 to study the incidence of cancer. The Tuberculosis and Chest Diseases Unit seconded staff for work in India on the treatment of tuberculosis under a scheme promoted by the World Health Organisation; and the Unit for Laboratory Studies of Tuberculosis has been closely associated with clinical trials in India, East Africa and Hong Kong. In 1961 the Council appointed a Committee on Tuberculosis Research in the Tropics. The chemotherapy of tuberculosis in Africa and India was the subject of a review article in the Report for 1958–59.

Again, there have been individual members of the Council's scientific staff in the United Kingdom whose normal duty has involved frequent periods of work overseas. Dr D. J. Lewis, for instance, has been attached to the Department of Entomology in the British Museum (Natural History) but has paid working visits on the Council's behalf to various parts of the tropics in furtherance of his studies of sandflies and blackflies, groups which include the vector species of leishmaniasis (kala azar) and onchocerciasis (river blindness) respectively.

So many species of insects are vectors of tropical infections, and sometimes themselves a menace to health, that medical entomology is a well established subject and one to which the Council has given much support. Certain molluscs are also important as vectors, for example the water-snails that harbour one stage in the life-cycle of the parasitic helminth causing schistosomiasis. This consideration led the Council, in 1955, to initiate a scheme for training a few young zoologists as investigators in medical malacology. Of those who have passed through this scheme, Dr D. S. Brown became a member of the external scientific staff, attached to the British Museum (Natural History) but working partly overseas.

Helminth infections are a major subject of investigation, at the National Institute for Medical Research and elsewhere with the Council's support. In the annals of the Council, medical helminthology and medical entomology will always be particularly associated with the names of, respectively, Professor R. T. Leiper and Professor P. A. Buxton, both in their day holding the chairs in those specialties at the London School of Hygiene and Tropical Medicine.

Restatement of policy

In May 1966 the Council devoted a special session to a review of its role in tropical research. It reaffirmed its conviction that biomedical research was indivisible and that no part could be neglected without detriment to the whole. It was concerned about the current weakness of United Kingdom support for medical research in tropical countries; and it was intimately aware of the difficulties of recruitment.

The Council reiterated its belief that the keystone of any organisation for the purpose must be a small cadre of biomedical research workers prepared to make their careers in studying the special problems of the tropics and to work primarily overseas. It was hoped

that these would attract, direct and supervise a succession of younger
(or less experienced) workers who would serve abroad for one or two
tours. It was recognised that such an overseas cadre could be maintained only if its members were offered the prospects of an assured
career with the Council, and only if the Council were allowed to
offer conditions of service appropriate to the circumstances of
expatriation.

The Council transmitted these views to the Department of Education and Science, seeking the support of HM Government in the
requisite action. The Department and the Treasury approved in
principle, but implementation of the scheme later encountered
serious technical difficulties relating to conditions of service.

Expeditions
It is convenient to consider here the part that the Council has
played from time to time in assisting expeditions, although not all
of these have been to tropical parts of the world. One does not
include, under this head, mere visits to foreign countries for purposes
of scientific liaison or for work at sophisticated centres of research.
An expedition involves an element of exploration, at least in that the
party must import its own scientific equipment and create its own
local facilities for research. Some expeditions promoted by the
Council itself, as well as the establishment of a few more or less
permanent research stations overseas, have been mentioned earlier
in this chapter.

There is no record of the Council's having in its earlier days given
support to expeditions carrying out scientific research, either as a
main or as a subsidiary purpose, although its advice was sometimes
sought on questions of diet and equipment. In the period since the
Second World War, however, the Council has supported expeditions
in a number of ways. For the most part it has been a question of
a small grant, often drawn from private funds, towards expenses
or equipment for the medical part of the programme. Many of
the expeditions have been organised by students, notably in the
University of Cambridge. Most of the expeditions are to tropical
countries, and the study of various tropical diseases and the collection of material for genetic and anthropological surveys have been
prominent among the subjects of study. During the 1960s the
Council's Serological Population Genetics Laboratory under Dr
A. E. Mourant provided a valuable service for the investigation of
blood samples, of possible anthropological significance, obtained in
the course of expeditions. A number of expeditions to mountainous
areas, for the study of high-altitude physiology, also attracted
Council support; and there has been a continuing interest in work
on adaptation to extreme cold.

Apart from a small grant to an individual for research in the
Antarctic in 1946, this latter interest dates from 1949, when the
Council participated (by the secondment of members of staff and the

award of grants for expenses) in the Royal Naval Arctic Cruise, during which a number of studies of cold physiology and protective clothing were made. Subsequently grants were made towards the expenses of the British North Greenland Expedition (1952–54) and to the Cambridge University Spitzbergen (Physiological) Expedition 1953. In 1957 it was agreed to second Dr L. G. C. E. Pugh for collaboration, with the United States Office of Naval Research, in physiological investigations on members of the Trans-Arctic Expeditions undertaken in connection with the International Geophysical Year. An informal association between the Council and the British Antarctic Survey (formerly the Falkland Islands Dependencies Survey) has existed since 1956, with the object of exploiting the opportunities for physiological research at the Survey's bases in Antarctica. Individual medical officers appointed to the Survey carry out parts of long-term programmes planned by the Division of Human Physiology at the National Institute. Physiological studies undertaken have included food intake and energy expenditure, body weight and skinfold thickness changes, water balance, continuous recording of skin temperature, peripheral blood flow and peripheral sensation, sleep rhythms and performance tests. The particular usefulness of the Antarctic research has been that there is a virtually captive group of subjects, with a captive observer, available for study over the period of a year.

It is, however, in the field of high-altitude research that the Council has made its major contribution to the support of an expedition. A full account of the Council's part in supplying scientific advice for the British Everest Expedition in 1953 is given in the Report for 1952–53. Dr L. G. C. E. Pugh of the National Institute for Medical Research accompanied the climbing party that went to Cho Oyu in 1952 to gain experience of high-altitude conditions; the information obtained, together with that available from other Everest expeditions (particularly the Swiss attempt of 1952), provided a basis for predicting the requirements of the 1953 Everest Expedition in respect of nutrition, acclimatisation and equipment, and the effects of supplementary oxygen on men at high altitudes. Subsequently the Council appointed Dr Pugh and Dr O. G. Edholm to maintain liaison with the organisers of the expedition and a High Altitude Committee was set up by the Council under the chairmanship of Sir Bryan Matthews to advise on questions relating to the supply of oxygen and the design of oxygen apparatus; the equipment eventually used with marked success on the ascent was based on their detailed recommendations. In the light of experience gained on the Cho Oyu expedition special protective equipment was designed, and major modifications were made to the traditional diet of Himalayan climbing parties. Pugh was a member of the successful expedition and was able to supervise a comprehensive programme of physiological investigations throughout its duration.

In his account of the Everest Expedition, Sir John (later Lord)

Hunt made full acknowledgement of the help given by the Council, its High Altitude Committee, and members of its staff. One of the latter who was particularly active in the design of oxygen and other equipment was Dr R. B. Bourdillon, Director of the Council's Electro-Medical Research Unit; in this work he had the collaboration of his son, Tom Bourdillon, a climbing member of the party.

Pugh later took part in another expedition to the Himalayas, led by Sir Edmund Hillary and sponsored by the Field Enterprises Corporation Inc. of Chicago, in 1960–61. This expedition had primarily scientific objectives and extensive physiological observations were made. In 1965 the Council gave some assistance to Mr M. Ward (another medical member of the Everest Expedition of 1953) for a survey of a high-altitude population during an expedition to Bhutan; this study was related to the International Biological Programme.

The Council's interest in problems of hot climates, especially in relation to requirements of the Services, is mentioned elsewhere (Chapter 16). Latterly the Council has supported, by grants and the services of staff, an investigation planned by Dr Edholm of the National Institute for Medical Research on the effect of the climatic environment on man; this was a contribution to the Human Adaptability Section of the International Biological Programme.

Chapter 11
Production and Evaluation of Medicinal Substances

Collaboration with industry—Patenting in the medical field—The British
Pharmacopoeia—Clinical evaluation of remedies—Evaluation of prophylactics

Collaboration with industry

The Council is, of course, not directly concerned with the commercial production of medicinal substances, although sometimes it may find it advisable to encourage or assist manufacture in its early stages. It is, however, very much interested in the important part that pharmaceutical firms take in research; and on appropriate occasions it collaborates with the manufacturers. Incidental to this aspect is the somewhat vexed question of the use of the patent law in the medical field. The clinical evaluation of the products, whether they be for therapeutic or for prophylactic use, is definitely a medical matter, and one in which the Council has played an important role. The biological standardisation and control of medicinal substances that cannot be assayed by chemical tests has been in a very special degree the province of the Council (Chapter 12).

The Council's relations with the pharmaceutical manufacturers were at first somewhat restricted by the firms' natural concern with commercial security and proprietary rights, as well as by the Council's own obligation to avoid giving any monopolistic advantage based on expenditure of public funds. Subsequently, however, many useful means were found of securing collaboration between the Council's scientific staff and the research departments of the manufacturers. The Association of British Chemical Manufacturers, and later the Association of the British Pharmaceutical Industry, was frequently the appropriate channel for dealing with the industry as a whole.

Considerable progress had already been made when the Council reviewed the question in its report for 1930–31:

> It has always been laid down and accepted as among the primary functions
> of the Council not only to promote the stages of scientific discovery as such
> within the medical field, but also to facilitate the 'availability' of the results
> of discovery in the interests of the public and the medical profession. It rarely
> happens that the discovery of a new substance or a new method allows imme-
> diate practical use to be made of one or the other. Very often much time and
> labour must be given, not seldom involving a new series of researches, before

the yield of a new substance can be brought into the phase of large-scale production, or a new method be adapted for widespread use. In these intermediate stages of work it is often necessary for rapid and economic progress that close co-operation should be established between the original scientific investigators and those whose work lies in finding the adaptations needed for large-scale production and use. The general social and political reasons that make it obviously desirable for State-supported work like that of the Council to be brought into the field of co-operative effort with British manufacturing firms are reinforced by the intimate relations of this kind of manufacturing to health and life within the country. Apart from any other reasons, it will be accepted as desirable for this nation, as for any other, that all the essential materials for good medical work should be readily procurable within the national boundaries.

The review also considered ways in which the Council had helped the industry, including the arrangements that had just been made for the clinical evaluation of new products and ways in which manufacturers had helped the Council's own programmes. The contribution made by British pharmaceutical firms to the general pool of knowledge was already growing rapidly, although it fell short of the vast research effort of certain foreign, and notably German, chemical manufacturers.

The importance of the industrial contribution, at home as well as abroad, has become well recognised in more recent times. Professor E. B. (later Sir Ernst) Chain put the case strongly in 1963: "Let us, once and for all, accept the indisputable fact which the history of drug research teaches us through innumerable examples . . . that the best results in the field have been obtained by close collaboration between industrial and academic laboratories."

The Council expressed its current opinion of the importance of the industrial contribution in a memorandum of evidence prepared in 1965 for a Committee of Inquiry into the Relationship of the Pharmaceutical Industry with the National Health Service, a body set up by HM Government in that year. Only extracts from this closely reasoned document can be given here:

> The participants in the total pharmaceutical research effort are academic workers, those in government-supported research establishments and industry itself. Original discoveries leading to totally new advances in therapy or prophylaxis may be made by any of the three groups. Thus prontosil, which opened up sulphonamide therapy, was discovered in a German industrial laboratory, whilst penicillin was discovered by academic research workers, and the first of the new hypotensive drugs resulted from an investigation in the Council's National Institute for Medical Research. In all three instances, however, the development of the initial discoveries, needed to make their full potentialities available to medicine, has depended largely on industrial pharmaceutical research.
>
> The Council hold the view that the policy of the Pharmaceutical Industry in investing heavily in research has proved to be wise in conception and, from the point of view of medicine, notably successful in the outcome. Viewed as a whole, the research that has been carried out in the industry has conformed to

the highest scientific standards and, to the Council's knowledge, it has been conducted with a full sense of responsibility to the community so far as concerns precautions to ensure the safety of products. The Council regards the results of industrial pharmaceutical research over the past 30 years as a notable contribution to biomedical science and as an essential factor in the great therapeutic achievements of this period.

Two major examples of the Council's cooperation with the pharmaceutical industry have already been mentioned—the production of insulin in the early 1920s, and research on penicillin in the wartime 1940s: one other instance, of recent date, must suffice. In 1959 the Council decided that cooperation with manufacturing firms would accelerate research following up the discovery, at the National Institute for Medical Research, of a "viral interfering substance produced by the action of a partially-inactivated virus on a susceptible tissue"; to this substance the name 'interferon' had been given. Three large pharmaceutical firms wished to cooperate. Agreements were accordingly entered into between these firms and the National Research Development Corporation, and between the Corporation and the Council. Different parts of the work to be done were allocated to the several laboratories, on the understanding that information would be exchanged, and that progress reports at regular intervals would be made to a joint scientific committee. All results were to be available for scientific publication, with no more delay than was necessary to secure patent protection. Patent rights were to be administered, on an agreed basis, by a body representative of the Corporation and the industrial collaborators. This was a long-term programme which exemplifies the type of cooperative arrangement that it is now possible to make.

During the Second World War, the Council joined with the wartime US Office of Scientific Research and Development in a common endeavour to secure the early production of an adequate supply of high-quality synthetic penicillin, or a therapeutic equivalent, at reasonable prices. The Office entered into contracts with American academic, industrial and governmental research workers to make a coordinated and concentrated effort to synthesise penicillin, including the exchange among the participants of information on purification, structure and synthesis. The Council had similar understandings with industrial firms and academic research workers in Great Britain. There was also provision for full exchange of information between the two countries. At Washington, on 25 January 1946, the arrangements were retrospectively embodied in a formal Agreement between Governments.

The actual collaboration, on an international basis, continued for nearly two years and ended on 31 October 1945. The programme did not achieve a commercially feasible synthesis of penicillin, and it thus failed of its main purpose. It did, however, yield a number of minor inventions, some of which proved to be of commercial value; the latter related particularly to 'adjuvants and precursors'—chemical substances capable of increasing the yield of penicillin in the fermentation processes—the 'biosynthetic' method of production that has necessarily remained in use.

An essential part of the international agreement related to the basis on which patent rights arising from the collaborative work were to be apportioned among the commercial interests. This was to be done by a 'Determination' made in concert by the two official agencies, applying defined principles. The agreement was hailed as a new model for international understandings on rights arising from collaborative programmes of research—but in the event it did not prove to be a shining example. In fact, the two agencies—each in consultation with its commercial contractors—in the end failed to agree. The complicated details of the dispute turned on what inventions did or did not fall within the scope of the Agreement, and on the ratings to be allotted to the several British firms as participants in the rights, according to an assessment of their respective contributions to the research achievement as a whole.

Patenting in the medical field
The commercial development of medical discoveries, and particularly any collaboration between manufacturing firms and academic institutions or governmental agencies, inevitably raises questions about the acquisition and subsequent use of patent rights. In the Council's early years these questions presented difficulties of various kinds. One was the existence of a strong objection to patenting on the part of many members of the medical profession. To some extent this was based on misconceptions, such as confusion with secret remedies (often misnamed 'patent medicines') and a suspicion of monopolistic price-raising; but a patent by its nature (and name) involves disclosure, and the law did contain safeguards against monopolies in medicines and foods. The real ethical objection was to medical men having "a proprietary interest in preparations which it may be their duty to recommend medicinally" (British Medical Association, 1904)—a contingency that would in reality seldom arise and could anyhow be easily avoided. There were, however, other objections that weighed more heavily with the Council. In its view, formulated in 1928, the whole concept of patenting was inappropriate in the biological field, where so much of medical research lay; and whereas the purpose of the Patent Law was to stimulate useful invention and encourage commercial development, it was feared that increasing use of the procedure in the sphere of academic and state-aided biomedical research would be inimical to the progress of discovery.

The Medical Research Committee was indirectly involved in a matter of patenting on the outbreak of the First World War in 1914. The British rights held by the German manufacturers of arsenical compounds used in the treatment of syphilis were confiscated as enemy property, and licences to make these drugs were granted to

British firms subject to their submitting the products to control by the Committee. This was a precursor of the programme of work on biological standardisation.

The Council was first directly involved in 1922, when—as mentioned earlier—the University of Toronto offered it assignment of the British patents covering the process of preparing insulin from the pancreas of animals in a form suitable for administration to diabetics. The offer was accepted by the Council on the ground that some authoritative body should be able to exercise control over the quality, strength and—if necessary—price of insulin manufactured in the United Kingdom. The Council not only accepted assignment of the main British patent and certain subsidiary patents from Toronto but also arranged for patenting an improvement devised by members of its own staff at the National Institute for Medical Research; the Canadian and United States rights in this improvement were assigned to the University of Toronto, and the Australian rights to the Commonwealth Government.

Non-exclusive licences to manufacture insulin under these patents were granted free of royalty to a number of British firms, subject to conditions on the quality of the material and the measurement of its strength in standard units. A clause giving the Council the right to fix a maximum price was never invoked, except formally by agreement, as competition between the firms rapidly brought the price to a reasonable level. Thereafter, the Therapeutic Substances Act 1925 created statutory powers for the control of insulin and other products that could be assayed only by biological methods. The purpose for which the insulin patents were held had accordingly disappeared, and in 1931 the Council decided to allow these patents to lapse instead of paying the renewal fees for the remainder of the normal sixteen years' period of validity.

The Patent Law had, indeed, not been used by the Council in this way without some misgivings and some murmurs of professional criticism. There were also doubts whether a patent which in effect claimed rights in the discovery of a natural biological phenomenon would have been held valid, at least under British law, if seriously challenged. As someone remarked at the time, the claim amounted to saying "What God intended the pancreas to do, I have invented". The patent, however, did not—and in law could not—cover insulin as a substance, or its natural action, but only the specified method of preparing it.

A much less agreeable aspect of patenting in the biological field was forced on the Council's attention in 1928 by an occurrence thus described in a contemporary memorandum of its views on patenting:

> In the past year the Council watched with anxiety the effect of the Patent Law upon the commercial development of an important discovery made in their own laboratories, namely, the production of vitamin D in highly potent form by the ultra-violet irradiation of ergosterol. This discovery came at an advanced stage in a long series of researches by many workers to which large financial

support had been given from public moneys. As is the usual practice in the medical field, this discovery was made free to the world by publication, and manufacturing firms were thus given the opportunity of bringing its benefits to the public. This action by manufacturers has, however, been hampered by the claims made under a British patent (No. 236197) which had been granted to a foreign worker, Professor Steenbock, of Wisconsin, U.S.A., some years earlier. This patent for a process of imparting anti-rachitic properties to foodstuffs by artificial ultra-violet irradiation, was drawn in wide terms which are now claimed as covering not only work of more recent date and greater importance, but also valuable practical applications which the latest discovery had made possible and easy.

Professor Steenbock had assigned the rights in his patent to the University of Wisconsin, and the latter exploited them commercially by granting licences to manufacturers, both under the original United States Patent and under patents obtained in other countries by virtue of the international convention. The Council's memorandum proceeded to comment on the claim in more detail:

What Professor Steenbock did in effect patent was a law of nature—i.e. that the natural product, vitamin D, is formed by the action of ultra-violet light upon certain natural substances: so far as is known, this is the only way in which this vitamin is formed in nature, whether in the body or in various foodstuffs and other organic materials. What he did in form patent was a process for artificially inducing this action to take place. But the process in itself contained nothing novel and required no ingenuity to devise, for with a knowledge of the natural law the application was ready to hand.

The Steenbock patent was based upon very imperfect knowledge of its subject matter: it covered the production of a substance of undetermined composition from an unknown constituent of certain complex materials by an action not then understood. The patent was nevertheless drawn in wide general terms so that it is now claimed as covering all the applications of the more definite discoveries of subsequent date.

It was considered doubtful whether an original British patent would have been granted in these terms—the American law gave greater latitude—and even after the grant of a British patent under the convention its validity could have been challenged in the courts; but the manufacturers preferred to pay the royalty for a licence rather than expose themselves to the uncertainties of expensive litigation. After all this, it was wryly amusing that in 1943 the original U.S. patent should be voided by the Federal Circuit Court of Appeals on the ground that it claimed rights over a natural action of the sun; by that time it was said to have yielded more than seven-and-a-half million dollars in royalties to the Wisconsin Alumni Research Foundation.

After discussing various other aspects of the general question, the memorandum summarised the Council's objections to the operation of the Patent Law in the field of biology and medicine as follows:

The discovery of new facts of nature in the medical field, concerned as they are with the body of man himself and the factors affecting it, may lead obviously and at once, without any intervening steps of ingenious invention, to valuable practical uses. There is not the same possibility of clear distinction between the discoverer on the one hand and the inventor on the other as there is in the inorganic field, where fundamental knowledge is far more complete and where much individual ingenuity is required to devise new practical applications. Those who seek to use the Patent Law in the medical field for personal or localised profit will be apt (as experience already proves) to claim proprietary rights in some particular use of a new discovery that follows it almost automatically, and may not in itself, considered as a practical invention, be particularly meritorious in the sense of deserving pecuniary reward.

Biological discoveries in their first phases are necessarily in the form of vague knowledge, and patents which may be sought by persons making useful application of them are likely to be drawn (as again experience has shown) in wide terms that really go beyond the knowledge of the moment. In the inorganic field patented inventions have to be, because they can be more exactly defined, and do not necessarily stake out claims by which further research by others in the same field may be discouraged or hampered.

Although resort to the Patent Law is open to everyone, it is in fact little used in the medical field, for reasons to which importance must be attached: in effect, therefore, the law works capriciously in favour of the few who break the tradition. Medical research is in general organised on a basis of free intercourse between workers: it is important that this should be preserved, but the introduction of rivalry in obtaining patents—even if only in defence against those who break the general tradition—would make this obviously difficult or impossible.

In conclusion, the Council urged "that the law should be amended to extend still further the special treatment already given by it to medical discoveries and, as in some other countries, to abolish altogether the right of patenting these". Admittedly there were certain difficulties, and the possibility of alternative courses that could have nearly equivalent effect was mentioned. In particular, the Council was aware "that a proposal is being made that there should be compulsory dedication of medical patents to some public official, body or department acting in this matter as a national trustee"; and to this proposal it gave qualified support.

A Departmental Committee reported in 1931, advising against any change in the law relating to medical patents. And the Board of Trade was not moved by further representations, in 1932, in the form of resolutions of a conference convened by the British Medical Association and attended by representatives of the Council and of the Royal Colleges.

Meanwhile the Council's policy, minuted in 1928 and reaffirmed in 1931, was to be prepared "to accept patent rights, in cases where this course seems to them desirable in the public interest, whether for the proper development of a medical discovery or for its protection against improper exploitation". The Council, however, would "not countenance patenting in any case where, by reason of an attempt to cover unexplored ground or otherwise, this step seems likely to hamper the freedom of research or to discourage further investigation". The Council did not intend to use any patent for

pecuniary gain either to its own funds or to its workers. The latter
were not allowed to patent except as the Council might direct; on
the other hand, they were not under any obligation to patent.

The subject was reopened in 1938, particularly as a result of the
Council's decision to promote research in chemotherapy on a much
increased scale. This made it probable that important new compounds would be produced by chemists working in the service of the
Council, and the whole question of relations with manufacturing
firms was raised in a new form. It had in any event become apparent
that synthetic chemicals were likely to bulk more largely in the
medical field than had been contemplated during the earlier discussions, which had turned largely on objections to the patenting of
biological inventions. If the Council were to embark on a system of
patenting, was this to be strictly confined to synthetic compounds or
would it extend to biological substances? In either event, what
arrangements should be made for administering the rights, both at
home and abroad? As already mentioned, no immediate agreement
could be reached; and the whole question soon fell into abeyance,
mainly as a result of increasing preoccupation with emergency work
relating to the Second World War.

By 1942, however, the subject of patents covering inventions made
by research workers in Government service had become important
for various reasons and was being considered by the Scientific
Advisory Committee of the War Cabinet. To this body the Council
presented a short memorandum, expressing *inter alia* its considered
view that, in the existing state of the law, "the only satisfactory
solution of the difficulties associated with patenting the results of
medical research is to be found in the establishment of a suitable
body of national trustees prepared to accept dedicated patents and
to administer them solely in the public interest". This was in effect
the alternative proposal to which the Council had given qualified
support in 1928, but now shorn of the provision—found in 1931 to
be unacceptable—that in the medical field the dedication of patents
should be compulsory. A similar proposal, but limited to inventions
arising from state-aided research, had been unsuccessfully advocated
by an Interdepartmental Committee in 1921; and there was a
precedent, although non-governmental, in the Research Corporation
registered in New York in 1912.

The post-war outcome was that in 1949, under the Development
of Inventions Act 1948, a National Research Development Corporation was set up under the general supervision of the Board of
Trade with the functions:

(a) of securing, where the public interest so requires, the development or exploitation of inventions resulting from public research, and of any other invention
as to which it appears to the Corporation that it is not being developed or
exploited or sufficiently developed or exploited;

(b) of acquiring, holding, disposing of and granting rights (whether gratuitously
or for consideration) in connection with inventions resulting from public

research and, where the public interest so requires, in connection with inventions resulting from other sources.

Some modifications were made by the amending Acts of 1954 and 1965.

The establishment of the Corporation was of course greatly welcomed by the Council. Its existence provided a means of dedicating patents to a body that would handle them as trustees acting in the public interest; and it also relieved the Council of the practical difficulty of administering patent rights. The arrangement likewise met the wishes of the British pharmaceutical industry by facilitating commercial development of the results of state-aided research, and particularly the results arising from scientific cooperation between the Council and manufacturing firms. Earlier, in 1942, the Therapeutic Research Corporation of Great Britain Limited, representing the common research interests of a number of firms, had made some suggestions to the Council with a view to effecting a change in the latter's attitude on the question of patents. Some misgivings, too, had been expressed by the Treasury lest the meagre use made of patenting in the medical field should be causing a loss of dollar-earning opportunities which the country badly needed. It had to be pointed out, in reply, that there were various reasons, other than any professional view, why medical patents were not more numerous; notably, the results of medical research were very often not patentable, consisting of discoveries of natural phenomena, the practical application of which might be possible by the use of processes having no particular novelty. Nevertheless, the rapid growth of work in chemotherapy was inaugurating a new era of medical research in which patentable inventions were becoming common.

The procedure adopted by the Council was that any of its workers making a potentially useful invention would be not only allowed, but if need be encouraged, to apply for a patent, first entering into a formal agreement to assign the ensuing rights to the Council or, on the Council's instructions, direct to the National Research Development Corporation. Official assistance was provided in making application, and if this were successful the subsequent course followed the terms of the agreement. This applied to new items of equipment as well as to medicinal substances and the like.

Patents held by the Corporation in respect of inventions by the Council's workers became increasingly numerous—115 patents or patent applications on the Corporation's active register at the end of March 1970—and some of them yielded substantial profits. In these profits the Council always declined to share, on the ground that motives of gain—even to its research funds—should not have the least suspicion of a role in shaping its programme. A point was reached, however, when it seemed unreasonable to deny some financial reward to the inventors themselves, when considerable profits accrued from their researches. Most of the research workers concerned were not members of the medical profession, and those who were did not necessarily regard patenting as unethical; in many other employments their claim to a share of the profits—sometimes even to the whole—would have been accepted without question. The principle was accordingly agreed; and it was thought that the Council and the directors of its establishments could ensure that the existence of financial incentives in certain directions did not divert members of the staff from scientifically more important but commercially less profitable lines of work.

So, with Treasury approval of the scheme, the Council minuted in 1961 "that awards should be payable to members of staff named in Council patents which had earned net royalties and also to those, whether or not they were members of staff, who could not be named as patentees but had contributed by their original work to the development of an invention". An Awards Committee was set up, with the Secretary of the Central Committee on Awards to Inventors as a member (the Treasury's suggestion), and with an assessor from the National Research Development Corporation. It was further minuted "that normally the maximum award should be £2000 tax free to any one individual for any one invention or series of related inventions all contributing to the manufacture of one substance or piece of equipment or the development of a new technique".

The British Pharmacopoeia

In 1925 the Council became involved in a question of public concern that related to the presentation of new knowledge rather than to its acquisition, and that in fact lay within the sphere of the General Medical Council (General Council of Medical Education and Registration of the United Kingdom). This statutory body was required by successive Medical Acts "to cause to be published under their direction" a *British Pharmacopoeia* containing descriptions of and standards for preparations and articles used in medical practice. Editions of this work appeared after long intervals and even then did not reflect the results of recent research. This was not surprising as the work was on each occasion compiled by a committee chosen by the General Council from among its own members, who were appointed primarily on other grounds and so included few, if any, experts in materia medica or therapeutics. Moreover, the avowed policy was to record and codify what was habitual in practice, rather than to give guidance. The opinions of expert bodies were indeed canvassed before a new edition was prepared, but it was said that these views were with almost equal regularity rejected and ignored; there was indeed a general attitude of opposition to change. Publication was therefore greeted in many circles with derision and protest. To make matters worse, the authority of the book extended to the Dominions and Colonies; objections were particularly vocal in Canada, where damaging comparisons with the corresponding United States publications were made. Opinions were being expressed in Whitehall that the responsibility should be removed from the General Medical Council altogether, although that would have required legislation.

The matter was brought to a head when a large group of "teachers and investigators in Pharmacology and Therapeutics" presented the Medical Research Council with a reasoned statement of the need for reform. This was transmitted to the Lord President, the Earl of Balfour, who personally saw the President of the General Medical Council, Sir Donald MacAlister—a dominating personality who had already held the position for over twenty years. Immediately thereafter the General Medical Council invited a number of bodies to send representatives to confer with the Pharmacopoeia Committee appointed to prepare the next edition of the book.

The conference was held on 23 February 1926, MacAlister being in the chair and having with him eleven other members of the Pharmacopoeia Committee (who observed strict silence throughout, except that the privately printed verbatim report indicates that at one point they murmured assent to some statement by their leader). The Ministry of Health, the Royal Society, the Medical Research Council and nine societies representing medicine, chemistry or pharmacy were represented by delegates. These presented a great weight of opinion in favour of drastic reform; in particular they urged that the preparation of the work should be entrusted to an expert body appointed for the purpose and assisted by a permanent staff keeping abreast of the subject between editions.

The outcome was a request from the General Medical Council to the Lord President that he should appoint a committee of inquiry to consider what action should be taken. By using the convenient machinery then available (Volume One), a British Pharmacopoeia Sub-Committee of the Committee of Civil Research was set up under the chairmanship of Mr H. P. (later Lord) Macmillan, KC, with four other members. This body advised that the work should be entrusted to an expert Pharmacopoeia Commission, of which the members should be periodically appointed by the General Medical Council on the recommendation of a Selection Committee consisting of representatives of the General Medical Council itself, the Medical Research Council and the Pharmaceutical Societies of Great Britain, of Northern Ireland, and of Ireland. This was accepted; the other necessary reforms were introduced; and a new edition of the *British Pharmacopoeia* is now issued once in five years, with an Addendum (or more than one) in the intervening period.

As mentioned elsewhere (Chapter 12), certain biological standards are maintained by the Council for the purposes of the *British Pharmacopoeia*, in respect of substances for which statutory standards are not provided.

Clinical evaluation of remedies
When a new remedy has given promising results in laboratory tests, it becomes necessary to submit it to clinical trial before it can be

launched as part of the recognised armamentarium of the medical profession at large. This decisive step is not always easily taken, as it involves considerations of several kinds. In the first place, the use of human subjects raises ethical questions for the clinician, such as have been discussed earlier (Chapter 2). In the second place, there are the scientific requirements of a test that will give an unequivocal answer; unless the effects are highly dramatic, as in saving life where death was previously inevitable, only trial under the conditions of a controlled experiment will serve the purpose.

At one time, also, a practical difficulty lay in the reluctance of clinicians—perhaps particularly in the British profession—to make trial of products for commercial laboratories, and especially to put their names to reports on these for publication. They presumably feared that direct association with the pharmaceutical industry, especially if any subsidy of the clinical work were involved, might lay their impartiality open to suspicion. Whether this attitude was justifiable or not, its existence is a historical fact.

It was in these circumstances that the Council in 1931, after receiving representations by the Association of British Chemical Manufacturers, decided to set up a Therapeutic Trials Committee. This body was charged with the operation of a scheme whereby new remedies could be submitted by academic or commercial laboratories, at home or abroad, for clinical trial; the nature and composition of the substance had of course to be stated, with particulars of the laboratory tests on which the claim for its efficacy was based. Those accepted were then to be allotted to clinicians, usually at more than one centre, for trial under prescribed or agreed conditions. Finally, a statement of the clinical evidence and the conclusions based on it would be published in the medical press as reports to the Committee by those who had made the trials. Where the clinical evidence was unfavourable to putting the remedy on the market, the report was communicated privately to the manufacturers and did not have to be published unless the Committee considered the negative finding to be of value in itself.

The Therapeutic Trials Committee was a large body, with a formidable representation of clinical, pharmacological and statistical expertise. It was also high-powered in the sense that the inclusion of men of eminence in medical practice gave a stamp of professional approval to the proceedings. The secretary throughout was Dr F. H. K. Green of the Council's headquarters staff; apart from what was said in annual reports of the Council, he twice (1944, 1954) published general accounts of the scheme—on the second occasion, a Bradshaw Lecture delivered before the Royal College of Physicians of London, in a context of scholarly discussion of the whole subject of clinical evaluation of remedies. Dr A. (later Sir Austin) Bradford Hill usefully discussed (1952) the proper relationship between the statistician and his clinical colleagues in the arrangement of clinical trials, a matter in which he played a great part on the Council's behalf.

Important drugs that were successfully launched into practical medicine by reports to the Therapeutic Trials Committee in the period 1933–39 included calciferol for rickets (J. C. Spence), digoxin for auricular fibrillation (E. J. Wayne), 'prontosil' and sulphanila-mide for septicaemia (L. Colebrook and others), and stilboestrol for menstrual disorders (P. M. F. Bishop and others). During the Second World War the Committee was allowed to lapse; it had become so large as to be unwieldly, and the whole procedure of the scheme occupied too long a time. Moreover, the success of the venture had made the clinical trial of commercial products respectable in pro-fessional eyes; manufacturers were thus enabled to make their own arrangements direct with clinicians, and the latter published reports of the trials on their own responsibility and with some saving of time. The operation of the official scheme had meanwhile set a standard for the methods of trial and the form of the report, although something more like a pilot trial now often sufficed.

The Council's subsequent policy was to set up special committees to organise trials of particular remedies or methods of treatment when this seemed to be advisable. Notably, there was the Peni-cillin Clinical Trials Committee, already mentioned. Among the sponsored investigations was the investigation at fourteen centres, coordinated by Professor R. V. Christie, of the value—and proper dosage—of penicillin in treating subacute bacterial endocarditis; in this instance, as there could be no thought of withholding a hopeful remedy from any patient, the invariably fatal outcome of the un-treated disease provided a valid retrospective control.

There followed a period during which trials of new drugs acting on the tubercle bacillus had a prominent part. The first of these remedies, already mentioned, was an antibiotic discovered in America in 1944 and named streptomycin. As the Report for 1945–48 said, this latest 'miracle drug' was hailed in the international press "in terms of hyperbole which too often omitted reference to its limitations and possible ill-effects"; and the ready availability of streptomycin in the United States, together with the wide publicity, "had the unfortunate and paradoxical effect of restricting the oppor-tunities for controlled tests of its value in that country". In Britain, however, there was in 1946 no practicability of substantial pro-duction; and the authorities were unwilling to permit the use of dollars for importing more than small quantities until controlled trials had confirmed the practical value of the drug and determined the magnitude of the attendant risks. It thus fell to the Council, at the request of the Ministry of Health, to organise careful clinical tests; and for this purpose two directing committees, concerned respectively with tuberculosis and with certain other conditions, were set up. The results confirmed that streptomycin had "a more powerful effect against the tubercle bacillus in the living body than any therapeutic agent hitherto tested". The tuberculosis trials were organised for the special committee, at a number of centres, by the

Council's Tuberculosis Research Unit (with Dr P. D'Arcy Hart as its director and Dr Marc Daniels as his deputy). In hitherto invariably fatal conditions such as tuberculous meningitis and miliary tuberculosis, it was unnecessary—and would have been unjustifiable —to include untreated controls; a proportion of patients restored to health was proof in itself that the remedy had value. Pulmonary tuberculosis, with its variable course and tendency to spontaneous improvement, presented quite a different problem; but in view of the shortage of supplies in Britain at that time, in relation to the large number of available subjects, it was permissible to make a rigidly controlled trial, comparing bed-rest plus streptomycin with bed-rest alone, in young adults with rapidly advancing bilateral tuberculosis unsuitable for collapse therapy. Patients satisfying the agreed criteria were allotted to one group or the other by random selection; and the X-ray findings were assessed by experts unaware of the groups to which particular patients belonged.

Later, similar strict assessments were made of other drugs or combinations of drugs. These newer remedies included the Swedish p-aminosalicylic acid (PAS) and the American isoniazid. The extensive series of tests was in continuous evolution for several years, and it included long-term follow-up observations. One of the major conclusions was that none of the existing chemotherapeutic agents should be used alone, because the rapid development of microbial resistance in that event might limit its action and prevent its successful use later in combined therapy.

In its report for 1948–50 the Council made this general comment:

> With the increased possibilities of specific drug treatment in tuberculosis, and the development of statistical methods in medicine, had come the realisation that a proper and rapid clinical assessment of promising new drugs is imperative. Medical history is littered with the remains of erroneously favoured remedies for this disease. Tuberculosis is protean in character, running a not easily predictable course, and subjective methods of assessment are bound to lead to gross errors.

It is further remarked that the experience gave the Tuberculosis Research Unit the opportunity to improve the technique of the statistical design and analysis of controlled trials, and so to increase the precision with which it was possible to define the value and limitations of different treatments. Trials of vaccines in prophylaxis against tuberculosis are mentioned later.

The Council has also arranged therapeutic trials of various other remedies in different diseases. These have included a number of new antibiotics in the treatment of infections of the respiratory and alimentary tracts. Mention has already been made of a special committee appointed jointly by the Council and the Nuffield Foundation to arrange for trial of the action of cortisone and ACTH in some of the diseases for which these hormones had been recommended. In this instance, a first result was to show that the claims made for cortisone as a remedy in early cases of rheumatoid arthritis had been pitched much too high—a finding on which one consultant made the comment: "Anyhow, it works in private practice."

Application of the methods of the statistically controlled trial were decisive in exploding the claims made for certain methods of treating such minor ailments as, in particular, the common cold. Here it was permissible to carry the principle of control to its ideal extreme, where neither the patient nor the doctor and nurses knew whether the remedy or an inert substance was being administered to particular subjects; this information was held by an independent party until the trial had been completed. In such a 'blind' test of an antihistaminic drug against the common cold in over 1500 volunteers, not only was the result no better in the treated group than in the control group, but the same side-effects were attributed by the subjects to the remedy and to the inert tablet—as Green said, "a vivid demonstration of the importance of psychosomatic factors as a complication in the assessment of remedies".

In 1962 the question of testing new drugs for toxicity came into prominence. Although testing for immediate toxic effects is an obvious routine step to be taken before introducing any new drug, it is more difficult to guard entirely against the possibility of cumulative or delayed results. Still more subtle is the relatively remote chance that a drug administered to a pregnant woman, without harm to herself, may be injurious to the foetus—as in the well known instance of the German thalidomide, which in fact drew special attention to the problem at this time.

The Council had to determine its attitude, and after full consideration decided that it must not become involved in the routine screening of drugs for possible toxicity; the responsibility for that should remain with the manufacturers. On the other hand, it was within the proper function of the Council to promote research into the methodology of toxicity testing and to this extent it had a general responsibility for the subject. It was thought that an effort should be made to produce a recommended pattern of testing for toxicity; and for this purpose the Council set up a Committee on Research on the Toxicity Testing of Drugs under the chairmanship of Sir Charles Harington. The Council also appointed an *ad hoc* committee under the chairmanship of Sir Robert (later Lord) Platt to advise on arrangements for bringing to light toxic reactions produced by drugs in man in the course of practice; some of the recommendations were implemented when in 1963 the Health Departments set up the Safety of Drugs Committee under the chairmanship of Sir Derrick Dunlop.

On the research side, the Council had its machinery in the Division of Biological Standards, and the complementary Division on Immunological Products Control, at the National Institute for Medical Research; in its Toxicology Research Unit; and in its Unit for the Experimental Investigation of Behaviour, which had in its programme a study of the effects of drugs on behaviour in animals.

While considering this subject in 1962, the Council also reviewed its policy with regard to therapeutic trials of the efficacy of drugs and minuted a restatement as follows:

> That full-scale co-operative therapeutic trials were likely to be necessary only when issues of major importance to medical practice arose and, consequently, that the Council must remain entirely free to decide whether or not to undertake the trial of a particular drug;
>
> "that usually when the therapeutic trials were clearly desirable on medical grounds, these could be arranged directly between the manufacturer and individual physicians; and
>
> "that in the case of new drugs which were only minor variants of existing types it was justifiable to leave the assessment of their therapeutic efficacy to the accumulation of experience in practice."

It was not only for new remedies that therapeutic trials were useful; many well established remedies have never been properly evaluated, even if there may be different schools of thought on which of two or more is preferable for a particular purpose. It has not been unknown, within quite recent times, for physicians in charge of adjacent wards in the same hospital to favour different treatments for an identical condition, without there being any objective measure of their comparative success.

Sometimes, indeed, the circumstances render a comparison extremely difficult to make. This is particularly true of methods of treating different forms of cancer. In that disease it is ethically impossible to withhold from a patient any form of treatment that may help his condition. Sometimes, moreover, two or more forms of treatment (e.g. surgery, radiotherapy, hormone therapy) may be used in combination; or it may be thought advisable to make a change in method during the course of treatment. In recent years, however, there has been a growing practice of comparing different combinations of well established treatments by means of controlled trials. In 1958 the Council appointed a Committee for the Evaluation of Different Methods of Cancer Therapy, with Sir Brian Windeyer as chairman. This body then delegated particular investigations to separate working parties; some reports have been published, and some of the inevitably protracted investigations are still in progress.

Evaluation of prophylactics

The assessment of preventive preparations, such as vaccines, presents a problem differing in several ways from that of therapeutic trials. The trial is made on healthy subjects merely exposed to the general risk of contracting the disease, not with patients who already have it. And as only a small proportion would in any event be attacked, the total brought within the trial must be relatively enormous; for if the effect of a good vaccine is to reduce the annual attack rate from, say, 2·0 to 0·5 per thousand, it is obvious that many thousands must be vaccinated to yield statistically valid proof of even such a dramatic result as a 75 per cent reduction. Moreover, as the possible attack may come soon or late, the follow-up period must usually extend for some years, during which all the subjects have to be kept in view; and this is the more true if it is desired to ascertain the duration of the protection, or the rate at which it deteriorates.

With these considerations in mind the Council has promoted a number of large-scale trials of prophylactics since the Second World War. In this it has had the cooperation of the Health Departments and of local medical officers of health, together with the invaluable help of the Public Health Laboratory Service. Three examples may be mentioned, beginning with the trials organised by the Council's Whooping-Cough Immunisation Committee, reports to which were published in 1956 and 1959. Pertussis vaccines were administered to 28 799 children; and after a first series had given poor results, a second showed that the vaccine could confer a substantial degree of protection over at least $2\frac{1}{2}$–3 years.

Secondly, the Council's Tuberculosis Vaccines Clinical Trials Committee organised trials of BCG and vole bacillus vaccines in adolescents. The background was that the Bacillus-Calmette-Guérin vaccine against tuberculosis was widely used and generally esteemed in other countries, but had never been submitted to properly controlled trial; there was therefore no real evidence of the part, if any, that it had played in reducing the incidence of the disease. The vole vaccine was one prepared by Dr A. Q. Wells, of the Council's staff, from a murine type of the tubercle bacillus. The work was organised by the Council's Tuberculosis Research Unit and began in 1950; reports were published in 1956, 1959 and 1963. Volunteers were sought among final year pupils at secondary modern schools, over two years, and these were clinically and radiographically examined to exclude those who already had signs of tuberculosis, inquiries being also made to exclude still others who had known contacts with the disease at home. The 56 700 included were tuberculin tested; the minority showing a positive reaction were not vaccinated, but kept in view. Of those who were tuberculin negative, some were vaccinated with one vaccine, and some with the other, while those in a third group were designated as controls. The follow-up showed that both vaccines very substantially reduced the incidence of tuberculosis, as compared with that among the controls (who had also been tuberculin negative at the outset); and that the protection was well maintained for several years.

In the third instance the Council's Poliomyelitis Vaccines Committee reported in 1957 on a trial of British vaccine made by the Salk method from inactivated viruses of the three main types. As mentioned earlier (Chapter 7), this differed from the American product in the substitution of another strain of virus for a more virulent one that had given trouble; it was also desired to try the vaccine on age-groups of children not covered by the American data. All but two of the numerous local health authorities in Great Britain agreed to cooperate, and the vaccinations were done in their clinics. In response to the call to parents in the autumn of 1955, nearly two million children born in the period of 1947–54 were registered, this being almost a third of the total in that age-group. Vaccine being then in short supply, there was no ethical question about a control group; 148 684 children, selected by months of birth, each received two injections. The follow-up showed that the incidence of paralytic poliomyelitis among the vaccinated, during the next year, was about a fifth of that among the unvaccinated.

A subsequent trial, of a poliomyelitis vaccine prepared by the Sabin method from an attenuated living virus and administered orally, exemplifies a different method. Here the criterion was the antibody response in the blood after a short interval. For this purpose only a few hundreds of children had to be tested, and no long follow-up was involved. The trials were made by 17 laboratories of the Public Health Laboratory Service; and the report, which confirmed the other, was published in 1961.

Chapter 12
Biological Standards

Biological assay and standardisation—International action on standards—
British legalisation on standards—The Council's responsibility for standards—
Immunological products control—Future policy on standards—standardisation
of laboratory methods

Biological assay and standardisation

The modern development of powerful therapeutic and prophylactic
agents has increased the need for accurate dosage, which in turn
must be based on a valid method of assay. For many substances, such
methods are not provided by the ordinary procedures of chemistry
and physics; they call for special techniques in which potency is
measured in terms of biological effects, compared with those of a
recognised standard preparation. This need has arisen in respect of
some of the older pharmacological substances and a few synthetic
compounds, and widely in respect of hormones, vitamins, antibiotics and immunological preparations. Biological standardisation
has thus become an important subject in its own right; and the
Council has been closely concerned with it from the beginning.

In its Report for 1919–20 the Council had, as for several years
following, a special section entitled "The Determination of Biological Standards and the Methods of Biological Assay and Measurement". This opened with a recapitulation:

> From the beginning of their work in 1914 the Medical Research Committee,
> in surveying the needs of the medical sciences, realized that in many directions
> progress was being delayed for want of fixed standards of measurement and of
> means for their ready application. Without accurate quantitative work little
> secure advance can be made in any branch of science, and the establishment
> of bases for this must usually require special and laborious researches. The
> rapid onset of war at that time made it impossible for the Committee to pro-
> mote any comprehensive scheme of work in this direction, yet war in itself
> brought immediate illustration not only of the need and value of biological
> standards of measurement but also of our grave national deficiencies in this
> respect.

In December 1916 the Committee had, in a Memorandum prepared by request of the Government's Reconstruction Committee
(Volume One), urged the desirability of taking action towards
setting up official standards of value and authenticity for certain
drugs such as arsenicals of the salvarsan type and for the numerous
biological preparations used in medical practice; and it expressed

the view that the existing absence of possibilities of control was "discreditable to our national position in the world of science and a source of grave danger to the community." The assessment of such products as antidiphtheria and antitetanus sera had been wholly dependent on German or American standards, the former no longer available. The Committee therefore urged "the establishment of a Government laboratory for biological standardization as needed for national purposes no less important than those of an analogous kind fulfilled by the National Physical Laboratory".

Early in 1919 the Committee was requested by the Local Government Board (about to be merged in a new Ministry of Health) to prepare a fuller statement of the need for a national system of biological standardisation, of the urgency of further research in preparation for this, and of the methods by which such a system could best be applied both as an indispensable aid to scientific work and for the practical purposes of national safety. The memorandum submitted by the Committee outlined the legislation that would be required, and again stated the need for a "National Laboratory for Biological Standards". In the following year a Departmental Committee was advising the Minister of Health on the administrative and legislative measures that might be necessary for controlling biological substances in medical use; and on this the Council was represented by Dr H. H. (later Sir Henry) Dale.

The outcome, for the Council, was that biological standardisation became a special function of the National Institute for Medical Research; and in that aspect it is mentioned in Volume One. The Council had indeed eagerly seized the opportunity of taking a lead in a subject that had become ripe for development just as its own organisation was getting under way. Such work has ever since formed an important item in the Council's programme, as a matter both of scientific policy and of official obligation. In brief, apart from questions of toxicity or sterility, the measurement of potency presents the central problem; as a basis for dosage, there must be a quantitative expression that can be related to a given weight or volume of the preparation. Many of these remedies, however, are not pure substances, and the composition of their active principles may not even be known; direct chemical tests being thus inapplicable, the methods of assay are necessarily biological. The crux is that such methods cannot themselves be adequately standardised; and so the principle of bioassay is to compare, side by side, the activities of the test preparation and those of a standard preparation of which the potency has been expressed in defined units. The principle dates from work on antitoxins by Ehrlich, in Germany, towards the close of the last century; but it had only a narrow application until some thirty years later.

Until 1914 the Germans held a monopoly, protected by world-wide patents, in the manufacture of the arsenical compounds salvarsan and neosalvarsan, used in the treatment of syphilis. On the outbreak of war these important drugs ceased to be available in the British Isles, apart from stocks in hand, and the Board of Trade therefore suspended the enemy rights in the British patents and granted manufacturing and import licences, respectively, to one British and one French firm. A condition of the licences was that samples of every batch produced should be submitted for biological tests by the Medical Research Committee. The testing was at first done by the Council's Department of Biochemistry and Pharmacology; but in time, after the war, the manufacturers were left to perform the tests in their own laboratories, submitting protocols to the Institute and being subject to occasional checks. Of this first example it may be noted that the object was to guard against undue toxicity rather than to measure therapeutic efficacy; and also that the authority for official control rested at that date on the conditions of licences granted under patent rights. The firms, incidentally, were helped by information that the testing scientists were able to supply.

Biological standardisation became an acute international problem with the introduction of insulin in 1921. Here was a substance produced naturally in the body and obtainable for medicinal use only in impure extracts of the pancreas of animals. In appropriate dosage it had life-saving effects in diabetes, but either too much or too little could be disastrous for the patient. It was therefore essential that the strength of every preparation should be expressed in accurate quantitative terms, and so biological tests had to be devised. In this work the National Institute for Medical Research played a very important part, but it also had a specific function in controlling the products of the British manufacturers. The authority for this again rested on patent rights; the original method of preparation had been patented by the discoverers on behalf of the University of Toronto, and the latter had assigned the British rights to the Council. The manufacturing firms that wished to participate received licences from the Council, without royalty but under conditions that ensured control in the public interest and prohibited sale under any but the proper name.

International action on standards

The subject soon began to broaden out, as there were already other medicinal agents in immediate need of standardisation and still more were likely to emerge from the research stage in the early future. International meetings to discuss the problem were held at Edinburgh in 1923 and at Geneva in 1925, and at these Dr Dale and Professor Thorvald Madsen of Copenhagen won agreement for the principle of comparative biological assay as the only means of measuring the potency of medicinal preparations of the kind in question. The adoption of an international unit for the potency of insulin indeed represented the final victory of Ehrlich's principle of calibration against a standard over the principle of standardising methods of test. Eventually, Dr H. W. Dudley at the National Institute devised a new method of purifying insulin and succeeded in producing a stable dry powder; this preparation was put forward by Dale at the 1923 conference and, after trial in various laboratories meanwhile, was adopted at the meeting two years later.

The other hormone urgently in need of standardisation was the oxytocic hormone of the posterior lobe of the pituitary body. This substance had been known for some time, but it had not been widely used in medicine until Dale's discovery of its very potent activity in stimulating contraction of the uterus. Thereafter, Dr Dale and Dr J. H. Burn compared different commercial preparations which were "all being offered with a presumption of equivalence in their biological activities", as Dale put it, whereas in fact the strongest sample was no less than eighty times as potent as the weakest; these results were published in the Council's series (Burn and Dale, 1922).

These two clear cases, together with immunological products and the arsenicals, provided a sufficient basis for international action. There was thus general acceptance of the policy that standards should be official, and that they should be made widely available under the auspices of the League of Nations; in 1924 the latter set up a Permanent Commission on Biological Standards, which continues in another form to this day.

The responsibility for setting up and safeguarding international standards was divided between the State Serum Institute in Copenhagen, of which Professor Madsen was Director, and the National Institute for Medical Research, represented by Dr Dale. To the former were allotted the immunological products, beginning with diphtheria and tetanus antitoxins; and to the latter went all the others, including insulin, pituitary extracts and arsenicals. This arrangement has continued ever since, the two Institutes between them having custody of standards for the whole world. The Council, for its part, entered into a formal contract with the League of Nations, and later with the World Health Organisation of the United Nations.

British legislation on standards
International agreement having been reached at a scientific level, it remained for the several countries to give statutory force to these methods of biological control of medicinal preparations. In the United Kingdom the Council made representations to the Government, and in 1920 a Departmental Committee was appointed by the Minister of Health, with Dr Dale and Dr C. J. (later Sir Charles) Martin as members representing the Council. The report of this body led eventually to the passage of the Therapeutic Substances Act 1925 (Volume One).

This measure was "to provide for the regulation of the manufacture, sale, and the importation of vaccines, sera, and other therapeutic substances . . . being substances of which the purity or potency cannot be adequately tested by chemical means". The Council was mentioned in the Act as appointing a member of an advisory committee to assist a joint committee of ministers in framing regulations; and the National Institute was later repeatedly mentioned in the Regulations as the custodian of this or that standard preparation. The Council was thus given a statutory responsibility for the preparation and custody of British national standards. In practice, the help afforded to the licensing authority went far beyond this: detailed scientific advice was given on the framing of the Regulations and on methods of control; the protocols of the manufacturers' tests were examined and occasional check testing was undertaken; and members of the scientific staff participated with medical officers of the Ministry of Health in the inspection of the manufacturers' premises and methods.

The substances listed in the original Schedule to the Act were: (1) a large class of immunological preparations; (2) arsenical drugs of the salvarsan type; (3) insulin; and (4) posterior pituitary hormone.

The Act came into force in 1927, and the first Regulations in 1931; by the latter date it had been found possible to make specific provision for a good number of the immunological preparations, and surgical catgut had also been added. The scientific work was well ahead, and standard preparations were available at the National Institute before the Act created an active demand for them. Consolidated Regulations were issued in 1952 and again, with many amendments to earlier provisions, in 1963. The Therapeutic Substances Act 1956 had consolidated the original measures with later legislative restrictions aimed at checking indiscriminate use of antibiotics and the consequent aggravation of the problem of resistant strains of bacteria.

The Council's responsibility for standards

The Council thus acquired in various ways a responsibility not only for all the British Standards but also for certain International Standards held either at the National Institute itself or in Copenhagen. To these were added some standards held for the purposes of the *British Pharmacopoeia*. Further, from time to time, standards have been set up for substances that are not produced commercially but are used in biological research; the availability of these standards avoids waste of effort on the part of investigators, who are enabled to put their observations on a quantitative basis.

In its Report for 1933–34 the Council referred to the much needed introduction of standards for the measurement of the different vitamins in terms of units of activity, in view of the large number of preparations that had been offered to the public without proper quantitative indications. International Conferences on Vitamin Standardisation were held in London in 1931 and 1934 under the auspices of the League of Nations, Dr Edward Mellanby being chairman of both. In the next Report there was a reference to the need to introduce standards for sex hormones, of which preparations were coming increasingly into therapeutic use. Later there arose an obvious need for the standardisation of a new class of therapeutic substances, the antibiotics; penicillin was scheduled under the Act in 1944. More recent additions to the list of standards held at the National Institute have included various preparations of human blood, certain enzymes, and certain substances used in research.

Dale was the Council's chief scientific adviser in the early days of biological standardisation, and he was largely responsible for initiating policy in this field, including the international aspect, and for directing the first phases of the work on the subject at the National Institute. As the task developed, however, it became necessary to create a special Department for it and to bring in another senior worker to take charge; and so in 1922 Dr (later Sir) Percival Hartley joined the Council's staff for this purpose—Hartley and Dale had earlier been colleagues at the Wellcome Physiological Research Laboratories. There has been a succession of distinguished heads of this department (or division) since his day, but it was Hartley who established its scientific work on a firm footing and who first developed the administrative procedures in conjunction with medical and other officers of the Ministry of Health. At a typical meeting with such officers, Hartley would open the discussion with an extremely lucid dissertation lasting for perhaps twenty minutes, on occasion perhaps forty; when he had finished there was little or nothing left for anyone else to say except to express agreement, so much was he master of his subject. Yet he constantly worried beforehand lest there might be some hidden flaw in his data or his reasoning—but there never was. Hartley was a biochemist and microbiologist, not medically qualified; he became a Fellow of the Royal Society and was knighted. He was an eager man, of medium height, rubicund in countenance with (at first) gingery hair and moustache. He was eminently sociable and could be a jovial companion on occasion, although somewhat irascible when worried; he had a keen sense of humour, where biological standards were not involved.

Hartley retired in 1946, and thereafter served for a term as a member of the Council. He died in 1957, and there is an obituary by Dale (1957). His successors have been Dr A. A. (later Sir Ashley) Miles, who became Director of the Lister Institute of Preventive Medicine; Dr W. L. M. (later Sir Walter) Perry, who left to be Professor of Materia Medica in the University of Edinburgh and is now Vice-Chancellor of the Open University; Dr D. G. Evans, who became Professor of Bacteriology and Immunology at the London School of Hygiene and Tropical Medicine and succeeded Miles at the Lister Institute; and Dr D. R. Bangham.

At first Hartley's was a one-man Department, including no other senior staff than himself. The policy was to have members of other departments undertake, or collaborate in, research on particular problems. Later the Department became more self-contained, with a substantial staff of its own. The methodology of standardisation has provided good scope for the application of statistical techniques; a pioneer study by Dr J. H. Gaddum, at that time a pharmacologist on the staff of the National Institute, was published in the Council's series in 1933.

Immunological products control

Legal control of commercial products covered by the Therapeutic Substances Act is exercised by the licensing authority, which is a joint committee of the Health Departments. The function of the Council's Department of Biological Standards, apart from the statutory one of holding the standards, is advisory and ancillary in respect of technical aspects. The policy has been to leave the actual laboratory work of bioassay as much as possible to the manufacturers, subject to occasional spot checks of the products offered for sale. It has nevertheless constantly been necessary, during the early days of any new or newly standardised preparation, for the Department to exercise actual laboratory control. The burden of this suddenly and greatly increased when British firms began to make the American (Salk) vaccine against poliomyelitis.

Here the problem was mainly one of safety, because the value of the preparation depended on the antigenic effect of an inactivated strain of the virus. Inadequate inactivation would make the vaccine a dangerous product, liable to cause the disease that it was intended to prevent; but too drastic measures to produce sterility might render the vaccine ineffective in conferring protection. Exploiting this margin was a delicate undertaking and it called for an elaborate system of testing before the material could be certified as fit for use. Yet the scale which the poliomyelitis menace had attained in Britain, much later than it had done in America and Australia, was such as to compel official action almost regardless of cost.

The Council could not set up the required organisation at the expense of research funds. Treasury approval was accordingly obtained for the cost to be borne on the vote of the Ministry of Health, on behalf of which the Council would operate the scheme. This was the origin of the Immunological Products Control Laboratory established in 1955. Space for it was found in the old building of the National Institute at Hampstead and a special staff was appointed. Since then, other control work for the Ministry has been added to the functions of the Laboratory. The whole scientific problem involved in the control of virus vaccines, inactivated or attenuated, was discussed by the Council in its Report for 1966–1967.

Future policy on standards

In 1964 the Council began to review its policy with regard to responsibility for biological standardisation and associated control services. The problem was formulated in the Report for 1963–65:

> When biological standardization was first accepted as an essential part of the control of certain therapeutic substances, it was assumed that it would eventually cease to be needed. The reason for this assumption was the expectation that, whilst newly discovered active substances of biological origin clearly needed the standardization procedure so long as they were available only in the form of crude preparations, the active principles would eventually be obtained in the pure state and would then be adequately assayed by chemical and physical tests. So far, this expectation has been realized for two groups of substances, namely the vitamins and the steroid hormones; these are available in a pure state and are all compounds of relatively simple chemical constitution, so that it has been possible to dispense with biological assays. For these substances, reference compounds (such as those provided by the Council-supported Steroid Reference Collection) instead of biological standards may be needed to facilitate the study of their physical and chemical properties. In other cases, for example insulin and many of the antibiotics, the substances can now be obtained in pure form but, owing to their chemical complexity or for other reasons, chemical and physical tests are still not an adequate substitute for biological assay. In still other instances, namely certain enzymes and immunological products, it seems probable that comparative assay against biological standards will always be needed. Moreover, it must be remembered that there is continued insistence on more complete testing and control of drugs of all kinds intended for use in man; this will inevitably tend to increase the demand for biological standards. Apart from these practical considerations, there is undoubtedly further scope for the application of the methods of biological standardization in research. So long therefore as the present rate of development of medical and biological research continues, the responsibility that the Council have assumed for the establishment, maintenance and distribution of biological standards is likely to become a commitment of increasing magnitude.

One difficulty was that any further major growth of this type of work might upset the scientific balance of the National Institute for Medical Research. In any event, no additional space could be provided for it in the building at Mill Hill, while the old one at Hampstead was thought to be nearing the end of its useful life. On the other hand, there was a historical and in part statutory commitment to the undertaking, and the Council's organisation was even in a world wide context uniquely fitted for the task. There was also an important research interest which the Council would not wish to discard, and there were strong reasons for keeping the two sides in close contact —the research work on standardisation and the more routine services implied in control.

Everything thus pointed to the desirability of moving the Division of Immunological Products Control to the Mill Hill site, in even closer touch with the Division of Biological Standards. A new building to house it would be necessary in any event, and the question naturally arose whether it might not be best to make this big enough to accommodate both Divisions. That would in effect, while releasing some space in the main building of the National Institute, create a separate, but contiguous, institute for biological standardisation and control—one recalls the proposal made by the Medical Research Committee in 1919 for a "National Laboratory for Biological Standards", spoken of as analogous to the National Physical Laboratory. This was one possible answer, but any solution would involve substantial cost. Urgency was added by the likelihood of still further increase in the volume of work through the development of a European Pharmacopoeia and the expected enactment of a Medicines Bill.

As recorded in the Report for 1967–68, the Council therefore set up, jointly with the Health Departments, a working party to examine the problem; and on this the British Pharmacopoeia Commission was also represented. The Working Party reported early in 1958, its main recommendation being that a Standing Committee on the Standardisation and Control of Biological Substances should be established jointly by the Council and the Health Departments to advise on the organisation of the work. Further recommendations dealt with the apportionment of costs between the Council and the Health Departments, and with arrangements for bringing the two Divisions together. The recommendations were accepted by the Council and the Health Departments. The proposals were implemented in 1972 when the National Institute for Biological Standards and Control came into being—housed in the Hampstead building and with Professor D. G. Evans back as overall Director.

Standardisation of laboratory methods
Although the bioassay of medical substances developed on the principle of calibration against standard preparations, the standardisation of methods as such was still useful for some purposes. In its Report for 1922–23 the Council said:

> The standardisation of pathological methods with a view to uniformity of results is another line of investigation; it includes the maintenance of central sources for the supply of standard types of pathogenic organisms and of standard diagnostic and curative sera, and the devising of standard technical methods for the performance of serological and other tests.

The several themes may be briefly exemplified.

In 1917 the Medical Research Committee appointed a Committee on the Standardisation of Pathological Methods (later simply Committee upon Pathological Methods, and precursor of the Council's Bacteriology Committee). This body undertook a number of studies of which the findings were published in the Special Report Series; these dealt with such subjects as the laboratory diagnosis of gonococcal infections, the Wassermann test for syphilis, the reaction of culture media, and the laboratory diagnosis of acute intestinal infections. There was also an international aspect, and Conferences on Serological Standards were held under the auspices of the League of Nations in 1921 and 1922, in London and Paris respectively. As a result of these meetings, the United Kingdom—in effect the Council—undertook to investigate the standardisation of methods for the serodiagnosis of syphilis, and also the standardisation of antidysentery, antipneumococcus and antimeningococcus sera.

The earliest of the Council's schemes under this heading was the Standards Laboratory, established at Oxford by the Medical Research Committee during the First World War. It was originally under the general direction of Professor Georges Dreyer, with Dr A. D. Gardner in charge. The purpose was to meet a demand for reliable serological reagents for the diagnosis and treatment of various infective conditions, including enteric and dysenteric diseases occurring in different theatres of war. The demand continued in time of peace, and the Standards Laboratory for Serological Reagents was accordingly maintained by the Council until it was eventually transferred to the control of the Public Health Laboratory Service; there was a research element that was of some concern to the Council, and a charge was made to meet the cost of the routine provision of supplies. A historical account of these 'Oxford' standards has been published by Bradstreet (1965).

An analogous service arose from the demands of the Second World War, namely a Blood Group Reference Laboratory for the supply of sera for identifying the blood groups of transfusion donors. Since the war the Laboratory has been maintained as an adjunct to the National Health Service; but it has been managed through the agency of the Council, under which it was originally established as an emergency measure. It is housed, now in a special building, at the Lister Institute.

In 1920 the Council formed a National Collection of Type Cultures, "from which biologists in general and bacteriologists in particular might obtain from a trustworthy source authentic strains of recognised bacteria and protozoa for use in scientific work". This provided a basis of reference for the identification and classification of species and strains of microorganisms. The need had not previously been fully met, although before the First World War the collection at the Pasteur Institute in Paris had been helpful to many workers in Europe, and more recently the American Museum of Natural History had established a Culture Bureau. Exchange arrangements were made with the latter; and cultures were presented by many workers both at home and abroad. The Collection was housed at the Lister Institute of Preventive Medicine, and Dr R. St John-Brooks was appointed to the Council's staff as first Curator.

For microorganisms the only practical form of 'type specimen' is a living culture, which has the advantage that subcultures can be made as required and despatched to other laboratories. It has the disadvantage that cultures are liable to various vicissitudes—death, mutation, contamination—although these risks have been reduced since the introduction of freeze-drying made it possible to keep cultures stable in suspended animation. During the Second World War it was in fact found that some items in the Collection had for one reason or another become useless for their purpose, and a long task of reappraisal and replacement had to be undertaken. This led the Council, with the aid of a special subcommittee, to review the functions of the Collection; and from 1944 the policy has been to concentrate on microorganisms of medical and veterinary interest, leaving responsibility for other kinds to appropriate bodies—the resulting scope was shown by the revised catalogue published by the Council in 1958. Meanwhile, in 1947, a national committee (for which the Council provided the secretariat) was set up to coordinate the activities of the various collections; there was also an international body. The Collection, with Dr S. T. Cowan as Curator, was eventually attached to the Central Public Health Laboratory at Colindale; and with the Service it passed from the Council's control in 1961.

A very different kind of reference material—not in fact biological except in significance—is kept in, and issued from, the Steroid Reference Collection, maintained by the Council since 1954 under the supervision of Professor W. Klyne. This was initiated in the Postgraduate Medical School at Hammersmith but has latterly been housed at Westfield College, University of London. The object is to provide specimens of some of the less common steroid compounds for comparison in identification tests by such methods as paper chromatography, including determination in urine and blood. The Council's interest centres on the steroids that are hormone metabolites; since the active principles of various sex hormones have become known as pure substances, chemical methods have replaced bioassay.

Chapter 13
The Public Health Laboratory Service

Origin of the Service—The situation before the Second World War—
Organisation of an Emergency Service—Deployment of the Emergency Service
—Vigilance against possible enemy action—Wartime role of the Laboratories—
New opportunities for research—Establishment of a permanent service—
Organisation—Staff—Finance—Work of the Service—Relations with hospital
aboratories—Achievement of independent status

Origin of the Service

The organisation of a Public Health Laboratory Service for England
and Wales, and its management on behalf of the Ministry of Health
for more than twenty years, was a rather unusual activity for the
Council. It is true that the Service has always engaged in research,
in addition to its primary routine; and it is advantageous from every
point of view that this should be so. It is also true that the officers of
the Council had more experience of administering laboratories than
had those of the Ministry. Later, the special reasons for maintaining
this particular enterprise on a countrywide basis made it unsuitable
for incorporation in a National Health Service organised on regional
principles. Nevertheless, it is unlikely that the Council would have
accepted such a responsibility except, at the outset, as a wartime
emergency function; it was likewise improbable that the arrangement would be permanent, although in fact the Council continued
its stewardship until circumstances were propitious for the creation
of a separate governing body. At no time was the cost of the service
a charge against research funds, being always met from separate
provision borne on the vote of the Ministry.

The idea of a countrywide chain of pathological laboratories was
not new, although earlier suggestions may not have considered the
requirements of public health to be distinct from those of medical
treatment. The need for laboratories for diagnostic work was stressed,
for instance, by some of those who submitted evidence to the Departmental Committee on Tuberculosis in 1912–13. Similarly, in an
essay published by Sir Clifford Albutt in 1921:

> Not only must laboratories be established in all colonies and stations—and, let
> me add, in every English country, a scheme which was provided for by Mr
> Lloyd George in the budget suppressed by the war—but these and other
> workers must be restored to the full stream of official recognition and
> reward.

The reference to budget provision is not strictly accurate, but on
4 May 1914 Mr Lloyd George had made the following remark in

the discussion of a financial statement in the Ways and Means Committee of the House of Commons:

> And here is another deficiency in our health service which has been exposed by the operations of the Insurance Act. There is no provision for the scientific diagnosis of disease. In Germany, in almost every town, and I think in France, you have pathological laboratories, which are of enormous assistance to doctors in ascertaining the real character of a disease when they are in any doubt upon the subject. There are a few boroughs in the United Kingdom where something has been done, even in London, but we propose to make a Grant for the purpose of aiding the local authorities to set up laboratories throughout the United Kingdom. The total of these services for the United Kingdom will be £750 000 in the first complete year.

A little further information was given in reply to parliamentary questions on 14 May, 16 and 24 June, and 2 July 1914. (In a written answer on 13 November 1912 Lord Charles Beresford had been informed by Mr Masterman that the Government had no present intentions of the kind.) After the war, nothing more seems to have been heard of the matter.

Contemporary published statements discreetly gave several reasons for instituting the Service, on an emergency basis, at the beginning of the Second World War. All of these had validity, but the really effective stimulus to official action was in those days not openly mentioned. This was the fear that, in the event of war, the enemy might resort to bacteriological methods of attack. In 1934 Sir Maurice (later Lord) Hankey, as Secretary of the Committee of Imperial Defence, consulted the Secretary of the Council on the subject; he in turn invited three bacteriologists—Professor J. C. G. (later Sir John) Ledingham, Captain S. R. Douglas and Professor W. W. C. Topley—to prepare a confidential assessment of the risks. The resulting memorandum was passed to Hankey, as was a further memorandum drawn up early in 1937 by Professor Ledingham, Professor Topley, and Professor G. S. Wilson, with Dr W. M. Scott and Dr F. Griffith of the Ministry of Health Laboratory.

Although the bacteriologists did not view the risks with much alarm, there was clearly a case for planning countermeasures to be taken in case of need. This led in 1936 to the formation of a sub-committee of the Committee of Imperial Defence, under Hankey's own chairmanship, to consider what should be done; this later became a committee of the War Cabinet, and the present writer was Joint Secretary throughout that stage. The proceedings, and indeed the very existence of such a body, were of course secret at the time.

The precautions recommended by the Committee envisaged the risks not only of deliberate bacteriological warfare or sabotage, but also of widespread epidemics arising from such other possible causes as mass movements of population and disruption of water supplies. The steps recommended included preparations for various hygienic measures, the stockpiling of certain immunological substances not usually available in quantity, and arrangements for the instant mobilisation of an Emergency Public Health Laboratory Service. The first of these tasks fell naturally to the Ministry of Health; the other two were allotted directly to the Council, and up to the outbreak of war the cost was met from civil defence funds. The provision of immunological supplies and also the maintenance of a register of pathologists and pathological laboratory technicians were purely transient tasks of wartime and are dealt with later (Chapter 16).

The situation before the Second World War

To understand fully the urgent need for public health laboratories, one must appreciate how lamentably inadequate was the normal provision of this kind in the period before the Second World War. Moreover, this was especially true of southern England, presumably the area of greatest risk in the event of war. The situation was summarised by the present writer (1943) in these terms:

Modern laboratory methods bring powerful aid to a Medical Officer of Health in the discharge of his responsibility for the control of infectious disease. In performing this important task he is clearly entitled to all the assistance that science can give; yet in actual practice he may count himself fortunate if he is able to call upon a thoroughly efficient public health laboratory service—staffed by trained specialists, adequately equipped and conveniently placed.

The difficulty, so far as Great Britain is concerned, arises incidentally from the way in which public health administration has developed. Executive responsibility rests primarily with local authorities, although general guidance is given by the appropriate departments of the central Government. The communities administered by these local authorities vary greatly in size and resources, ranging from large cities to small or sparsely populated rural districts. Each authority employs its own public health staff, and only the most important can afford to include in this a complete laboratory service.

Most local authorities are thus compelled to rely on such assistance as can be obtained from laboratories intended primarily for other purposes. Many university laboratories, for instance, undertake routine work for neighbouring local authorities, but this function is naturally subordinate to the claims of teaching and research. The work done is of a high technical standard; but it cannot easily extend to the provision of a complete service, including constant availability for personal consultation and for participation in field investigations. Similarly, many hospital laboratories make examinations for public health purposes, but their main work is of a different kind. They are interested in the individual case, with a view to its diagnosis and treatment, rather than in the herd from the standpoint of preventive medicine; their methods are those of clinical pathology, consisting largely of work which is not bacteriological in nature.

In other cases the Medical Officers of Health have to depend on laboratories run on commercial lines and often situated at a distance which precludes personal consultation and may involve serious deterioration of specimens in transit. Or again, the work may be done locally by persons who do not possess the necessary specialised training and experience. In the extreme case laboratory aid may be practically non-existent.

Wilson (1948) has, retrospectively, described the evils of the

postal system from the point of view of a public health bacteriol-
gist. For different reasons the Council had, in its Report for 1923–24
(referring back to that for 1918–19), strongly criticised the arrangement whereby many university departments of pathology were
expected to earn money by undertaking routine work.

The remedy was clearly to provide laboratories to serve groups of
local authorities, each laboratory handling a volume of work that
would justify an adequate establishment. In ordinary times, however, this would have required a series of agreements between
authorities, raising innumerable points of prestige, advantage and
finance. Or it could perhaps have been achieved by the intrusion
of the central government, had the latter in those days been prepared to meet the whole cost. There were in fact strong reasons
in favour of a national basis, one being mobility of staff in times of
stress in particular areas, and another being facility in tracing
epidemic sources across administrative boundaries. Above all, the
laboratories would constitute an epidemiological intelligence service
covering the whole country, for it is often from laboratory reports
that the earliest and most precise information is obtainable. There
were also possibilities of further developing the system whereby
certain types of examination could be referred to specialists, such
as the staff of the small central laboratory then maintained by the
Ministry of Health.

For emergency purposes a public health laboratory service could
be planned only on a national basis—and in the event the country
found itself provided with one almost overnight. The particular
form of emergency envisaged never materialised, but by the end of
the war the service had come to be recognised as an indispensable
part of the permanent machinery for safeguarding the public health.
The gain would have been greater still had the service extended to
the whole of Great Britain, but in Scotland the emergency arrangements were different and transient.

Organisation of an emergency service

The Report for 1938–39, briefly recorded that the service, mobilised
on the outbreak of war, consisted of three central and sixteen subsidiary laboratories in England and Wales under the Council's
direct control; and that ten emergency hospital laboratories on the
outskirts of London, together with six existing university laboratories in the Midlands and North of England, were associated with
the service for public health work. Similar arrangements were made
in Scotland by the Department of Health in consultation with the
Council.

All this was not achieved without much preparatory organisation,
starting more than two years beforehand. The main plan had been
conceived by Professor W. W. C. Topley; and it was elaborated by
him in consultation with various colleagues, some of whom were
later actively engaged in the enterprise. Topley and other bacteri-

ologists also collaborated with the Council's office in giving the plan administrative shape.

As the Report for 1939–45 put it, "The general principle was to utilise existing resources as far as possible, and to a large extent the Service came into being only on paper until the signal for action was given." The Ministry of Health Laboratory in London was to close down, and its small staff provided a nucleus. Otherwise, bacteriologists and technicians for the new laboratories were to be drawn from departments normally engaged in teaching or research. In this way, a staff complement was drawn up in which each member had an allotted place; and meetings were held to explain and discuss what was to be done.

Laboratory accommodation was earmarked in universities, public schools and other institutions. The science departments of schools were often found to be particularly suitable, and visits to many of these in southern England were paid by the organisers with a view to selection. The cooperation of headmasters and science masters was perhaps the more readily given because nothing had to be done except in the event of war, which most of them regarded as unlikely. In two different cases, the concepts of bacteriology were so alien to the scholarship of clerical headmasters that the purpose was envisaged as being to manufacture poison gas—but even so it seemed that they had no objections.

Arrangements were made to borrow some of the initial equipment from institutions that would be sending staff, notably the Ministry of Health Laboratory, the London School of Hygiene and Tropical Medicine, and the Lister Institute. Further equipment was purchased and stored. Provision for transport had also to be made, in addition to the private cars that staff would bring with them. The nucleus of the store comprised six specially purchased vans, each ready loaded with the essential equipment for one laboratory. Only under this head of equipment and transport was any significant expenditure incurred in advance.

The 'war book' of the operation was complete in good time; everyone knew what he or she had to do; final orders were ready for issue. So, on the outbreak of war, it was almost a matter of pressing a button for the Emergency Public Health Laboratory Service to be mobilised at its appointed stations.

Deployment of the emergency service

The Report for 1939–45 describes the deployment of the Service, and its further development during the war in more detail than the scale of the present work permits—but some day the Service should have its own history.

Dr W. M. Scott of the Ministry of Health Laboratory was made Director of the Service. He was at first stationed in the central laboratory at Oxford, which had been designated as the technical and intelligence headquarters of the Service; but it was later found to be administratively more advantageous to attach him to the Council's wartime office in the London School of Hygiene and Tropical Medicine. When Dr Scott, with his colleague Dr F. Griffith, was killed in an air-raid in 1941, Professor G. S. (later Sir Graham) Wilson, who had earlier taken charge at Oxford, was appointed in his place. A full list of the laboratories, with the names of their directors, is given in the Report cited above.

A notable feature of the Service was the provision of reference laboratories to which specimens could be sent from anywhere in the country for certain special types of examination. These were variously placed, either in laboratories of the Service or in different institutions. Their respective subjects were: Vi-agglutination tests and Vi-phage determination of strains in enteric infections; typing of group A streptococci; typing of salmonellae; and the chemical examination of water, milk and sewage. In addition, bacteriologists both within and outside the Service were nominated as specialist referees for particular purposes.

Vigilance against possible enemy action
There was also a Bacterial Sabotage Reference Laboratory at the National Institute for Medical Research, where Mr P. Bruce White examined suspected material of possible enemy origin. This vigilance against bacteriological warfare or sabotage remained a potentially important responsibility of the Emergency Service. The military, the police and others had received instructions to report suspicious actions or findings to the nearest laboratory of the Service; the laboratories made any necessary immediate inquiries and sent the report, with the suspected object or material, to the Reference Laboratory.

Bruce White, a non-medical bacteriologist on the Council's regular staff, threw himself into the work with zest. Nobody could have been better fitted for the task; not only was he highly competent to discover any noxious factor in the specimen, but he enjoyed the detective role and persisted towards a complete identification of the object long after he knew it to be bacteriologically harmless. That most of the suspicions soon proved to be not only baseless but fanciful appealed to his appreciation of the absurd; he had indeed a strong sense of humour, so deadpan that one was often in doubt whether he was serious, was pulling one's leg, or was guying himself.

As a real risk was involved, it would have been unwise to discourage the public from reporting; but, predictably, many of the incidents merely illustrated the extent of human credulity and ignorance. Common objects of natural history were seen, even by countryfolk, as if for the first time. Detached components of articles of commerce aroused wild conjectures—and were not, in fact, always easy to identify precisely. Any unfamiliar object thrown over a garden fence by a passing boy was thought to have been dropped from an aircraft. One lady ascribed such an origin to some kapok dust which she carefully collected from her windowsill after the tenant of the flat above had flapped some item of bedding in the outer air. Examples of that kind, and some of more reasonable suspicions, could be multiplied many times. It must suffice to say that the results of all examinations were negative. No evidence of enemy attempts at bacteriological warfare or sabotage was ever found.

The Council did not wish to be concerned with the study of bacteriological warfare from an offensive angle, even although such methods would not be used except in retaliation—and granting that information of value for defensive purposes might be obtained. Dr P. G. (later Sir Paul) Fildes, of the Council's staff, was seconded to the Ministry of Supply for work on this aspect.

Wartime role of the Laboratories
In fact, the Service was never called upon to deal with any major emergency directly due to the war. On the other hand, the laboratories were increasingly asked to undertake all the public health bacteriological work required by local authorities in their vicinity (in return, at that stage, for a contributory payment based on peacetime expenditure for like purpose); and many of them made investigations for military establishments. In this way, most of the laboratories soon became fully employed; and, as the Report says, "many medical officers of health experienced for the first time the value of the scientific aid which a Service of this kind could bring to the diagnosis, control and prevention of infectious disease".

Some of the problems did indeed arise from wartime circumstances. Thus, outbreaks of diphtheria in village schools were related to the admixture of evacuees and local children. Infectious diseases occurred in the residential and day nurseries that sprang up. Canteens and communal feeding centres presented questions of food hygiene. The military required advice on the purity of water supplies for new camps. The pasteurisation of milk under wartime regulations needed laboratory control. And the use of imported foodstuffs of unusual kinds, such as dried egg, involved added risks of food poisoning.

It was the aim of the Service to maintain a high level of laboratory work, using the most modern methods and calling when necessary on the specialised reference centres already mentioned. Stress was also laid on the availability of staff for personal consultation by medical officers of health, and for participation in field inquiries when desired. Information of epidemiological concern was regularly reported to the intelligence centre, thus greatly assisting the control of widespread outbreaks and the discovery of remote sources of infection. A confidential 'Weekly Summary', a multigraphed document based on reports received, was circulated so that all laboratories might have a general picture; and copies were of course sent to the Ministry of Health and its regional medical officers.

The epidemiological intelligence was enhanced in value because the Service was not content with merely recognising species of organisms, but required an exact definition of the serological or bacteriophage type to which they belonged—and here the reference laboratories played as essential role. This subspecific identification was an invaluable aid to tracing the ultimate sources of carriers of infections causing particular outbreaks.

New opportunities for research
To these routine functions was added the regular participation of the staff in research. As the Report for 1939–45 puts it:

> The benefits of such a system are by no means static but should be cumulative in effect. The Council have naturally regarded the Service not merely as an instrument of routine but as a weapon of research. Organised investigations into epidemiological problems are capable of yielding important additions to fundamental knowledge as well as information of immediate utility. The object is not only to apply existing knowledge, but at the same time also to increase that knowledge and thus constantly to improve and extend the methods of preventive medicine.

The constitution of the Service opened up opportunities of a new and most valuable kind for what was called "group research". By this was meant research on the same subject simultaneously undertaken at one or more laboratories—even many or all of them. Subjects of group research by the Service during the war were nonpulmonary tuberculosis, cerebrospinal meningitis, combined active and passive immunisation against diphtheria, distribution of different types of diphtheria bacillus, the incidence of cross-infections and complications in scarlet fever, neonatal diarrhoea, the bacteriology of dried egg, infective hepatitis, and the infection of cattle with *Brucella melitensis*. The subjects of individual and team research in the same period would greatly extend that list; and, in all, more than seventy scientific reports and papers were published.

Many of these research publications, together with current intelligence, appeared in the *Monthly Bulletin of the Emergency Public Health Laboratory Service*. This periodical, first issued in November 1941, was given a wide free distribution to laboratories and medical officers of health. From October 1943 it was combined with other matter and became the *Monthly Bulletin of the Ministry of Health, London.*

Establishment of a permanent service
It was not surprising that, before the end of the war, the value of a Public Health Laboratory Service for the normal needs of the country was fully recognised. In 1944, accordingly, the Government decided that the Service should be continued on a permanent basis. This decision later received statutory sanctions when Parliament passed the National Health Service Act 1946, which included the following Section:

> 17. The Minister may provide a bacteriological service, which may include the provision of laboratories for the control of the spread of infectious diseases.

and the Minister may allow persons to make use of services provided at such laboratories on such terms, including terms as to the payment of charges, as the Minister thinks fit.

This provision took immediate effect, covering the action already taken, when the measures received the Royal Assent on 6 November 1946 (although the major provisions of the Act did not operate until an "appointed day" two years later).

The Council had in July 1944, with the approval of the Lord President, accepted the invitation of the Ministry of Health to remain responsible for the Service (in England and Wales) for five years in the first instance—a period that was in the event several times extended, although latterly with some reluctance. The task was admittedly outside the ordinary peacetime functions of the Council, but good reason was given in the Report for 1945–48. "The fact that the Council had been primarily responsible both for the initiation and for the development of the Service, together with the hope that its continued administration by a research organisation would best stimulate investigation in the field of epidemiology, prompted them to accept this responsibility."

There was a constitutional implication that at first caused no embarrassment in practice. In this matter the Council was acting as agent for the Ministry of Health, through which the necessary funds were provided, and thus outside the usual ministerial jurisdiction of the Committee of Privy Council for Medical Research. Eventually, as will be seen, difficulty did arise from an adventitious discrepancy in remuneration between members of the Service (aligned with the National Health Service) and bacteriologists on the Council's own research staff (aligned with the universities)—a problem presenting no solution that the Treasury would permit.

Apart from a few reserved questions of general principle, the administration of the Service was from February 1950 delegated to a Public Health Laboratory Service Board, appointed by the Council with its Second Secretary (the present writer) as chairman. This was a convenient arrangement, as the same person had charge of the administrative action to be taken in the Council's office, and was likewise of sufficient standing to deal directly with the higher authorities—the Ministry of Health and the Treasury—in the Council's name. The Board otherwise consisted of one member of the Council, two former members, one bacteriologist from the Council's research staff, the Chief Medical Officer of the Ministry, and a medical officer of health; the Director of the Service attended meetings, as also did two assessors from its senior staff and one observer from the Ministry.

Organisation

At the end of the war the word 'Emergency' was dropped from the title of the Service, and the latter was—without any break in continuity—moulded as quickly as possible into its permanent form.

Members of the staff who had been seconded during the war either returned to their former employment or elected to take appointments with the Service; and further members of staff were engaged, including a number of bacteriologists demobilised or retiring from the Forces.

Dr G. S. Wilson relinquished his chair at the London School of Hygiene and Tropical Medicine in order to continue as Director of the Service. He held the post on its new footing for close on twenty years, retiring late in 1963; he was then succeeded by Dr J. W. (later Sir James) Howie, from the chair of bacteriology in the University of Glasgow. The Director had his office in the Council's headquarters building.

Some of the original constituent laboratories had been closed early in the war period; others were now moved to different localities and some new ones were added. At first most of them were housed in temporary accommodation provided by local authorities, universities or hospitals; a few were in huts or converted houses. Gradually, as permission and finance were obtained, new buildings were put up —commonly in association with hospitals. A standard type of public health laboratory building was designed to the Director's specification, but there was of course much diversity to suit local circumstances. The concept of the ideal laboratory was thereafter progressively developed in the light of experience.

An event of the greatest importance followed the Government's decision to discontinue the production of smallpox vaccine as a public activity, and to rely for supplies on the Lister Institute. The building of the Government Lymph Establishment at Colindale, on the north-western outskirts of London, thus became available and was provided to the Service for a Central Public Health Laboratory. After suitable adaptation, the building was occupied for its new purpose in 1946. Some additional accommodation was built in the grounds; and eventually a much larger building was erected, coming into use in 1953. The Central Public Health Laboratory became virtually an institute of public health bacteriology, attracting visitors and visiting workers from all over the world. Its first Director was Dr Robert Cruickshank, later Professor of Bacteriology in the University of Edinburgh; and his immediate successor, in 1958, was Lieut-Colonel H. J. Bensted.

In addition to a routine diagnostic laboratory serving the adjacent part of Middlesex, the Central Public Health Laboratory comprises most of the reference and special laboratories of the Service. At the close of the Council's period of responsibility in 1961, these numbered ten. There were reference laboratories for cross-infection (incorporating earlier ones for streptococcal and staphylococcal infections respectively), disinfection, dysentery, enteric infections, salmonella infections, and virology. In addition, there were an Epidemiology Research Laboratory, a Food Hygiene Laboratory, the Standards Laboratory for Serological Reagents and the National Collection of Type Cultures—these last two were transferred by the Council to the Service as noted in the preceding chapter.

Elsewhere than at Colindale, four other units were brought into being on various dates: the Mycological Reference Laboratory (London School of Hygiene and Tropical Medicine), the Venereal Diseases Reference Laboratory (London Hospital Research Laboratories), the Tuberculosis Research Laboratory (Institute of Preventive Medicine, Cardiff), and an Epidemiological Research Unit (Cirencester, Gloucestershire).

By 1961 there were 59 ordinary constituent units of the Service, each with the title 'Public Health Laboratory'. Nine of these were classified as regional laboratories and were situated at Bristol, Cambridge, Cardiff, Leeds, Liverpool, Manchester, Newcastle, Oxford and Sheffield. Regional laboratories are mostly staffed by from three to five medically qualified workers, together with junior bacteriologists under training (see later). Each acts to some extent as the parent laboratory of a group of area laboratories, helping the latter in epidemiological or other special inquiries, and providing staff substitutes during periods of leave or illness.

At the end of the war, some pre-existing laboratories that had been associated with the Emergency Service reverted to their former status. In the course of time, however, most laboratories maintained by local authorities were handed over to the Service and so became constituent units. At first there were parts of the country in which the Service could not operate directly, notably Lancashire and Kent, but the cover was gradually extended—although it has never become quite so complete as was at one time contemplated, the Treasury having in 1952 placed a 'ceiling' on the number of laboratories. Some small gaps have been filled by the device of associating hospital laboratories with the Service, the latter making a contribution towards the cost.

Staff

Appointments were made to the permanent Public Health Laboratory Service three years before the National Health Service was established in 1948. Salary scales were accordingly fixed *ad hoc*, with the approval of the Ministry of Health, consistently with the Council's usual standards. When higher rates of pay for hospital pathologists came into force, with eligibility for distinction awards at consultant level, it became imperative for the survival of the Service that its staff should be given equal treatment. It was indeed scarcely conceivable that two groups of bacteriologists with equivalent qualifications and responsibilities should receive different pay from the same Ministry; and it was at least certain that such a situation could not last—indeed the first signs of a 'brain drain' were quickly apparent. Nevertheless, it was not until after much argument that the point was conceded by higher authority; and only later was it accepted as a principle that subsequent pay awards for the National Health

Service must automatically apply. This inevitable conclusion had the unfortunate result of creating a dichotomy in the Council's employment; but this was the lesser of two evils, as the Council's administration of the Service was not expected to last indefinitely.

The structure and functions of the Service, however, demanded a more hierarchical staff organisation than was appropriate to the hospitals. There was a Director of the Service as a whole, and each constituent laboratory had its director. There was also an administrative need for an overall Director of the Central Public Health Laboratory (who might be the director of one of its components); and it came in time to be recognised that the holder of this post should deputise for the Director of the Service in the latter's absence.

The medically qualified staff consisted almost entirely of bacteriologists, with a few epidemiologists for special posts. Except in the specialised reference laboratories, little use was made of science graduates, because the strong epidemiological bias of the Service places those without knowledge of clinical and preventive medicine at too great a disadvantage. The other categories of staff were technical, clerical and maintenance (including transport).

Except for occasional senior men of suitable experience transferring from other employment, the recruitment of bacteriologists to the Service has been almost entirely from young medical graduates who have held their initial 'house' appointments. They are accepted as trainees and retain that status, on a rising salary scale, for five years. During the first year they are attached to the pathological laboratory of a teaching hospital to get all-round experience; during the second they are placed in an area laboratory of the Service to learn the nature of the work; during the third they attend the courses for the Diploma of Bacteriology, in London or Manchester, with all fees paid. In the fourth and fifth years they work in a regional laboratory of the Service and are allowed increasing responsibility.

Members of the technical staff are recruited from boys and girls leaving school when 16–17 years old and having reached a sufficient standard of education. They undergo an apprenticeship system of training for five years, and at appropriate stages take the examinations of the Institute of Medical Laboratory Technology.

In the final year of the Council's responsibility, the medically qualified staff numbered 126, other scientific staff 34, and the technical, clerical and maintenance staff 965.

Finance

Although there was statutory power to levy payments, the policy was to provide the help of the Service free of charge. This was no more than logical in the context of legislation providing full medical care for all at the expense of central funds. Moreover, any system of recovering costs from local authorities would have been practically unworkable and would have severely restricted the effectiveness of the Service. A relatively small amount of work was done outside the normal scope of the free service, and for this charges were made.

The total provided in the Civil Estimates for the cost of the Service in the financial year 1961–62 (during which the Council transferred its responsibility) was £1 506 390, including £82 000 for capital purposes. This was borne on the vote of the Ministry of Health and was accounted for separately from the ordinary expenditure of the Council.

Work of the Service

The routine work is described in the Yearbook of the Service as being "essentially bacteriological, virological and epidemiological". From about 1956, facilities for virological examinations have been widely developed in the Service. Apart from certain tests closely associated with bacteriological and virological investigations, chemical and biochemical tests and histological examinations are not performed.

Specimens are not accepted from private persons but only from medical practitioners, veterinarians, dentists, public health inspectors, and others acting on behalf of medical officers of health or official bodies. The routine specimens fall under the main heads of 'medical' and 'sanitary'. The former are specimens (e.g. sputum, faeces, throat swabs, blood samples) taken for diagnostic purposes from persons suspected of suffering from infectious disease (excluding certain categories falling within the ambit of the hospital service).

'Sanitary' specimens are those submitted for the bacteriological examination of water, shell-fish, watercress, sewage, milk and cream; of processed foods such as ice-cream, artificial cream, and canned foods; and of imported products such as various forms of meat, fish, processed egg, coconut, and fertiliser. The Service normally examines only material as offered to the consumer, but it will of course also examine specimens taken at any stage in production or distribution as part of the investigation of suspected food-borne infection. The Service is ready to give free advice to food manufacturers and processors to assist them in securing the bacteriological safety of their products.

The number of specimens examined is only a rough and partial index of the work done, but in 1961 it was 2 181 832.

The epidemiological side of the work includes not only the investigation of outbreaks of infectious disease but studies of the distribution and behaviour of infective agents throughout England and Wales, and various aspects of the immunisation programme. Field trials of vaccines or other protective agents are carried out from time to time; the trials of whooping-cough vaccine and of poliomyelitis vaccines, made by the Service in collaboration with the Council, established the value of these prophylactics. Supplies of certain immunological agents are distributed through the Service on behalf of the Ministry of Health; and there is also the issue of standard serological reagents for diagnostic purposes, as already mentioned.

Research work of more generalised aim is also actively carried on by the staff of the Service, on the lines described in an earlier section —but of course with a constantly changing subject content.

Relations with hospital laboratories

In the early planning days of the Service, stress was laid on the difference between public health bacteriology and hospital bacteriology, the latter considered as a branch of clinical pathology. This was perhaps to emphasise the valid contention, then not always admitted, that the bacteriological needs of public health could not be fully met by the examination of specimens in hospital laboratories. The hospital bacteriologist was concerned to assist the physician in the diagnosis of the individual case; his work took him no further outside his laboratory than to the ward. The public health bacteriologist, on the other hand, was concerned to assist the medical officer of health in controlling infectious disease in the community, and he had to consider not only the individual patient but also contacts, possible carriers and non-human sources of infection; he must be prepared to go out into the field to collect the specimens that he wanted.

Yet bacteriology is a single subject, and it was natural that, during consideration of post-war arrangements, the possibility of integrating the two sides should come under professional discussion. One school, headed by Topley, was anxious that what had been gained in wartime for public health bacteriology should not be jeopardised by striving for some greater but probably unattainable ideal. Another school wished to press for a unified national bacteriological service. There were in fact three propositions, which could not all be reconciled. The case for retaining public health bacteriology on a national basis was overwhelming; the arguments for unifying the two sides of bacteriological work were strong; the removal of any specialty from the impending regional organisation of the hospitals was practically impossible.

In the event, administrative separation has not prevented close working arrangements between public health and hospital bacteriologists. It soon became settled policy that whenever new laboratories were required for the Service they should be sited close to important hospitals, and preferably in the grounds of the latter. In many instances buildings were erected to house the two laboratories under the same roof, to their mutual advantage in many ways.

Sometimes collaboration has been quite informal. In an increasing number of places, however, it has been arranged that the public health laboratory should assume responsibility for the hospital bacteriology in addition to its primary function; this has been particularly welcome to hospital pathologists whose chief personal interest has lain in the morbid anatomy or chemical aspects of their work. In such cases the hospital authority contributes part of the salary of the director of the public health laboratory, and part of its other costs in accordance with an approved formula; this obviates tedious cross-accounting for work done.

The second Director of the Service, Sir James Howie, expressed its attitude in such matters as follows (1965):

> These arrangements have been most beneficial; but they do not represent either a universal pattern or a new P.H.L.S. policy aimed at taking over the work of hospital laboratories wherever this can be secured. In many places, for a variety of good reasons, joint arrangements are not either practicable or desirable. Everywhere, however, it is the hope of the P.H.L.S. that relationships between hospital laboratories and those of the P.H.L.S. will be complementary and mutually helpful. Many hospital laboratories, although not operating a formal joint agreement, collaborate with the P.H.L.S. by providing regular information about their isolations of significant microbes and by exchanges of scientific and technical staff for training.

Achievement of independent status

By 1954, the Council had become anxious to see the establishment of a separate form of control, always envisaged as ultimately desirable. The embarrassment of discrepant rates of remuneration for staff, particularly as regards eligibility for distinction awards, had grown to be acute. A further difficulty was that the Council had responsibility for making the Service function, but without power to reconcile the prescribed general policy with the resources provided— these being at that time incompatible. Also, for personal and other reasons, the formula of delegation of powers to a Board under the chairmanship of an officer of the Council was losing its convenience.

The Council was, nevertheless, by no means willing merely to abandon its foundling to whatever fate might be decided in Whitehall, but was concerned that the arrangements should be fully appropriate to what it knew to be the needs of the Service. Thus, the Council recorded on 15 October 1954 a desire for a solution that would "preserve a Service which they had created and which provided them with valuable opportunities for research in this field of preventive medicine".

The Council disliked an early suggestion that the Service should become a sort of outlying department of the Ministry of Health, directed from the headquarters of the latter. This would have treated the Service, perhaps logically enough, as a great extension of the former Ministry of Health Laboratory; but there were formidable objections. It was, in particular, essential for the staffing of the Service that it should offer bacteriologists and technicians the same rates of pay and conditions of employment as were available in the hospital laboratories of the National Health Service. As it happened, there was then also strong political reason for avoiding any increase, however formal, in the total size of the Civil Service. An alternative idea that part of the administration should be delegated to hospital authorities in the Regions of the National Health Service was thought to be dangerous, as running counter to the whole principle of the organisation. The Treasury took the Council's view, and the suggestion was ruled out.

The Council's own proposal was for a Public Health Laboratory Service Board, established as a corporation and analogous in status to a Regional Hospitals Board of the National Health Service, but with jurisdiction in its special sphere throughout England and Wales. This solution was accepted in principle, but legislation was considered to be necessary for giving it effect; this inevitably caused further delay, during which the Council from time to time extended the period during which it was willing to retain control. The conclusion was recorded in the Council's Report for 1958–59.

In the event, the Public Health Laboratory Service Act 1960 became law on 28 July 1960, and by an order of the Ministry of Health came into force on 1 August 1961. The purpose was to establish a Board for the "administration of the bacteriological service provided by the Minister of Health under section seventeen of the National Health Service Act 1946"; this was enacted by Section 1, which left it to the Minister to decide what precise administrative functions the Board should exercise. Section 2 transferred the staff of the Service from the employment of the Council to that of the new Board, with continuity of rights. Section 3 transferred to the Ministry all property held by the Council for the purposes of the Service. The Schedule to the Act incorporated the Board, and prescribed that it should consist of a chairman appointed by the Minister and such other members as the Minister might think fit; these were to include, inter alia, "not less than two persons appointed after consultation with the Medical Research Council".

The Minister invited Sir Landsborough Thomson, who had been chairman of the old Board but was now retired from the Council's staff, to be the first chairman of the statutory Board, from 1 August 1961. Three years later he was succeeded by Dr E. T. C. Spooner, Dean of the London School of Hygiene and Tropical Medicine, a former member of the Council who had had associations with the Service from its pre-war planning stage.

The Council retained a link with the Service through its nomination of two members of the statutory Board. It continued, in addition, to have close working contacts in both scientific and administrative matters. Members of the Service remained eligible for research grants from the Council for purposes outside the ordinary run of work; and certain joint undertakings were maintained. The Service still made full use of the Council's central store, adjacent to the Colindale site. The Council leased office accommodation to the Service in its own headquarters building; and it seconded a senior member of its administrative staff, Mr D. V. T. Fairrie, to be Secretary of the Board. He was afterwards succeeded in this position by another member of the Council's staff, Mr J. D. Whittaker.

Part III
War Medicine

Chapter 14
The First World War
(1914–18)

The outbreak of war—Research for peace and war—Reorientation of the
Committee's programme—Army Medical Statistics—The treatment of
wounds—Wound shock—Diseases of the war—Medical problems of chemical
warfare—Medical problems of flying—Information services—Collections—
The civilian front—The war in retrospect

The outbreak of war
The outbreak of war on 4 August 1914 found the young Medical
Research Committee little prepared to cope urgently with a new
situation. After an initial year spent mostly in planning for conditions of peace, it had just begun to be active; and it had secured
the whole-time services of a Secretary only a few months before.
Fortunately, it had also appointed the nucleus of a research staff,
which provided it with a spearhead for its scientific effort. It had
acquired a building for a central institute, but this was not yet fitted
to the purpose—nor, in the event, was it to be ready until six years
later. The Committee had drawn up a nation-wide scheme of grant-
aided research; but this could not be submitted for ministerial
approval until nearly three months after the outbreak of war and
much of it was, in the changed circumstances, destined to remain
unfulfilled.

It is indeed remarkable that, despite this handicap, the untried
and as yet little known organisation was able so quickly to deploy
its potentialities in support of the national effort. An early beginning
was made, as the Report for 1914–15 shows, and the proportion of
resources so directed naturally increased as the war went on. The
greater part of the Committee's special wartime activities was
devoted to assisting the Army Medical Service, although there were
also civilian problems of an emergency kind. Relations with the
Royal Navy were relatively slight, and there was until late in the war
no separate Air Force. As was said in the Report for 1914–15:

> The Committee found early and repeated occasion for the rapid organisation
> of pathological work in connection with military objects and for the safeguarding
> of the health of the large part of the male population enlisted in H.M. Forces.
> For these emergency schemes, approval was obtained from the Chairman of
> the Joint Committee from time to time without reference by him in each
> emergency to the Advisory Council.

The contemporary annual reports, drafted by Walter Fletcher,
constitute by far the best record of the Committee's attitude and

actions during the First World War. Office documentation for the period is fragmentary; and there is no personal recollection with which to fill the gaps or to interpret bald statements. In its Report for 1915–16 one finds the Committee in philosophical vein:

> This inevitable change in the scope of their work has never appeared to the Committee to need justification even upon formal grounds of technicality. The Medical Research Fund exists for the advancement of the medical sciences by which ill-health and disease may be reduced among the population, and it would seem to be a negation of that purpose to use the fund in any important degree for work aimed at a distant future of peace, during a time when so large a part of the whole population is exposed to the special risks arising from war, whether during active service abroad or in the performance of other work at home.
>
> The question is indeed hardly one within the decision of the Committee. Few, if any, of the scientific workers available for medical research of any kind would have been found free or willing to undertake or continue work remote from present national necessities, when the alternative presented itself to them.
>
> Nor can the Committee regard this disturbance of their former schemes as having been in any real sense a diversion from their main objective. Medical problems, brought into sudden urgency by war, have their solutions, which, when once gained, remain for all the future of peace. The Committee are able to recognise that the conditions of war, with the special opportunities they give for disciplined study and for repeated observation, have already allowed in some directions a more rapid progress of medical knowledge in a few months than had been seen in as many previous years. Instances of this may be noticed in the results of study of infected wounds and of antiseptics, in the recent growth of our knowledge of typhoid and allied infections, and of cerebro-spinal fever, while abundant hope of similar gains may be found already in many other branches of medicine.

Research for peace and war

The theme was further developed in the Report for 1916–17 in allusion to the distinction drawn, in those wartime accounts of current investigations, between schemes for research framed before the war and work in connection with the war:

> To maintain this distinction between the two groups may be convenient for purposes of reference and of historical continuity. It has now, however, become almost wholly meaningless from any point of general view, whether national or scientific. In their scientific methods and results it will be seen that the two sets of investigations meet inseparably at very many points, while in so far as knowledge has been increased by either of them the national good has been equally advanced. To a nation at war any gain in the store of medical science is a matter of vital concern, whether it comes to aid the present workers at home or the future generation, or to add efficiency to the fighting forces.
>
> In former Reports the Committee have pointed to this insignificance of the distinction between military or other opportunist schemes of enquiry and those framed under the less urgent stimulus of peace. They would draw attention again to the value in permanence which may spring from the study of problems emerging, as in war time, from unusual and temporary conditions. The occasions of war have called imperatively for enquiries into the proper treatment of wounds and of their various infections, into the control of epidemics

like those of cerebro-spinal fever, into the physiological meaning of surgical 'shock' and collapse, into the nature and treatment of functional nervous disorders, and indeed into almost every corner of the whole field of medical science and practice, whether for Europe or the tropics, and into every branch of surgical manipulation and contrivance.

These problems have been set by immediate naval and military needs, but the disturbances in civilian life have offered others of equal urgency in the medical sphere. The stress of industrial work has thrown into sharp relief our ignorance of its proper physiological regulation for the common good and has done much to stimulate a belated study of the natural laws of fatigue and of right living. The unfamiliar limitations in food supply have forced us to gain clearer knowledge of many biochemical and dietetic groups of facts long ago within easy reach, though not attained.

It is to be remarked, further, that the conditions of war have provided, not only insistent demands for the application of the scientific method, but many exceptional opportunities at the same time for its easy and fruitful use. The mere collection of men in large numbers under military rule, for instance, has allowed observations to be made and recorded which have yielded information otherwise almost unprocurable. To give only one example, it will be found in the present Report that a study has recently been made of the kidney efficiency of no less than fifty thousand young men considered to be in good normal health and leading active lives in a training camp. This survey had immediate import- ance as part of an enquiry into the kidney deficiency found to result from life in the trenches in a small percentage of men, but at the same time it will be found to have given new information upon a scale never obtained before, or easily obtainable, with regard to the health of the young male population of the country.

To one example of this kind others might easily be added to show that the conditions of war may actually bring aid as well as stimulus to enquiry. There is another direction, moreover, in which medical research during war time may find unusual opportunities for advance. It has often been pointed out that medical investigation at the great civil hospitals, which are its chief centres in time of peace, is commonly directed to the study of disease in the advanced stages which are presented there for relief or palliation, rather than to the detection and study of the early stages of onset which a patient, if he is aware of them at all, accepts for the time as private or unimportant. But it is in these early stages that disease may always be most easily checked and often most fruitfully studied. To the medical services of the armed forces, and no less in the medical supervision of the armies of workers at home, prevention of disease is more important than cure, and the bias of effort will always and rightly be towards general and preventive measures rather than towards individual and remedial efforts when prevention has failed. In these preventive efforts, research work ought always to find both encouragement and opportunities. If instances are sought, they may be found in many parts of the work the Committee have to report for the past year. The rapid and organised study of the condition of so-called irritable heart of soldiers could hardly have been made in any civil hospital in peace conditions, yet it has given results valuable alike to medical knowledge and to the preventive work of the service. The study of kidney deficiency in slight degrees and early stages among young men which has just been mentioned is another case in point. The efforts towards prevention of T.N.T. poisoning and the study of its causation and early recognition have led at least to some gains in knowledge and have certainly secured a high degree of success in prevention; yet the study of toxic jaundice at the bedside or afterwards has led neither to fresh knowledge of its nature nor to any new hopes of its cure.

The links between the enquiries, which may be labelled 'military' or 'civilian' by the accidents of their origin, are often intricate and curious in detail, even if they only illustrate the commonplace that no piece of sound knowledge has isolated value. It has been necessary to study the treatment of men suffering from the effects of the poison gases which the barbarism and treachery of the enemy introduced to warfare. In this the administration of oxygen which is a daily commonplace in any civilian hospital was required. Service conditions called, however, for the extreme of efficiency and economy in the apparatus, and there was revealed at once, or rather freshly illuminated, the wastefulness and inefficiency which for many years have marked our habitual hospital methods of oxygen supply to pneumonia and other patients. The application here of physiological principles—long ago established by English work but too little applied in England—will now, we may believe, bring permanent benefit back from the trenches to the Hospitals and sick rooms at home. Nor is this the only story of oxygen in the war. The supply of oxygen to flying men at high altitudes, where it is needed as in the more familiar case of mountain-sickness, has called for the application not only of mechanical ingenuity, but of physiological principles, which it may be noticed have been founded almost wholly upon scientific work done in French and in British laboratories in the last half century. Of the studies and devices thus called out by these new needs in the upper air it is already clear that some will bring long needed improvements to the apparatus and methods used in the depths of mines for the rescue of life.

Reorientation of the Committee's programme

In May 1915 the Minister responsible for National Health Insurance laid before Parliament, as a White Paper, an "interim Report on the Work in connection with the War at present undertaken by the Medical Research Committee". The same ground, and more, was covered in the First Annual Report of the Committee, bringing the account up to the end of September 1915. The earlier of these publications shows that even within about nine months the Committee had accomplished a substantial redeployment of its resources to the immediate needs of the war emergency.

The building at Hampstead acquired by the Committee for its central research institute had immediately been lent to the War Office for use as a military hospital (Volume One). The supply of pathologists for work in military hospitals in the United Kingdom had been organised by the Committee. Various members of the Committee's own staff had been commissioned in the Forces for special duties; in particular, the Department of Bacteriology under Sir Almroth Wright had found a new focus for its activities in a laboratory at Boulogne. The arrangement for members of the staff thus joining the Forces was that any difference between their usual salaries and their military pay was made up by the Committee.

The task of the Statistical Department in compiling and analysing the medical statistics of the Forces was a major undertaking that is described in a separate section below. The Committee's work on testing salvarsan preparations, formerly obtained from abroad, has already been mentioned (Chapter 12). Also relating to the treatment of venereal disease were the arrangements made by the Committee for the performance of Wassermann tests at a central laboratory. At Oxford, the standardisation of emulsions and sera for agglutination tests in the diagnosis of typhoid and paratyphoid infections was the beginning of a permanent scheme, to which reference has already been made (Chapter 12).

Colonel Sir William Leishman, a regular officer who was a member of the Committee, had been appointed Adviser in Pathology to the British Expeditionary Force in France. He was invited by the Committee to indicate the chief directions in which it appeared to him desirable that special inquiries should be instituted at home. A memorandum containing his suggestions was circulated by the Committee to all suitable centres of research, and various investigations were initiated by pathologists who selected particular points.

The despatch of investigators to Galicia and Egypt, to study cholera and bilharziasis respectively, has already been mentioned (Chapter 10). The White Paper also refers to the beginnings of investigations that continued throughout the war, but these can be better followed up under separate headings below; they included enteric infections, cerebrospinal meningitis, neurological injuries, and new antiseptic methods in the treatment of wounds.

Army medical statistics

At the beginning of the war the Committee offered to place its appropriate resources at the disposal of the War Office for medical statistical purposes. The Army Council accepted the offer, and in its Report for 1914–15 the Committee was able to say that it was conducting the whole compilation of statistical information about sick and wounded from Home and Expeditionary Forces. It expressed the purpose as follows:

> In the view of the Committee the compilation and analysis of these medical statistics, in the circumstances of the present time, will have a general value in providing information in various directions with regard to the health and stamina of the male population of these islands, in addition to its particular value from the special points of view of military requirements and of the Army Medical Service. It is hoped that the organisation of the work during the War will allow a much more rapid and complete manipulation of the material after its conclusion than would have been possible otherwise. The Committee may also allow themselves to believe that this work by their staff has given material assistance to the War Office in checking by contemporary observation and report the manner in which the regulations with regard to records have actually been followed in widely different places and conditions during the recent times of emergency and pressure.

The undertaking involved a great expansion of the Committee's Statistical Department, under Dr John Brownlee, for which a house in Bloomsbury had been rented. Clerks and typists were engaged for

work both at the centre and in military hospitals in the United
Kingdom; and Mr M. J. C. Meiklejohn was appointed as staff
officer in charge of this organisation. The work quickly grew in
volume and complexity and the Report for 1915–16 records its
transfer to the British Museum, near by, where basement accommodation recently completed for the Copyright Department was
made available by the Trustees. Before long the clerical staff had
grown to over a hundred.

On 4 December 1916 the Committee submitted to the Director-
General, Army Medical Services, a printed "Memorandum on the
Compilation of Medical and Surgical Statistics of the War, undertaken by the Medical Research Committee (National Health
Insurance) at their Statistical Department". This document summarised the history of the undertaking and gave an account of the
work, the latter mainly in quotation from the Report for 1915–16.
It then asked that the War Office should relieve the Committee of
the main part of the greatly increasing expenditure, which could not
properly, or even possibly, be borne by the Medical Research Fund.
As a result, the War Office agreed to bear the cost of the routine side
(typing and stationery), as distinct from that of scientific supervision by the Committee's staff.

As the Report for 1915–16 says, "the experience of the South
African War had shown the grave disadvantages of deferring the
collection of statistics until the final collection of the original documents". These documents were the hospital records, and any patient
might pass through half-a-dozen hospitals or lesser units (field
ambulances, casualty clearing stations, hospital trains, hospital
ships), some overseas and some at home; the need was thus for
extraction of the essential particulars and their despatch to a centre
where everything relating to one patient would be brought together
on a single card. An ideal system could have been devised in advance,
had the magnitude of the task been envisaged, and immediate use
could have been made of punched cards (for which machinery was
obtainable). As it was, the scheme was a little late in coming into
operation, and it was found that in the early months the record-
keeping at emergency hospitals had left much to be desired. Despite
this initial handicap efficient methods were established.

The project was far from being limited to the collection of information that would be useful after the war, whether for scientific
investigation or for the verification of pensions claims. The data
were available at once for the assessment of causes of illness or injury
and of the results of treatment, thus affording guidance in further
practice. So, in addition to the purely statistical work, Brownlee's
Department undertook the sorting and classification of the medical
case-sheets that were called in from military hospitals by the War
Office, and Dr Matthew Young was appointed to take charge of
this work. Apart from the extraction of information from these for
the general card index, supplementing or correcting the data from

admission and discharge books, these case sheets greatly facilitated the rapid supply of information sought for special purposes by medical officers serving abroad. It is recorded in the Report for 1915–16 that Young had already provided summary reports upon large groups of cases of particular kinds at the request of the consulting physicians and surgeons to the Forces.

Even so, the system did not provide this type of information with the speed that was sometimes desirable, as "when some new problem of disease or casualty presents itself for prompt solution". It also did not allow any easy or rapid transference of information about a given patient between the various medical officers concerned with his treatment in a succession of hospital units, although at any point in the chain it might be of great importance to have information about the immediate past or the later history of a case or groups of cases. The Report for 1915–16 records that:

> Towards the means introduced by the Army Medical Department to meet these needs, the Medical Research Committee have been permitted to contribute largely. In the early months of war an informal system began to take shape when the Secretary of the Committee arranged to secure, by a post card system, voluntary information from medical officers in this country, which was supplied to individual officers abroad who sought it for special reasons. This has gradually developed into an organised and official system for the collection and interchange of information.

Major T. R. Elliott was appointed to represent the Committee in France, in this and other parts of its work.

At the close of 1919, a year after the Armistice, this branch of the Committee's Statistical Department was moved from the British Museum to Dudley House, Endell Street, London, where mechanical analysis of information from punched cards was continued. The weight of the records, cards and machinery was so great, however, that it had to be widely distributed as a measure of safety, with the result that the total floor-space proved to be inadequate. This circumstance inevitably retarded the work, a large part of which now consisted of answering questions about individual cases, chiefly from the Ministry of Pensions, but also from military departments, insurance committees, and various dominion, colonial and foreign governments. The Council's Report for 1919–20 states that over 11 000 replies of this kind, many of them based on prolonged search, had been sent during the year. Nearly half of the inquiries were concerned with claims made by soldiers for which no support could be found in their military documents; about 90 per cent of such claims were found to be supported by the medical facts recorded in the Statistical Department, and only a very small minority of cases were they actually disproved. The Report goes on to say: "It is plain that all the work of the Department upon this side should pass at the earliest convenient time from the direction of the Medical Research Council, and conferences upon this subject have been held already between representatives of the War Office, Pensions Ministry and the Council."

The transfer was effected on 1 February 1921, and in the following month the work was moved to ample accommodation at Burton Court, Chelsea. Dr Matthew Young remained a member of the Council's staff, but his services were lent to the Ministry to advise on medical statistical questions, to complete the extraction of statistics for *The Medical History of the War*, and to keep the Council in touch with the medical and scientific interests of the work. In its Report for 1920–21 the Council devoted a special section to a brief history of the whole undertaking from 1914 onwards. This had to record that the final transfer was marred by some high-handed unilateral action on the part of the Ministry, which at the time called for condemnation in more forthright terms than were used by the Council in its official publication.

The treatment of wounds

In its Report for 1914–15 the Committee stated:

> No subject for research has seemed of more urgent importance than that of the pathology of infected wounds considered with a view to their effective treatment. It is not an exaggeration to say that the recent experience of septic wounds inflicted under the conditions of the European battlefields has revealed previously unsuspected difficulties in treatment which the resources of modern surgery have not been able to overcome.

Sir Almroth Wright and his team at Boulogne gave their chief attention to this question, and the provisional results emphasised the value of physiological methods as contrasted with antiseptic treatment by artificial bactericides. The irrigation of wounds by a hypertonic salt solution, without antiseptics, was in fact widely adopted. Meanwhile the Committee supported further investigations of the action of particular antiseptics, including new preparations, that might be suitable for the type of treatment required. These included hypochlorite preparations such as 'Dakin's solution'.

In the following year the Committee reported that "The idea that the dirty and often extensive wounds of warfare can be cleansed as a routine surgical procedure by the direct application of a strong antiseptic has already been abandoned." The requirement was an antiseptic that could be continuously applied and that would, like the hypertonic salt solutions, facilitate the physiological processes of the body. It was noted, however, that care in the method of application by the surgeon could be more important than the choice of fluid. Many pathologists and others took up this subject, and here it must suffice to name Dr H. D. Dakin for his work on chloramine compounds and Professor C. H. Browning for his on aniline derivatives of the acridine series ('flavines'). This study of antiseptics was a major research project of immediate practical utility. Concurrently, the treatment of wounds advanced in other directions. Experience showed the value of early and drastic surgical procedures, and administrative changes were made in order to implement this policy in the field.

Another important problem was that of the anaerobic organisms causing gangrene in wounds—the so-called 'gas gangrene' bacteria. This occupied the attention of many bacteriologists, and in March 1917 the Medical Research Committee appointed a coordinating Committee upon Anaerobes, with Professor William Bulloch as chairman and Dr Muriel Robertson as secretary. On the eve of the Armistice a serum for the prevention and cure of wound-gangrene had been produced, containing antitoxins against the three species of anaerobe concerned.

Another question of disinfection arose towards the end of 1915, when it was found that there were great difficulties in maintaining good sanitary conditions on board hospital ships bringing sick and wounded from the Mediterranean, and in avoiding secondary infections among patients, staffs and crews. The close confinement of up to 400 patients, including many with dysentery or paratyphoid fever, imposed a stringent test. On behalf of the Committee, Dakin devised a simple apparatus for the electrolysis of sea-water, enabling the ship to produce its own supply of sodium hypochlorite solution in ample quantity and at a low cost. This was first tried in the Cunard liner *Aquitania*, in use as a hospital ship, both for general disinfection of the wards, latrines and bedpans, and for the purification of drinking water and in the dressing of infected wounds. The formerly grave number of secondary infections was at once strikingly reduced, practically to zero, and the deodorant effect of the solution also gave great relief.

After the war, much of the new information about the treatment of wounds, the infecting organisms and methods of disinfection was brought together in a report in the Council's series by Captain S. R. Douglas, Dr (later Sir) Alexander Fleming and Dr Leonard Colebrook. Apart from antiseptic measures, the Committee organised special study of particular types of injury; and for this purpose various questionnaire forms, with convenient anatomical diagrams, were printed for distribution to military hospitals. One group, for instance, comprised gunshot wounds of the chest; and the collection of general information was supplemented by intensive investigation of selected cases.

A very important group consisted of the neurological injuries, and at one time about fifty specialists were working on a common plan under the Committee's scheme. These injuries called for special study with a view to improving treatment of wounds that often presented particular difficulty in their long-term effects; but at the same time many of the cases provided opportunity for adding to knowledge of the physiology of the nervous system. The records and experience were later collated by the Council's Nerve Injuries Committee to provide the material for two classical reports, published in 1920 and 1924 respectively.

Many other investigations relating to wounds were set on foot—for example, some work on skin-grafting. And associated with the large number of cases for surgical treatment was a greatly increased demand for radiographic services. This entailed the employment of many inexperienced helpers at military hospitals, and in 1915 the Committee made suggestions to the War Office about training staff in measures of protection against damage to themselves by X-rays.

Wound shock
As the war progressed, a problem lying somewhere between surgery and medicine assumed increasing importance, namely that of traumatic 'shock'. The term 'shock' had been in familiar surgical and medical use, long before the war, for conditions of failing circulation and generally depressed vitality due to the severity of an operation or to rapidly spreading toxaemia caused by an infection. A relatively recent addition to the conditions thus described had been 'anaphylactic shock'; and it is not irrelevant that Dale and Laidlaw in their first description, in 1910, of the actions of the base now called 'histamine' had drawn attention to the suggestive resemblance of its effects to those of anaphylaxis. (This war had also brought into use the term 'shell-shock', to describe the concussive effects of explosions or even psychological disturbances due to the din and stress of battle.) A better understanding of the nature of traumatic shock was likely to be a valuable guide to measures that would tide many patients over the too often fatal phase of 'shock'. The clinicians at first believed that the condition was new to surgical experience, and attributable to the extensive shattering wounds which had been rendered common for the first time by the use of shells filled with high explosives; the physiological approach was destined to give a different answer.

Clinical inquiries were directed by Colonel (later Sir) Cuthbert Wallace, and physiological work was undertaken especially by Professor W. M. Bayliss and by Dr H. H. Dale and Dr P. P. Laidlaw. Bayliss was soon joined by Professor W. B. Cannon from Harvard, and Dale by Professor A. N. Richards from Philadelphia. (Richards later had the distinction, remarkable for a scientist without medical qualification, of being appointed by the United States Government and the National Academy in Washington to be Chairman of the Committee of Medical Researches in relation to the Second World War.) A preliminary account of results was prepared for the Committee in an interim memorandum, *Surgical Shock and Allied Conditions*, and this was communicated to workers in the field in February 1917. The Committee also appointed a special investigation committee on shock to coordinate further studies. This had a very strong membership, with Professor E. H. Starling as its first chairman and his colleague Bayliss as successor, while Dale acted as secretary throughout; there was also liaison, through Cannon, with an equivalent American committee.

At one stage in the activities of the Shock Committee, there was some clash of opinion between the physiologists who favoured a theory that depletion of the alkali reserve of the blood plasma was the essential cause of wound shock, and others who attributed the condition to a toxaemia due to products from the massively injured tissues and affecting the circulation. Eventually, a joint experimental study resulted in an agreed acceptance of the latter view and the recommendation of treatment which it implied.

The Shock Committee's investigations thus led it to typify a condition of progressive circulatory deficiency as the chief element in the kind of shock most often seen in battle casualties, probably attributable to the absorption of substances having an action like histamine; and the immediate practical outcome was to suggest treatment to replace the blood lost from effective circulation through the physiological causes involved in shock, just as when blood is actually removed from the body by haemorrhage. Attention was thus directed to finding the most efficient artificial substitute for blood, and laboratory work by Bayliss had indicated a solution containing an osmotically active colloid, gum acacia. This was found in practice to be increasingly successful in saving life; and the procedure was free from the difficulties and risks which at that date attended transfusion with actual blood.

Seven reports of the Shock Committee were printed for official distribution. After the war, these and two others were published by the Council in its Special Report Series.

Diseases of the war

The Committee's work on typhoid and paratyphoid fevers was largely directed to their differential diagnosis, and to the supply of standardised preparations for the purpose. Reference has been made to this, and to work on cholera and on bilharziasis, in earlier chapters.

Dysentery called for much investigation, especially with regard to infections incurred in the Mediterranean and eastern theatres of war; both bacillary dysentery and amoebic dysentery were involved. Again there was the question of differential diagnosis, not only between the two diseases but between the various types of bacillary infection. The Committee, in addition to promoting special investigations, organised assistance in the large amount of pathological laboratory work required for dealing with the numerous cases arriving in the United Kingdom from Gallipoli and elsewhere.

The treatment of amoebic dysentery presented particular difficulty, and there were important gaps in knowledge to be filled. There was also a dearth of pathologists experienced in protozoology and arrangements were accordingly made for a few trained biologists, skilled in microscopic work but not medically qualified, to become rapidly practised in the elements of routine diagnosis. In this project Mr Clifford Dobell worked for the Committee in collaboration with Lieut.-Colonel (later Sir) Andrew Balfour and Dr C. M. Wenyon of the Wellcome Research Bureau. The scheme was extended at Cambridge under the auspices of the Royal Society, with which the Committee continued to cooperate. Pharmacological investigations were made in the Committee's Department of Bio-chemistry under Dale, especially on the use of emetine and bismuth iodide in the treatment of carriers.

By the end of hostilities in those theatres of war that were the chief sources of dysentery, a great deal of new information had been amassed about the epidemiology, diagnosis and treatment of both kinds of dysentery, and about the bacteria and protozoa concerned; and Dobell had made a wide study of the amoebae pathogenic for man. Many scientific papers were published, and eight early numbers of the Special Report Series were concerned with dysentery.

Before the war, there was a small outbreak of cerebrospinal meningitis, or 'spotted fever', in the United Kingdom every year; but the concentration of large bodies of troops in billets and camps presented favourable opportunities for the propagation of the disease and large epidemics occurred. They were especially serious because of the high case-mortality rate, and the Committee gave the military authorities every assistance in its power for investigation and measures of control. Dr M. H. Gordon was appointed to the Committee's whole-time staff in 1915 to organise and direct the bacteriological work done for the Committee. It was found that the meningococci present in the cerebrospinal fluid of cases were of different sero-logical types—four main types, of which two were particularly abundant. This was of great practical importance in preventive measures, as it appeared to be necessary to place in quarantine only those carriers showing the type of organism causing the currently prevalent epidemic. It was even more important in treatment, as curative sera homologous with the respective type of infecting organ-ism were found to be efficacious. In the Report for 1917–18 it is stated that "It has become increasingly probable that the chances of recovery depend upon the early administration of curative serum prepared to correspond with that type of meningococcus actually infecting the patient." For both these reasons, a supply of diagnostic sera and arrangements for the rapid performance of tests were essen-tial, and the Committee's workers were able to give much help in these respects. Incidentally, the bacteriological work undertaken for this practical purpose gave rise to fundamental studies of bacterial growth which were undertaken at Cambridge under the direction of Professor F. G. (later Sir Frederick) Hopkins. Other practical investigations were concerned with methods for freeing the nasal passages of 'carriers' from infection, including the use of fine dis-infectant sprays. Staff Surgeon P. G. (later Sir Paul) Fildes had ex-ceptional opportunities for studies of the carrier condition while conducting the nasopharyngeal examination of large numbers of new entries to a naval hospital.

The Committee was able to assist in the investigation of a small outbreak of spirochaetal jaundice (Weil's disease) among the troops in France in 1916; and it was able to provide advance information about work on this condition in Japan and the United States. In the same year the Committee helped the work of Captain J. W. (later Sir John) McNee on trench fever, a form of 'pyrexia of uncertain origin' that was causing serious morbidity in France; some apparatus was provided, and also the collaboration of Mr J. E. Barnard in the ultramicroscopic photography of blood specimens sent home. McNee and his colleagues were the first to demonstrate the infective nature of this disease, unknown before the First World War, and not reappearing on any significant scale in the Second. The crucial experiments on human volunteers, proving that the infection was louse-borne, were made under War Office and American auspices.

The disastrous 'pandemic' of influenza in the autumn of 1918 caused the Committee to expand such work on this disease as it had in hand, and to coordinate it with studies promoted by the Royal Navy and the Army. An account of observations made in British hospitals in France was published by the Committee in the following year.

In 1915 the Committee was asked by the Director-General, Army Medical Services, to assist in the investigation of a condition variously known as 'acute nephritis (epidemic dropsy)', 'acute (trench) nephritis', and 'trench (war) nephritis', which was another common cause of illness among the troops in France. Arrangements were made for the reception of cases in two of the military wards at St Bartholomew's Hospital, in order to concentrate material for study. Later, the Committee sent Dr Hugh MacLean to France as a chemical pathologist; although there seemed to be a strong probability that the disease was of infective origin, there was the alternative possibility—subsequently excluded—that it was a toxic condition due to exacerbation of some latent deficiency in kidney function. To investigate this point it was necessary to establish a base-line, and MacLean assessed the kidney efficiency of 50 000 fit young men, thus collecting (as already mentioned) a mass of data never before available. He then returned to St Thomas's Hospital in London, where a ward was set aside for cases of trench nephritis to be investigated from the point of view of clinical chemistry. A full report of MacLean's work was afterwards published by the Committee, which in its own Report for 1918–19 remarked that: "The general results of the investigation have a much wider interest than their original military application."

Early in the war the Committee arranged a scheme, under the general direction of Sir James Mackenzie, for the investigation of cardiac disorders of military importance—'soldiers' heart'. Beds were reserved in the military wards at University College Hospital, London, for the reception of certain groups of cases under the care of Captain (later Sir) Thomas Lewis. In 1916 the work was transferred to the Hampstead Military Hospital (the Committee's own building), so that larger numbers could be studied and treated; Lewis had meanwhile joined the Committee's staff. The aim was that as many cases as possible of the so-called 'irritable heart of soldiers' might rapidly be restored to fitness.

In 1917 the Committee published a report on this work, to make available without delay the new information about the pathology of 'DAH' (disordered action of the heart) and the best method of dealing with cases. Essentially the system was to separate out the numerous patients showing disordered cardiac action without organic disease, and to treat them by means of graduated exercise until normal function was restored. In 1917 the work was moved to a larger military hospital, at Colchester. In its Report for 1917–18 the Committee said that:

> The records show a remarkable reduction in the average stay in hospital of soldiers suffering from complaints in this group, as the result of the system which has been introduced. This reduction, as applied to the cases treated at the Colchester hospital alone, and when the average stay in hospital is compared with that found prevailing before the introduction of the exercise system, is at present saving an expenditure of approximately £50 000 a year, an amount closely equivalent to that of the whole of the Medical Research Fund which the Committee are privileged to administer.

The Army Medical Service opened similar centres at other places.

Medical problems of chemical warfare
The enemy's resort to poison gas in France in 1915 introduced a new weapon into warfare and a new type of casualty for the medical services. Retaliation inevitably followed, and chemical warfare was developed on both sides; gas-filled shells largely replaced windborne clouds of gas, and the original chlorine was succeeded by more sophisticated substances. The medical problems thus became more urgent and more difficult. The subject is first mentioned by the Committee in its Report for 1915–16.

Initially, the Committee's part was mainly the collection of information about casualties by its Statistical Department, as described above, but a few special investigations were promoted. At Cambridge, Mr (later Professor Sir) Joseph Barcroft and others worked on a new method of treating gassed patients; and at Oxford Dr J. S. Haldane collaborated with Lieut.-Colonel J. C. Meakins of the Canadian Army Medical Corps in physiological studies of the aftereffects of gassing. Later, the Committee's Departments of Biochemistry and of Applied Physiology became involved in the improvement of treatment, including the use of oxygen.

In January 1918 the Director-General, Army Medical Services, in consultation with the Medical Research Committee and with the concurrence of the Controller of Chemical Warfare, appointed a Chemical Warfare Medical Committee. Professor A. R. Cushny was chairman, with Dr J. S. Edkins as secretary and a membership that included a number of leading physiologists. The task was to prepare reports on information from all sources, to propose further coordinated medical investigations, and to advise the DGAMS generally on medical scientific aspects of chemical warfare.

The Chemical Warfare Medical Committee had existed for less that a year when its active work was suspended by the Armistice. It had already issued a number of reports for official distribution, and it issued several more, in which were gathered together such earlier results as seemed most deserving of permanent record. Research work on anoxia and on oxygen treatment, originally undertaken in relation to chemical warfare, continued on a broader basis into the years of peace.

Medical problems of flying
The Report for 1916–17 records that the Air Board had accepted the proferred aid of the Medical Research Committee towards the investigation of "important problems of a medical kind that present themselves in some special disabilities associated with flying, and especially flying at high altitudes". Grants were made by the Committee for several items of research: at Oxford, Dr J. S. Haldane took part in physiological studies, and Professor Georges Dreyer devised special apparatus for supplying oxygen to flying men in the air.

The services of Captain Martin Flack, of the Committee's Department of Applied Physiology, were provided for whole-time work on the physiological condition of pilots who showed disability in flying at higher altitudes (by the standards of that era). The Committee's building at Hampstead, having been vacated by the removal of the cardiac work to Colchester, was assigned to the Air Board as a hospital for officers of the Royal Flying Corps and the Royal Naval Air Service; it thus became the scene of investigations into conditions specially associated with flying.

In March 1918, the Medical Administrative Committee of the Air Ministry, in consultation with the Medical Research Committee and with the concurrence of the Air Council, appointed an Air Medical Investigation Committee, with Dr (later Sir) Henry Head as chairman, Lieut.-Colonel M. Flack as secretary, and a distinguished membership. The terms of reference were:

(a) To prepare reports for submission to them [the Medical Administrative Committee] with a view to their distribution to those concerned. (b) To make suggestions for further co-ordinated medical investigations that may seem desirable. (c) To advise generally in respect of the scientific medical aspects of aeronautics.

Members and officers of the Medical Research Committee were at this time concerned, by request, with some general problems connected with the establishment of a separate medical service for the new Royal Air Force. Following rearrangements in this respect, and at the suggestion of the RAF, the Medical Research Committee reconstituted the Air Medical Investigation Committee as one of its own advisory bodies; and various investigations were continued for a time. Wing-Commander Martin Flack took a permanent commission in the new service in order to devote himself to further research in this field; but his career was cut short by early death.

The Air Medical Investigation Committee was responsible for a series of reports that were given official distribution during the war and were afterwards accorded full scientific publication in the Council's Special Report Series.

Information services
Mention has been made earlier in this chapter of the information that the Committee was able to feed back to the Forces from its Statistical Department, and also of its official distribution of various memoranda and reports by its special investigation committees. In addition, the Committee was from time to time able to bring to official notice items of 'intelligence' gleaned from the foreign medical press, and particularly from scientific papers published in enemy countries. During 1915, for instance, the Committee communicated to the Army Medical Service translated extracts giving German and Austrian experience of outbreaks of disease in the Near East that might be relevant to the medical needs of British troops in the Mediterranean area, or on the Western front if diseases were transferred thereto by enemy movements. Towards the end of the war it became possible to organise this work on a regular and more effective basis; the Committee became responsible for a monthly *Medical Supplement* to the official *Review of the Foreign Press*, and the first number of this was issued in January 1918 (see Volume One). It was found very useful by British medical officers; and in its Report for 1918–19 the Committee cites a message of appreciation by the Chief Surgeon to the US Forces.

Collections
In addition to the statistical and other information that would be available for the official history, two other collections were assisted by the Committee. One was a collection of pathological specimens, for the instruction of future medical officers and others, illustrating the casualties and diseases of the war. The collection included wet specimens showing the nature and sequelae of wounds and diseases; dry specimens showing injuries of bones; X-ray plates and skia-grams; and wax models illustrating the plastic surgery of the face. This work was directed for the War Office by Professor (later Sir) Arthur Keith at the Royal College of Surgeons of England.

The other project was a collection of pathological drawings, largely from life, for a similar purpose and available for reproduction. The Committee made grants for two medical artists allotted to this task, one of them working in France under the general direction of Major T. R. Elliott.

Unfortunately, the eventual fine collection of specimens and drawings at the college was totally destroyed by enemy action during an air-raid on London in the Second World War. All that survived was a special collection of 56 drawings by Henry Tonks, FRCS (who gave up the teaching of anatomy to become Slade Professor of Fine Art); this was fortunately away on loan at the time of the bombing.

The civilian front

As early as 1915 the Committee was giving some support to investigations of physiological fatigue in factories, and was assisting the Health of Munition Workers Committee set up by the Ministry of Munitions of War. By the following year, the Department of Applied Physiology under Dr Leonard Hill was inquiring into the ventilation, heating, lighting and general hygiene of old and new workshops at Woolwich Arsenal. Other investigations related to the dietaries provided by canteens at munitions factories, and to avoidance of the hazards of noxious dusts and vapours arising from industrial processes. In particular, Dr Benjamin Moore and others investigated sickness due to TNT poisoning, including fatal cases of a toxic jaundice. These wartime studies were the forerunners of a programme of work on industrial health that has already been described.

It is not until the Report for 1916–17 that one finds a special heading for research work bearing directly on the economic and medical problems of the nation's food supply in time of war. That is largely because the Ministry of Food and other departments were being advised by the Food (War) Committee of the Royal Society, on which were members of the Medical Research Committee and its staff. A few research grants in this field were nevertheless being made.

Dr (later Sir) Edward Mellanby, working for the Medical Research Committee, undertook research on the physiological action of alcohol at the request of the Central Control Board (Liquor Traffic); other studies were also made, and three special reports were issued. It has been related in Volume One how the Medical Research Council became responsible for a booklet on alcohol originally published under the Board's auspices.

Wartime work on the standardisation of arsenical drugs has been mentioned earlier (Chapter 12).

The war in retrospect

About a year after the Armistice the Medical Research Committee, as such, issued its final Report—that for 1918–19. This opened with an important Introduction, from which some forward-looking passages have already been quoted in Volume One. These passages were preceded by some retrospection of the scientific gains of war-time research:

The stimulus and the special occasions of war have led to great progress in many parts of medical science. This has not only given direct aid in the practical conduct of war, but has led also to many permanent gains in scientific knowledge. . . . Already it is plain that many results of research, begun at first with purely military objects, are directly applicable to medical work in civil life. The studies made, for example, of the nature of wound 'shock', and of the best modes of replacing lost blood, have already during the past year found fruitful application in the surgical theatres by some of our great hospitals; the fresh studies of the organs and mechanism of respiration which arose from the need for better prevention and treatment of the effects of poison gases have revealed, and helped to remove, unsuspected gaps in our knowledge, and the results will bring certain benefit to the daily work of the physician if he avail himself of them; the laboratory studies of wound infections and of the causes of wound gangrene have not only gained some of their immediate and practical objectives, but have led to advances both in basic knowledge and in manipulative technique that will stand as permanent gains in this part of science. To these many other instances might be added.

If the advances made in war time are to be continued and multiplied in peace it may be well to note what the conditions have been that have allowed so many important contributions to medical science to be made during a time of such disturbances and stress. First, we may point with pride to the fact that our country has never been found wanting at any time in men of originality and insight, fitted to advance knowledge. The demand for them has too often been absent or cold and the support given to them has been casual and inadequate; but the supply has never failed. Second, the war has presented problems of immediate practical significance and of absorbing interest, and it has given opportunities for inquiry on the largest scale. Lastly, the men fitted for the work have received—perhaps for the first time in the history of war, or indeed of peace—a large measure of public support. It has been increasingly realized during the war, if not in its earliest stages, that only a true knowledge of nature can guide physical activities rightly, and that research work is a vital necessity for success in warfare which is a contest of activities. This truth has been brought home in a thousand lessons, and as its realization has gained ground during the war, so men fitted for the work of inquiry have been increasingly permitted to perform it. What from this point of view appears now as a fortunate accident, namely, the constitution of the Medical Research Fund so shortly before the war, allowed some practical support to be given from the first to medical investigation, as such, directed to war purposes. The Committee may perhaps be allowed to think, in reviewing the past five years, that the independent aid of this Fund which they were put in a position to bring forward, had an important influence in promoting the general cause of medical research. It helped to accelerate the movement which has advanced throughout the war, in both naval and military and in the civilian services, towards widely using the services of officers in suitable cases for new investigation as distinguished from routine technical work. Before the end of the war it may be said that most of the men best fitted for original inquiry were given opportunity for it, and given pay for it from public funds, whether by way of commissions in the Navy or Army or Air Force or of research grants from the Committee out of the Medical Research Fund, and that in the main this national system of medical research was welded into a coherent intellectual service by appropriate arrangements made between the different disbursing authorities.

Finally, it may be said that the Committee looked forward "to the future appearance of a worthy historical retrospect in an official Medical History that may give some adequate record of the scientific work done in and for the Medical Services of the country during the War"; and to that project it was giving all the aid in its power. Twelve volumes dealing with medical services eventually appeared, and these are an important source for detailed reference over a wider field than that which the Committee was itself directly concerned; the volume on pathology is especially rich in references to research work.

Chapter 15
The Second World War
(1939–45)

Comparison with 1914—The Council's initial policy—Certain problems in anticipation—Wartime research in retrospect—Historical sources—Wounds and injuries—Wound infection—Burns—Injuries to the nervous system—Traumatic shock—Wartime diseases—Malaria and rickettsial fevers—Basic therapeutic requirements—Nutrition in wartime—Calcifying factors in the diet—Vitamin studies—Service rations—Protein requirements and malnutrition—Special diets—Wartime health in industry—Scientific liaison

Comparison with 1914

When the Second World War broke out, on 3 September 1939, the Council was in a very different position from that of the original Committee twenty-five years earlier. It was well established, well tried, and well known. It had a substantial scientific organisation of its own, and it had acquired a prestige that gave it undisputed national leadership in medical research. Moreover, the situation had been forseen; the Council had been involved in planning, and to some extent in actual preparations, for at least two years before the event.

The lessons of the First World War had been learnt; and much new knowledge in medical science had been gained in the interval and was ready to be applied to wartime needs. Some of the old problems had been solved, or for various reasons did not recur; others remained, but they could often be approached with improved methods; fresh problems also arose.

The Council was not again called upon to undertake the collection of Army medical statistics, as this time the requirements had been foreseen and were met on a Service basis. On the other hand, the Council's help was sought by the Services over a wider scientific field than before; it was not limited to questions of wounds and disease but extended also to what came to be known as 'personnel research', relating to human efficiency under extreme climatic conditions or in relation to the use of weapons and equipment. Problems of flying were naturally of outstanding importance, and cooperation in their study between the Council and the Royal Air Force had already been developed before the war began. The enemy did not in the event resort to bacteriological methods of warfare or sabotage, as had been thought possible, but precautions against the potential hazard had nevertheless to be taken (Chapter 13).

There was also more to be done by the Council on the civilian front. This was partly because the population of the United Kingdom was certain to be much more closely involved in warlike operations; and owing to the greatly increased scale of the air attacks that were expected, and that did in fact take place, civil defence raised problems of its own. The Council was also more directly concerned with questions of nutrition, which in the First World War had been dealt with largely by a special committee set up by the Royal Society. Further, the Council now itself controlled the organisation for research on the health and efficiency of industrial workers.

For convenience of length, two topics have been relegated to another chapter. These have nothing in common except that they had no counterparts in the earlier war—personnel research for the armed forces, and certain civilian emergency services of a technical nature (Chapter 16).

The Council's initial policy

The Council was from the beginning of the war anxious, no less than its predecessor a quarter of a century before, to use its resources as fully as possible in support of the national effort; as noted above, it was already committed in various directions. It realised, however, that its organisation could not be immediately deployed in a new direction, but that problems would present themselves gradually as the war developed. The process was all the slower because for several months, the period of the so-called 'phoney war', the enemy refrained from launching any massive land offensive on what again became the Western Front, or any sustained air attack on the United Kingdom. In this situation there was a distinct risk that research workers employed or aided by the Council, and especially the younger men, would become impatient and offer themselves individually for types of war service in which their special abilities could not be used to the greatest advantage. In this way the research potential might have been frittered away before the full demand upon it had materialised; and there might also be, as was pointed out in the Report for 1938–39, an unnecessary sacrifice of "the fruits of promising research unrelated to war".

The Council accordingly stated its policy and made it widely known to those concerned. On 20 October 1939, it minuted that as a matter of general policy ordinary research work should be continued during the war as far as possible, subject to the demand for investigations into special problems which may arise. This policy was reaffirmed in a minute of 12 July 1940, when the war was in a much more critical phase, with the elaboration that teams of highly qualified investigators should be kept together for work on normal or special subjects as occasion might demand, although sympathetic consideration should be given to any specific proposals by members of the staff for diversion of their energies to new subjects of research directly related to the war.

Certain problems in anticipation

The Report for 1938–39 covered only the first four weeks of war and was written not long after the end of that period. There had been

HCMR—U

time to think in advance, during the preceding two or three years
of threatened hostilities, but the validity of speculations about the
medical problems that would arise had still to be put to the test
of reality—a position which, as it happened, largely persisted for
several further months. After a retrospective survey of what the
Medical Research Committee was called upon to do in the First
World War, the Report went on:

> It will be asked what contribution medical investigation can make in the present
> war. At the moment this question is almost impossible to answer. Although
> substantial knowledge has been gained in the twenty years that have elapsed
> since the last war, it is quite certain that many of the old problems of shock,
> of wound infection and of the hygiene of warfare will again claim great at-
> tention.

The problem of wound shock, the Report went on to say, would be
tackled with much better understanding of its nature; and greatly
improved methods of transfusion would be available for treating the
condition. In the case of wound infection, "probably the largest
single cause of death among wounded men reaching hospital in the
last war", modern chemotherapy was expected to be of outstanding
benefit. This would be notably so in the case of infections with
haemolytic streptococci treated with sulphonamide compounds, of
which the value had been well established in time of peace; in the
case of gas-gangrene infections, the relative curative effects of sulphonamide compounds and antitoxin had still to be assessed. The treatment of such diseases as pneumococcal pneumonia and cerebrospinal
meningitis with sulphapyridine and sulphanilamide could be con-
fidently predicted to make spectacular reductions in case mortality,
as compared with 1914–18; for cerebrospinal meningitis a fatality of
1·4 per cent had lately been recorded, in England in time of peace,
as compared with anything up to 90 per cent in earlier days. It
would, however, be necessary to establish the best methods of
avoiding the ill-effects that these drugs were capable of producing.

Wartime research in retrospect
The next Report covered the whole period of the war, 1939–45,
during which annual publication had been suspended. The development of wartime activities was thus described in retrospect,
as a whole, and not from year to year as in 1914–18. It was
pointed out in the Introduction to the Report that activities related
to the war were of two kinds. First, there was a great increase in the
demands made on the Council by Government Departments and
the Fighting Services for advice in the application of the latest
scientific knowledge to practical affairs; in some cases the assistance
sought went much further, laying on the Council administrative
tasks of a kind that such a scientific organisation could best perform.
Second, the actual research work became increasingly directed to
problems to which wartime needs had given special prominence;

and many of the investigations were designed to give quick answers
to immediate practical questions as they arose. On this, an important
comment is made:

This type of *ad hoc* investigation, however, can be based only upon information
and methods already available, and more complete answers often have to
await the acquisition of greater fundamental knowledge. Thus, there comes a
time when the research worker has to decide whether to confine his interests
to giving limited answers or to delve deeper, and inevitably more slowly, to
obtain a fuller grasp of the principles involved. So it is that, although war
acts at first as an intense stimulus to certain branches of medical research, in
the long run it tends to lose its effect as an incentive to discovery. The late war
was in this way beginning to lose much of its stimulating influence on medical
research when it ended.

The principal objectives that had been in view throughout the
war were retrospectively formulated in the following terms:

The response of medical science to the challenge of war has three main objectives. First, it must be directed to maintaining the health of the armed forces
and of the civilian population, particularly in the prevention of infective disease
and of malnutrition. Second, it must study methods for rapidly restoring the
wounded and sick to full health. Third, an object which became very prominent
in the late war, it must find the conditions required for the highest possible
efficiency, safety and comfort of fighting personnel and of industrial workers in
all the circumstances and tasks of war. Obviously these aims of application must
also be those towards which new research under war conditions is chiefly
directed.

Historical sources
The history of British medical research in the Second World War is
compactly given in two overlapping publications. The Council's
single large report covering the six years of war was published in 1947
under the special title *Medical Research in War*. Its compilation and
editing was the work of Dr F. H. K. Green of the Council's headquarters staff. He was likewise joint editor, with Major-General Sir
Gordon Covell, of the volume on medical research in the official
history of the war. *Medical Research in War* is accordingly the chief
source drawn upon for the present chapter and the next; quotations
not otherwise attributed are from it, and it has also been freely para-
phrased.

It was particularly with a view to the official history that the
Council was asked by the Ministry of Health, in 1942, to advise on
a system for recording statistics of hospital patients, involving the
use of a standardised classification of diseases and injuries. The
Council accordingly appointed a Committee on Hospital Morbidity
Statistics, on which the interested departments, services and professional bodies were represented; Sir Ernest Rock Carling was
chairman and Dr A. H. T. Robb-Smith secretary. A revised and
amplified classification, regarded as provisional, was published in
1944 and widely adopted in the United Kingdom.

Wounds and injuries

In its Report, the Council opened its summing up under this head as follows:

> Great as were the improvements in the treatment of wounds in the first world war, in the second these improvements were still more remarkable. The outstanding advances were the development of the blood transfusion services so that resuscitation of the injured with blood or blood products was possible even in the battle zone, the use of sulphonamide drugs and later—and much more effectively—penicillin to prevent or treat wound infection, and the more widespread recognition of the desirability of dressing wounds or burns as infrequently as possible, and then only with strict precautions to prevent extraneous infection.

The advisory services and the special investigations undertaken by the Council for wartime purposes were organised by a series of committees appointed for the purpose. These committees were based on the Council's headquarters, where their activities were coordinated; and their chairmen and secretaries were usually persons closely associated with the Council's work. From the first, too, the Medical Departments of the Services were represented on these committees and their subcommittees, thus securing integration of thought not only between the research side and the Services but also between the several Services themselves. As the Report for 1939–45 says, the committees "were accepted as advisory authorities by the Medical Departments of the Fighting Services at all stages of the war". The committees had immediate access to the Council's research organisation whenever new investigations were required; or in appropriate circumstances the Service representatives could arrange for observations by medical officers in the field.

Of prime importance among these wartime bodies, although not actually the first to be set up, was the War Wounds Committee, which stood centrally to the general problem of casualties. Its successive chairmen were eminent surgeons who had both served on the Council, Sir Cutherbert Wallace and Sir Ernest Rock Carling; its successive secretaries were Professor W. W. C. Topley, a member of Council, and Dr F. H. K. Green of the headquarters staff. As time went on, the Committee proliferated a number of specialised subcommittees; these dealt severally with anaerobic wound infections, burns, chest injuries, crush injuries, vascular injuries, and the collection of pathological specimens. Further, the Committee was flanked by a number of separate committees dealing with such subjects as brain injuries, nerve injuries, traumatic shock, blood transfusion, and penicillin clinical trials; there was also one on air-raid casualties, appointed jointly with the Ministry of Home Security and the Ministry of Health.

The intensification of hostilities in France and the Low Countries in the summer of 1940 suddenly produced large numbers of wounded, many of whom had of necessity to be treated by surgeons with limited war experience. The first task of the War Wounds

Committee was thus "to issue detailed suggestions for the treatment of certain types of war injuries and their consequences, based on past war experience and the latest available information, making it clear that such suggestions were provisional and liable to be changed or extended as the result of further experience". It was also decided to try "to collect and collate the results of different methods of surgical treatment, and to arrange for the rapid dissemination of useful new knowledge".

As in the First World War, the Council took part in arrangements for forming a national collection of pathological specimens illustrating the injuries and diseases of war. This was supplemented by a collection of colour photographs, for which purpose the Metal Box Company Ltd had placed the services of a photographer (Mr P. G. Hennell) and the firm's technical facilities at the disposal of the Council. The Royal Society of Medicine accepted the Council's invitation to be responsible for permanently housing, and making available for reference, a master-set of selected pictures.

Wound infection
On the research side, the problem of wound infection was of special importance. In respect of gas-gangrene and other anaerobic infections, "there was an urgent need for a planned and co-ordinated scheme of combined clinical and bacteriological research to demonstrate the respective places of surgery, antitoxin and drugs in prophylaxis and treatment". As there is little opportunity for investigating this kind of infection in time of peace, the research work done in 1914–18 "was resumed almost as a consecutive story (and in some instances even by the same workers) during the war of 1939–45". Similar combined studies of other wound infections were also required. Dr Leonard Colebrook of the Council's staff had, at the beginning of the war, been seconded as Consultant Bacteriologist to the Army with the rank of Colonel. He had been one of Sir Almroth Wright's men who worked for the Medical Research Committee during the earlier war; and, in a very different sphere, he had had recent experience in the use of sulphonamide drugs against infections.

As already indicated, the diagnosis and treatment of infections with anaerobic organisms of the gas-gangrene group received early attention. Notes on the subject was issued in 1940 (MRC War Memorandum No. 2); a revised edition appeared later. Experimental research on different aspects of the problem was undertaken at the National Institute for Medical Research, the Lister Institute, the Middlesex Hospital, the Central Emergency Medical Service Laboratory at Watford, the Radcliffe Infirmary at Oxford, the University of Cambridge, the University of Leeds, and elsewhere. The work included, as a main objective, the attempt to produce a prophylactic toxoid, following the striking success of a similar preparation for tetanus; but this was not brought to fruition before the end of the war, although valuable clues were gathered.

Gas-gangrene, fortunately, is one of the rarest forms of wound infection, but it is important because of its severity. The study of the prevention and treatment of other wound infections during the war covered a wider field and was attended by much greater clinical success. "A lesson learnt in previous wars, which nothing in the experience of 1939–45 has contradicted, is that the most effective way of preventing infection by the bacteria introduced into wounds at the time of injury is by early and adequate surgical operation." The experience gained by surgeons as to the best operative techniques was collated by the War Wounds Committee. Particular attention was at first paid to evaluating the 'closed plaster' treatment used in the Civil War in Spain, but the serious limitations of this technique later led to its being abandoned.

The value of sulphonamide drugs against streptococcal and other infections had been firmly established before the war (Chapter 3). Wounds, however, offered a relatively new field for their application; and the assessment of their potentialities was a major subject of investigation. They were found to be useful in controlling infection by susceptible bacteria in superficial wounds, and valuable in preventing the systemic spread of infection from a local focus. Later in the war, penicillin became available and was soon shown to have some outstanding advantages over the sulphonamides. It acted against a wider range of organisms and was able to do so under less favourable conditions; and its use involved much less risk of ill-effects. The use of penicillin in the treatment of wounds was the subject of MRC War Memorandum No. 12, published early in 1944.

The main attack on the treatment of war wounds with penicillin was made early in 1943, when sufficient quantities for a field trial were first available. The trial was made in North Africa by medical officers who had been trained in the techniques at Oxford, and Professor H. W. (later Lord) Florey and Brigadier Hugh Cairns, who had done so much of the pioneer work at Oxford, went out there for part of the time. The value of penicillin in dealing with gram-positive organisms in septic conditions had already been amply shown in England, so the problem was to find whether it could be effectively used in the field, and how the limited supplies could be best employed.

The answer, in brief, was that penicillin should be used as early as possible after wounding, as the amounts required when serious infections had become established were too great. A new scheme, on these lines, was accordingly devised for the impending invasion of Sicily; and further experience was gained in Italy. By the time of the Normandy landings, in 1944, there was sufficient penicillin for all who needed it, and arrangements for much more extensive use were accordingly made. The War Wounds Committee and the Pencillin Trials Committee of the Council cooperated with the Medical Departments of the Fighting Services, and with the Emergency Medical Services at home, in planning a large-scale investigation of the value of penicillin and other drugs in the treatment of wound infections in casualties evacuated to Great Britain. The results were highly encouraging, and were so much better than anything in earlier experience that the absence of untreated controls was of little moment. The success was of course partly attributable to the high quality of the war surgery—itself enchanced by the surgeons being able, with penicillin, to suture even the most severe wounds without the danger of major sepsis.

Other subjects of investigation included the cross-infection of wounds in hospital, the physiology of wound healing, the technique of emergency amputations (MRC War Memorandum No. 5), the treatment of war fractures, and injuries to blood vessels (MRC War Memorandum No. 13).

Burns

An extensive research programme on the pathology and treatment of burns was promoted by the Council. This was urgently necessary because the tannic acid treatment, generally favoured before the war, was found to be unsuited to the typical burns involving the hands and faces of air-crews. This treatment was later found to have disadvantages in other respects, and the whole subject was thrown wide open. The War Wounds Committee appointed a Burns Subcommittee; and the Council set up a small Burns Research Unit at the Radcliffe Infirmary, Oxford, under the direction of Dr J. M. Barnes. Also at Oxford, Professor R. A. (later Sir Rudolph) Peters and others made biochemical studies of the toxaemia of burns. Peters and his colleagues worked also on chemical burns, first for the Ministry of Supply and later for the Council, and discovered an effective antidote to lewisite and other arsenical poisons—subsequently named 'BAL' (British Anti-Lewisite) by the Americans.

Injuries to the nervous system

A separate Brain Injuries Committee, under the chairmanship of Professor E. D. (later Lord) Adrian, directed attention to the need for keeping accurate and detailed case-histories of patients with wounds involving the brain, and drew up plans for further investigation. Among other things, a glossary of the relevant psychological terms was published (MRC War Memorandum No. 4); and a memorandum on head injuries in air-raid casualties was drawn up by Professor (later Sir) Geoffrey Jefferson for circulation to medical officers concerned. At the Head Injuries Centre at Oxford, directed by Brigadier (later Sir) Hugh Cairns, Dr Dorothy Russell of the Council's staff studied the effects of different antiseptics on brain tissue. A sub-committee, which later became the Nerve Injuries Committee under the chairmanship of Brigadier G. Riddoch, was early in the field with a comprehensive follow-up scheme for cases of injury to the peripheral nerves. To assist medical officers to recognise the effects of injury to individual nerves, a copiously illustrated memorandum was presented to the Committee by Professor J. R. (later Sir James) Learmonth of Edinburgh and was published (MRC War Memorandum No. 7). Later, the Committee was responsible for a volume on peripheral nerve injuries, which was edited by Mr H. J. (later Sir Herbert) Seddon and published for the Council (Special Report Series No. 282, 1954).

Traumatic shock

The problem of 'shock' and haemorrhage in battle casualties had received much attention during the First World War. The opportunities for studying the condition had been uncommon in peace-time but with the outbreak of new hostilities it was certain to be again prominent. The Council accordingly at once appointed a Committee on Traumatic Shock, with Professor G. E. Gask as its first chairman; and a memorandum prepared by this body, in cooperation with the Army Medical Service, was published in 1940 (MRC War Memorandum No. 1).

During the intensive air attacks on London and other cities in 1940, a condition previously unrecognised in Britain was frequently found in persons who had been buried for some hours under heavy debris. In this, the state of shock involved damage to the kidneys, so that the initial symptoms were followed by a frequently fatal uraemia. The concept of a 'crush injury syndrome' arose mainly as a result of observations by Dr E. G. L. Bywaters and his colleagues at the British Postgraduate Medical School, London. Experimental research bearing on the subject was undertaken by workers for the Council at various centres. Shock following industrial injuries was studied at Sheffield by Mr F. W. Holdsworth and Professor H. N. Green.

In the Council's Clinical Research Unit at Guy's Hospital, London, Dr R. T. Grant and Dr E. B. Reeve made observations on shock in air-raid casualties; and when the building was itself badly damaged by enemy action, the Unit was temporarily transferred to the Royal Victoria Infirmary, Newcastle upon Tyne. Here Dr Bywaters, mentioned above, took charge after Dr Grant had gone abroad; and it is of interest that the renowned philosopher Ludwig Wittgenstein did wartime service as a technician in the Unit.

In 1942, Professor W. C. Wilson of Aberdeen was seconded to the RAMC for special research duty in North Africa, as mentioned later (Chapter 16), and among other things he made a detailed clinical study of shock in men severely wounded at the battle of El Alamein. Towards the end of 1943 the Shock Committee concluded that more extensive observations were required to assess the relative significance of blood loss, tissue damage and other results of serious injury in the causation of shock; and that sufficient clinical material could be found only on the battlefield. The Council and the War Office accordingly arranged to send "British Traumatic Shock Team No. 1" to Italy early in 1944; and this was led by Dr (Lieut.-Colonel) R. T. Grant, seconded from the Council's staff to the RAMC.

Much fresh knowledge resulted from all these investigations, and from others undertaken in the Dominions and the United States, and with their forces in various theatres of war. A drastic revision of MRC War Memorandum No. 1 was accordingly undertaken in 1944, and a new edition was published before the end of that year.

Wartime diseases
Looking back, in its Report, the Council said:

> Outbreaks of infective disease have always been a special menace in war and, indeed, up to the time of the opening of the present century they had often been a decisive factor. On the other hand, it is no exaggeration to say that in the recent war epidemics of infective disease were, with very few exceptions, reduced almost to strategical insignificance. It was consciousness of the part that had been played in the past by disease in wartime that made all concerned with the maintenance of health determined to apply existing knowledge to the utmost, and to extend that knowledge.

Thus, some infectious diseases that had been a serious menace to the armed forces during the First World War now proved to be relatively easy to control. This was partly due to different conditions of warfare, but mainly to the advances that had meanwhile been made in methods of therapy and prophylaxis. The new agents included the sulphonamides and other drugs, penicillin in the later stages of the war, and serological preparations of different kinds. In some instances peace-time conditions had not provided massive opportunities for trial; but, in the words of the Report, "most of the diseases thought to be controllable proved to be so in the recent war to an impressive degree", although sometimes not until further investigations had been made. The prophylactic use of toxoid in the Army, to take one example, dramatically reduced the incidence of tetanus.

On the other hand, some familiar diseases presented new problems under the conditions of war. In the civilian population of Great Britain, a reversal of the favourable prewar trend in mortality from tuberculosis was soon apparent; and at the request of the Ministry of Health, in the autumn of 1941, the Council set up a Committee on Tuberculosis in Wartime, under the chairmanship of the Viscount Dawson of Penn and with Dr P. D'Arcy Hart as secretary. This Committee, whose report was published in 1942, initiated a survey of the position; and it made various practical recommendations, among which the controlled use of mass radiography for early diagnosis played a large part. In England, the survey was directed by Professor G. S. (later Sir Graham) Wilson and Dr D'Arcy Hart, making full use of the Emergency Public Health Laboratory Service; parallel schemes operated in Wales and in Scotland.

Infective hepatitis and the allied condition of homologous serum jaundice occurred in outbreaks of unprecedented scale, constituting a substantial drain on manpower, both civilian and military. A research problem of a formidable kind was presented; and at the beginning of 1943, in response to a request by the Ministry of Health, the Council appointed a Jaundice Committee, under the chairmanship of Professor L. J. Witts, and organised a Jaundice Research Team. The clinical, epidemiological and virological investigations were mostly made in Britain, the team being housed in the Department of Pathology, University of Cambridge; Professor S. P. (later Sir Samuel) Bedson acted as general director. Contact was maintained with investigators working on the subject in America.

Malaria and rickettsial fevers

The campaigns in South-East Asia and the Pacific made malaria one of the major medical problems of the war. Except where operations were static, the ordinary measures of mosquito control were inappropriate; efficient mosquito repellants were not yet available; and new synthetic drugs, with some advantages over the older quinine, were just beginning to emerge.

The search for new antimalarial drugs had for some years before the war been part of the Council's programme in chemotherapy. This work was beginning to show promise by the time that war broke out; but workers in Germany were ahead with two new drugs, 'plasmochin' and 'atebrin', which were already on the market. As a short-term measure it was therefore decided to manufacture these drugs, previously protected by patents; the British manufacturers' products proved to be identical and were given the non-commercial names of pamaquin and mepacrine. The former was suitable only for treatment in hospital; but the latter was widely used for prophylaxis in the field, despite some drawbacks, during the early stages of the war. The dependence on synthetic drugs sharply increased when the Japanese occupation of Indonesia in 1942 cut off a large part of the world's supply of quinine, just when the extension of hostilities in the Pacific area was beginning to increase the demand.

In 1943 the Council appointed a Malaria Committee under the chairmanship of Major-General (later Sir) Alexander Biggam. This body concerned itself chiefly with the immediate practical problems of therapy and individual prophylaxis, and it served as a focal point for the work on these aspects. The investigations were made by an Army Malaria Research Unit temporarily established at Oxford, and by medical officers elsewhere at home or overseas, notably in North Africa. Throughout, there was close liaison with the American Board for the Co-ordination of Malarial Studies; and there was also very valuable cooperation with Brigadier (later Sir) Neil Hamilton Fairley and his colleagues in the Australian Army Medical Research Unit at Cairns, Queensland.

Some of the work at Oxford and London on the toxicity of mepacrine involved the use of human volunteers, to whose services the Report pays tribute. Volunteers were also needed, later in 1943, for new experiments in London by Major K. Mellanby and colleagues; the persons on whom drugs were to be tried had to be bitten by infected mosquitoes, and this depended on the skill of Mr P. G. Shute in breeding and infecting the insects in large numbers.

Meanwhile, the search for better antimalarial drugs had been intensified by a closely integrated effort in which British academic laboratories collaborated freely with commercial firms. The joint programme was based on important discoveries already made in the laboratories of Imperial Chemical (Pharmaceuticals) Ltd and later culminating in the development of a highly effective new malarial suppressive named 'paludrine'.

As had been expected, louse-borne epidemic typhus fever became an important disease of the war, particularly among troops in the Mediterranean area. Laboratory studies of the disease were accordingly given a major place in the wartime programme of the National Institute for Medical Research. Close touch was kept with workers in the Army Medical Service; and investigation was concentrated on aspects not already being intensively studied in Canada and the United States. Particular attention was paid to possible chemotherapy; two new sulphonamide compounds gave encouraging results experimentally, but did not fulfil their promise when used in the field. The trials were part of the work of a British Army Typhus Research Team headed by two workers from the National Institute, Major M. van den Ende and Major C. H. (later Sir Charles) Stuart-Harris. The team worked in Algiers in 1943 and in Naples in 1944, and a full account was eventually published.

At the request of the War Office, later in 1943, the Council appointed a Typhus Research Committee, which had Major-General L. T. Poole as chairman. Its primary function was to coordinate the research work at the National Institute and in the Army, and to establish liaison with investigators of the Allied Nations. At this stage, the development of work on typhus vaccine and on the use of new delousing powders was well advanced.

Almost at once the Committee had to extend its scope to meet an urgent request from South-East Asia Command for assistance in dealing with a new menace, the outbreak of mite-borne scrub typhus among the British troops in Burma. This disease of the Far East is due to another species of *Rickettsia* and is conveyed, mainly to rodents but also to man, by the larvae of trombiculid mites inhabiting the ground vegetation. Troops operating in the jungle were thus exposed to infection, and the number of cases soon became alarming; there was also a substantial death-rate. Earlier attempts to produce a vaccine had been unsuccessful; but it was decided to make a fresh endeavour, by new methods, at the National Institute for Medical Research. This yielded a vaccine of high rickettsial content which gave a fair degree of protection in mice; and in view of the urgency this was put straight into mass production by the Wellcome Foundation Ltd, for the Ministry of Supply. Large quantities were despatched to South-East Asia, but the campaign ended before the efficacy of the vaccine under field conditions could be assessed.

Meanwhile, it was essential to improve preventive measures. These consisted of the use of protective clothing and mite repellants, the appropriate siting of camps, and instruction of the troops. A key part was played by a Scrub Typhus Commission, sent by the Council to South-East Asia early in 1944. The Field Director of this Commission was Dr R. Lewthwaite of the Colonial Medical Service (Institute for Medical Research, Kuala Lumpur); and the other members were Dr K. Mellanby, released from the Army to the Council's service, and Squadron Leader C. D. Radford, RAFVR. Dr Lewthwaite later collaborated with American workers in clinical trials of the first successful drug treatment for typhus.

Another rickettsial infection, the louse-borne 'trench fever', had caused heavy morbidity among the opposing armies in Europe during the First World War. This disease scarcely reappeared during the Second World War, probably in part because of the more open conditions of warfare and in part because of more effective methods for preventing bodily infestation with lice.

Work on antilouse measures, directed by Professor P. A. Buxton at the London School of Hygiene and Tropical Medicine, was supported by the Council. This led to the development of an efficient body-belt of cotton, impregnated with lethane, which gave protection of some duration while allowing the underclothes to be washed. Later in the war, however, the Swiss preparation DDT was found to give the best answer, and its large-scale production was undertaken.

Basic therapeutic requirements

Before the war, the Committee of Imperial Defence had instigated measures to avoid a repetition of the situation that had been created in 1914 by the peace-time dependence on Germany for certain essential drugs. In these measures the Council was associated with the Ministry of Health and with an organisation that later became the Directorate of Medical Supplies of the Ministry of Supply. In the first place, arrangements were made to accumulate adequate reserves of such drugs in advance, and eventually to promote the production of British equivalents, under Government licence where patent rights were involved. The Council was largely concerned with these arrangements for production, dealing either through the Association of British Chemical Manufacturers or directly with particular firms. The principle was adopted that the British preparations should be sold under non-proprietary names. Except where chemical identity with the prototype was certain, clinical trials were arranged before the substitutes were used on a large scale.

Immediately after the outbreak of war, the Council's part in these matters was deputed to a Therapeutic Requirements Committee (at first called the Drug Formulary Committee) set up in consultation with the Ministry of Health; and in agreement with the Ministry of Agriculture and Fisheries the veterinary use of drugs was brought within the purview of the same body. The latter was under the chairmanship of Professor L. J. Witts of Oxford, and had Dr C. H. Hampshire of the Pharmacopoeia Commission as its secretary.

As the war progressed, the task became more complex and the need for economy increased. The main sources of many natural substances were cut off, first in Europe and then in Asia; and the cessation of whaling caused a shortage of sperm oil derivatives used in the manufacture of creams, now needed in increased quantities for various medical purposes. Within the United Kingdom, moreover, there were competing claims for raw materials; alcohol, glycerin and mercury were required for munitions and phenolic compounds for plastics. Other important chemicals were, for different purposes, controlled by the Ministry of Food or, the Petroleum Board. There were also restrictions on production owing to shortage of labour and plant.

It was therefore necessary to recommend drastic changes in the prescription of medicines. Serious deficiencies had to be countered by the use of alternatives or substitutes, and existing stocks conserved for the purposes for which they were vitally necessary—for example, the limitation of quinine to the treatment of malaria. Many substances included in prescriptions as flavours or vehicles, had to be omitted or reduced. This affected preparations used in the dressing of wounds and skin diseases; and even "tooth-pastes and cough mixtures acquired a wartime austerity".

The work of the Committee consisted essentially in the pooling and application of knowledge, and many of the recommendations were brought together in a publication entitled *Economy in the Use of Drugs in Wartime* (MRC War Memorandum No. 3) issued early in 1941 (second edition 1944).

Problems of supply were complicated by the continuing rapid advance of research in chemotherapy. An outstanding example was the emergence of new, and for some purposes better, compounds of the sulphnamide group. As the Report says, "The problem was strictly comparable with the progressive improvement of aircraft and weapons of war, and it gave rise to the same difficulty in production programmes". Guidance on the use of new compounds was given where required; and the Committee had the advice of many experts in preparing *The Medical Use of Sulphonamides* (MRC War Memorandum No. 10). This "was one of the most successful and widely read medical publications of the war, and it had a great effect, not merely in improving practice, but in popularising the new outlook on pharmacology, and in accelerating the acceptance of scientific standards in the control of treatment".

The Report concludes its account, under this head, with the following passage on the lasting gains that were thought to have resulted from an activity dictated by conditions of wartime expediency:

The more permanent effects on prescribing produced by the Committee's activities during the war remain a subject for speculation. In general, they were the acceleration of changes which would have come more gradually in peace-time, an acceleration which was the result of expert direction and the avoidance of vested interests or unsupported tradition. Single substances and active principles were used instead of tinctures and mixtures; the many hospital pharmacopoeias, each with their favourite prescriptions, which are chiefly of historical interest, were replaced by the National War Formulary of the Ministry of Health, and the use of foreign or proprietary names was discouraged. Synthetic chemicals were substituted for galenical drugs.

Nutrition in wartime

The advent of war gave an opportunity for practical application of the newer knowledge of human nutrition, with a thoroughness and urgency that had earlier been lacking; it also raised special problems requiring immediate study. The Council was also called upon for certain regular advisory duties related to the administration of food rationing. The general setting is described in the Report as follows:

> The feeding of the population of the United Kingdom, often under conditions of appalling difficulty due to the enemy sea and air blockade, was one of the outstanding achievements of the war. Despite the irksome restrictions of rationing, the fatigues and disappointments of 'queueing', the inevitable limitation of the variety of foodstuffs to be purchased, and the reduced supply of fats and of animal protein, it is a fact that the diet of the nation as a whole was not only maintained at an adequate level in face of the enemy's fiercest efforts to starve us into surrender, but was planned more logically, distributed more equitably, and contained a higher proportion of certain health-producing food substances than ever before. Thus, while everyone was deprived of many dietary luxuries and variants, it is equally true that everyone had a fair share of the available foods, and that certain important nutrients were for the first time allocated on priority to those who needed them most, without regard to their economic circumstances. Research workers in nutrition had the satisfaction of seeing adopted, as measures of urgency under blockade conditions, a number of improvements in the national dietary for which they had pressed in vain for many years beforehand. Moreover, the time-lag between the gaining of knowledge was materially reduced by the establishment of a much closer association between scientific experts and the Government.

The overall official authority in this field was the War Cabinet Committee on Food Policy, over which the Lord Privy Seal presided. For its assistance, he appointed in 1940 a Scientific Food Policy Committee under the chairmanship of Sir William Bragg, then President of the Royal Society (two years later Sir Henry Dale, who had meanwhile become President, was made chairman). The nine members were experts on nutrition, agriculture or economics, and under the first head included Sir Edward Mellanby, Secretary of the Council; Dr B. S. Platt of the Council's staff was one of the secretaries. The Committee constantly referred to the Council, and through it to its expert committees, for advice on questions of human nutrition and food technology. It reported frequently to the War Cabinet Food Policy Committee, and its recommendations often resulted in major changes in the emphasis of the country's food management as well as having an important bearing on the subsequent policy of the Ministry of Food.

The main work of the Scientific Food Policy Committee was done early in the war; but it was apparent that the practical application of the national food policy would raise questions affecting the health of the population, and so it was decided that the Minister of Health should be responsible for advising on these. He accordingly appointed a Standing Committee on Medical and Nutritional Problems, under the chairmanship of his Chief Medical Officer. This body included nominees of the administrative departments and of the research councils. On particular points, the Council and its special committees were frequently called upon for advice.

A valuable source of information was a monograph, by Dr R. A. McCance and Dr Elsie M. Widdowson of the Council's staff, entitled *The Chemical Composition of Foods*. This gave the results of twelve years of work in determining the organic and mineral constituents (vitamins having been assessed by others) of most of the foodstuffs eaten in Great Britain, analysed both in the raw state and as prepared for the table. The first edition was issued by the Council in 1940 (MRC Special Report Series No. 235).

The same two workers, at their own suggestion immediately after the outbreak of war, undertook an experimental study of rationing in advance of the introduction of any compulsory system. They and some colleagues at Cambridge voluntarily subsisted for periods of weeks or months on rations that were considered minimal for the maintenance of general fitness and well-being. In some respects these rations approximated closely to those enforced two years later, and in others they were more restricted than was actually found necessary even under the worst conditions of blockade. The four volunteers who underwent the full experiment were all very fit at the end of three months and satisfactorily passed severe physiological tests. The results were communicated confidentially to the War Cabinet and the departments concerned, but were withheld from publication until 1946 (MRC Special Report Series No. 254). The knowledge provided a reassuring basis for rationing and dietary planning. On the personal side, this tribute was paid in the Report:

> The Council recognise that to submit to a personal experiment of this kind, at a time when food rationing had not been generally introduced in this country, required a very high degree of individual discipline on the part of the volunteers and they here pay tribute to the self-sacrifice and persistence of those who engaged so meticulously in this important and timely investigation.

Calcifying factors in the diet

A matter of outstanding importance in determining the national dietary was the adequate provision of the calcifying factors essential to the proper formation of the teeth and bones. This was a well known requirement in normal times, and not only for the young;

but it acquired special significance because it might not have been met under conditions of rationing.

The practical solution was the eventually compulsory use of 'national wheatmeal' flour for the baking of bread; this was a flour of 85 per cent extraction, midway between the 70 per cent of peace-time white flour and the 100 per cent of wholemeal. The consequent reduction in the amount of imported wheat liberated a large tonnage of vital shipping. On the other hand, the process left the flour with a greater proportion of the phytic acid content of the grain; and it had been shown by Mellanby and D. C. Harrison, in a paper published in 1939, that phytic acid reduces the absorption of calcium from the alimentary canal. This discovery disclosed the danger that the large amount of phytic acid might make the natural calcium content unavailable to the body. Fortunately, it also pointed to the remedy, which was to add more calcium to the flour—as it were, to overtop the enhanced inhibiting effect of the phytic acid. This simple health-saving process was known to the obscurantists as "putting chalk in our bread".

As had long been known, chiefly from earlier work by Mellanby, the body's utilisation of calcium depended also on a sufficiency of vitamin D in the diet. This further requirement might not have been satisfied after the rationing of butter, as margarine (made from vegetable fats) was deficient in this respect. Here the remedy lay in the compulsory fortification of margarine with vitamin D from other sources.

Vitamin studies

Early in the war the Council was consulted about a lack of uniformity in tables currently used by the Ministry of Food and by the Ministry of Health, purporting to show the vitamin content of various foodstuffs. Miss E. M. Hume, a member of the Council's staff and of the Accessory Food Factors Committee, was deputed to investigate the discrepancies, which she found to be large and to affect many items. A subcommittee was therefore appointed to compile tables that might command general acceptance. There was a further demand, by both departments, for tables showing all the constituents of foodstuffs. The information was gradually compiled by the subcommittee in collaboration with medical officers of the Ministry of Health; vitamin and other nutritive values for raw foods, and for foods that had altered in composition during the war, were particularly required to supplement the information in existing publications. The values determined were brought into official use as they became available; and in the last year of the war the final tables, incorporating the results of much work in various laboratories, were published under the title of *Nutritive Values of War-time Foods* (MRC War Memorandum No. 14).

Owing to the shortage of foodstuffs rich in vitamins, it became advisable to reassess the minimal requirements of vitamins A and C.

This was done for the Committee in two critical experiments made at the Sorby Research Institute, Sheffield, on batches of volunteers who were mainly conscientious objectors to military service. The first experiment lasted for rather more than two years, and the second for about a year and a half. Both yielded values that could be recommended as a basis for nutritional planning.

Other studies included an investigation of the deterioration of vitamin A, in some chemical circumstances, when used (with D) in the fortification of margarine. Much work was done, under the aegis of the Committee, on the possible use of food yeast as a supplementary source of proteins (and B vitamins) in a deficient diet. A summary of the results, including those of human trials by Dr T. F. Macrae and others at Cambridge, was published in 1945 (MRC War Memorandum No. 16).

In 1943 the Ministry of Food sought assistance in formulating principles under the Defence (Sale of Food) Regulations "for imposing requirements as to . . . labelling food of various kinds and for restricting the making, in advertisements of food, of claims . . . of the presence of vitamins or minerals". A Vitamin Claims Subcommittee was accordingly appointed, with Professor R. A. (later Sir Rudolph) Peters as chairman and Dr Katherine H. Coward as secretary. The eventual recommendations were endorsed by the main Committee and forwarded by the Council to the Ministry.

Service rations

Much advice was given to all three Service Departments on the question of ration scales. A special question was the adequacy of the vitamin content of emergency canned rations, stored under various conditions, and determinations were made by Dr S. S. Zilva, Dr L. J. Harris and Dr T. Moore of the Council's staff. Advisory help with regard to Army and Royal Air Force feeding arrangements was given by Dr B. S. Platt, also of the staff. Assistance was likewise given, by Dr Platt and others, to the Ministry of Labour in improving arrangements for feeding industrial workers in factory canteens; and a later study of this question was made by Dr R. B. Buzzard for the Council's Industrial Health Research Board.

A special problem was involved in planning very compact rations for use by commandos and airborne troops. Another was that of the emergency rations to be provided in case of shipwreck, whether of naval or mercantile vessels, and also for flying personnel brought down into the sea. In 1941, at the request of the Admiralty, the Council appointed a Committee on the Care of Shipwrecked Personnel, under the chairmanship of Surgeon Vice-Admiral Sir Sheldon Dudley and with Dr Platt as secretary. The most important item was water, and many trials were made on volunteers to determine the minimal daily intake needed to preserve health and the best way in which water could be rationed in lifeboats to secure maximum survival. The Council particularly commended Dr

W. S. S. Ladell and others at the National Hospital for Nervous Diseases, London, and Dr R. A. McCance, Dr D. A. K. (later Sir Douglas) Black and others at Cambridge, for their fortitude in submitting themselves to these trying experiments. The Committee's recommendations on water, food rations and other matters were published in 1943 as *A Guide to the Preservation of Life at Sea after Shipwreck* (MRC War Memorandum No. 8); the Admiralty made an extensive distribution of this pamphlet, and it achieved the largest circulation among all the Council's wartime publications. The findings were also helpful to workers for the Council in southern Iraq who were studying the salt and water requirements of forces in tropical climates, with particular regard to the prevention of heat effects.

Protein requirements and malnutrition

Early in 1943, after consultation with the Ministry of Health, the Council instituted a survey "to obtain evidence of the nutritional state of the people of Great Britain in the fourth year of war". The haemoglobin content of the blood was chosen as the main index because of the simplicity of the test for application to large numbers of people, and because serious continuing deficiency of iron or protein is reflected in diminished values—that is, in anaemia. The chairman of the directing committee was Dr A. N. (later Sir Alan) Drury, with Dr P. L. Mollison and Dr D. P. (later Sir David) Cuthbertson as successive secretaries. The general situation revealed was reasonably good, but a need was shown for some improvement in the haemoglobin levels of young children, pregnant women and the poorer members of the population.

Early in the following year, the Council set up a Protein Requirements Committee, under the chairmanship of Professor H. P. (later Sir Harold) Himsworth and with Dr Cuthbertson (succeeded by Dr A. Neuberger) as secretary. During the preceding ten years, research on protein metabolism in health and disease had been so actively pursued in various countries that "the subject was beginning to approach that of the vitamins in complexity". The immediate task of the Committee was to apply the new knowledge to practical problems of wartime.

Arrangements were made by the Committee, in consultation with the chemical advisers to the manufacturers, for the production of protein hydrolysates of potential value. Similar arrangements were made, with the help of the Ministry of Supply, for the preparation of essential amino acids in concentrated form. The technical difficulties were in some instances formidable; and the products had to be tested both in the laboratory and in clinical use. The hydrolysates found their application in the closing stages of the war, as described in the Report:

At the beginning of 1945 it became apparent that starvation on an unprecedented scale would be encountered on the liberation countries previously occupied by the enemy. In expectation of this, the Committee collected and reviewed the available information on the treatment of starvation, and was thus in a position to help when the Netherlands Government officially requested the aid of the Council in regard to it. Members of the Committee proceeded to Holland to study the condition and needs of starving populations in the regions then liberated. They made recommendations to Supreme Headquarters, Allied Expeditionary Force, and were requested to make the necessary arrangements to deal with the medical aspects of the problem.

With the liberation of North-West Holland:

Simultaneously, and quite unexpectedly, the appalling conditions in German concentration camps were disclosed, and these provided a situation demanding urgent measures for the treatment of starvation of extreme degree, and of the fevers and other illnesses associated with it. Supplies of the special materials for treating starvation were diverted to Germany, and the trained medical students, together with a special team of research workers directed by Dr Janet M. Vaughan, were sent to Belsen camp. Much valuable information was obtained, on the basis of which the War Office directive for the treatment of prisoners-of-war liberated from Japanese prison camps in the Far East was constructed.

Special diets

At the beginning of 1940, the Council was asked by the Ministry of Food, the Ministry of Health and the Department of Health for Scotland to appoint an expert committee "to advise from time to time on the question whether it is necessary on medical grounds to modify or supplement rations in the case of invalids or other persons on special diets". The Food Rationing (Special Diets) Advisory Committee was accordingly set up, under the chairmanship of Sir Edward Mellanby and with Professor H. P. Himsworth as secretary (eventually succeeding to the chairmanship). After the war, Dr M. L. (later Sir Max, later Lord) Rosenheim was appointed deputy secretary and then secretary, carrying the main burden until the end of rationing. At meetings the Ministry of Food was represented by an observer in the person of its scientific adviser, Sir Jack Drummond, or one of his deputies. The Report records that:

The Committee, as an advisory body, was free to comment on policy and was independent of the executive; it was thus able to serve as a court of appeal, and to give opinions which were generally accepted as disinterested, to the several departments it advised. The success of such a relationship depends, nevertheless, upon a high degree of co-operation and trust between the advised and the advisers, and the members of the Committee wish to place on record their appreciation of the confidence, support, and help which they received from the Government departments with which they were associated. Not only were matters referred to them without prejudice, but no relevant information was withheld and, when such information was not available, every facility to procure it was placed at their disposal.

The full Committee met to consider general principles, and individual cases in so far as these raised new issues. Owing to wartime difficulties of travel, much of the business had to be transacted by correspondence, while the handling of individual applications was delegated to particular members. Applications were referred through the machinery of the Ministry of Food, beginning at the Local Food Offices, and findings were notified through the same channel in reverse. The average interval between receipt of the application at the local office and notification of the decision to the applicant was nine days; and during this period the Local Food Executive Officer was empowered to allow extra rations if these were urgently requested. Appeals and complaints were referred by the Ministry to Professor Himsworth or, in Scotland, to Professor L. S. P. (later Sir Stanley) Davidson.

A much fuller account of the Committee's wartime work than is possible here can be found in the Report for 1939–45. In summary:

> Three general principles were adopted: first, that illnesses qualifying for extra rations should be precisely defined and the concession strictly limited to that precise group of patients; second, that extra rations should be granted only on the grounds of proven therapeutic necessity; third, that when it was impossible to satisfy all of several competing claims, the concession should be granted to those groups with the better prospects of recovery or which, by means of special rations, could be kept at work in full vigour.

The first principle was essential for proper administration and it encouraged confidence in a reasonably uniform standard of certification. The second principle inevitably involved some hardship, but its enforcement was unavoidable when the requirements for invalids had to be weighed against the needs of the general population. The Committee had to reject applications in cases where satisfactory alternatives to dietetic therapy were available; and it had to disallow traditional dietaries for invalids and convalescents which had no known effect on the ultimate outcome of the disease. More distressing was the necessary refusal of extra rations on compassionate grounds, mainly to the incurably ill or very old. In a few instances, nevertheless, it was indicated to the Ministry that its prerogative of clemency might well be exercised—for example, that of a child dying of leukaemia who craved for sweets. The Report laconically concludes its discussion of this theme: "By the same principle were decided applications for special rations from eccentrics, from gourmets, from devotees of strange dietary cults, and from persons who believed that their social or public position could legitimately be taken into account."

The third principle was a grim necessity. In the autumn of 1941, at a very grave stage of the war, about 50 per cent of the nation's milk supply was going to persons with priority claims, while in the general population the individual consumption of animal protein from other sources was under 30 grams a day—and the country sorely needed the energy of every able-bodied worker. The Committee had reluctantly to advise the Ministry that "until the supply of milk was such as to provide a full allowance of milk daily to the working population, it would be against the interests of the national health to allow extra milk to mental defectives and hopeless invalids at the expense of the already restricted supplies to active workers". Later it became necessary to apply the principle to all rationed foods. The conditions for which the Committee had to consider extra rations included diabetes mellitus, 'spontaneous' hypoglycaemia, the steatorrhoeas, the anaemias, tuberculosis, liver disease, severe burns and chronic suppuration.

A general problem was that of alleged 'food sensitivity'. Thus, there were innumerable applications for extra butter by people claiming to be sensitive to margarine; it was indeed hard to believe that there could be so many cases of such an allergy, especially as they nearly all occurred in a limited section of the population. It was accordingly advised that extra butter should be allowed only when sensitivity to margarine could be demonstrated by prescribed tests; one of these was that the applicant should be able to distinguish butter from margarine when the taste was disguised. As soon as the requirement was made known, the number of applicants declined abruptly; and of the few who presented themselves to the appointed specialists, none showed clear evidence of margarine sensitivity and only one was able to distinguish margarine from butter.

Similarly, the numerous complaints of sensitivity to the 'national wheatmeal' flour, on the part of persons not subject to the recognised allergy to wheat flour in general, were found to have little substance when put to test. There were also complaints of sensitivity to rye, barley, oat or potato flour that might have to be used to eke out the supply of wheat; but "many applications claiming sensitivity to these diluents came from parts of the country where only pure wheat flour had been issued".

In the period immediately after the war, the rationing of the main energy-producing foods—bread and potatoes—increased the responsibility of the Committee as an advisory body. It continued to fill a most important need until rationing drew to a close, and it was not discharged until 1954.

Wartime health in industry
Apart from strictly medical aspects, physiological and psychological problems of industry had urgently demanded attention during the First World War; and between the wars a mass of accurate scientific data had accumulated, largely from studies by investigators under the Council's Industrial Health Research Board. Many of the resulting recommendations had been implemented by progressive employers, with good effect, but regrettably little of this knowledge had been assimilated by industrial leaders in general and by the mass of workers.

One of the first tasks in the Second World War was accordingly to publicise the information already available. This was done, in 1940, by issuing "a summary of research findings capable of immediate application in furtherance of the national effort" (IHRB Emergency Report No. 1). This was supplemented later in the war by three pamphlets dealing briefly, in a readily understandable way, with the several problems indicated by the titles: *Ventilation and Heating: Lighting and Seeing; Absence from Work: Prevention of Fatigue;* and *Why is She Away? The Problem of Sickness among Women in Industry.* Nevertheless, as the Council's Report puts it:

> The fear that the lessons learnt in 1915–17, regarding the deleterious effects of excessively long hours of work on health and output, might be forgotten under the stress of a new and even fiercer struggle for national survival proved to be well-founded—as was shown by what happened in industry in the months following the evacuation from Dunkirk. At that time the call was for more and more munitions to replace those lost upon the Continent, and to prepare for the next stage of the conflict. The response of industry was commensurate with the urgency of the situation, and for many weeks both men and women in war factories voluntarily endured excessively long working hours without holidays The result, as might be expected, was that although initially there was an exceptionally high level of output, it could not be maintained, and the ill-effects of the almost superhuman effort voluntarily endured were soon reflected in an increased amount of sickness absence. These facts were clearly established in a series of surveys made by workers for the Board, of which the results were published.

The foregoing was only one of many special investigations made by the Board's investigators in the course of the war. These involved the application of well tried methods to new problems—or, more often, to old problems in different or intensified form. Thus, in the field of air hygiene (Dr T. Bedford and others), there was the ventilation of air-raid shelters and of buildings under conditions of 'black-out'; there were also particular difficulties in factories where noxious dusts or fumes were apt to accumulate. Experimental work on airborne infection and air purification was undertaken at the National Institute for Medical Research.

Similarly, with regard to industrial illumination (Mr H. C. Weston), the requirements of black-out introduced new difficulties. The investigations were helpful to the drafting of the Factories (Standards of Lighting) Regulations 1941. Dr Dora Colebrook made a carefully controlled study of treatment by ultraviolet rays ('artificial sunlight') introduced in many factories as a corrective to work under black-out conditions; the results disclosed no assessable benefits, and even the subjective views of the workers were by no means unanimous.

On the psychological side, investigations were made into hours of work, absenteeism and cognate problems as presented in the wartime environment (Dr S. Wyatt and others), and also into the selection and training of personnel and the prevention of accidents (Mr E. Farmer and others). Experimental work on fatigue and on the design of display panels and controls for precision instruments was done by the Council's Applied Psychology Research Unit at Cambridge; this had bearings on industrial problems, although under-taken primarily for the Flying Personnel Research Committee. Studies of neurosis among factory operatives in the engineering industry were made in Birmingham (Dr T. Russell Fraser and others) and in London (Dr Elizabeth Bunbury and others).

A substantial increase in the Council's programme of research on industrial hazards and diseases, in the course of the war, was largely part of long-term planning, but immediate attention was naturally given to problems directly related to the war effort. Diseases due to inhaled dusts, including especially the pneumoconiosis of coalminers (Dr P. D'Arcy Hart), were prominent among the subjects of study. So also was industrial toxicology (Dr D. Hunter and others); the known hazards of manufacturing certain explosives, for example, were accentuated by wartime environmental circumstances, and many substances new to industry were being made on a large scale.

In addition, research work on wound infections, burns and trau-matic shock, mentioned earlier in this chapter, had its bearing on treatment following industrial accidents as well as on that of casual-ties due to enemy action.

Scientific liaison
As the Report says, "In normal times medical research is little concerned with subjects of a secret nature, and early publication of findings is the best means of keeping workers informed of the progress of others, wherever situated, whose investigations are following similar lines". In wartime this easy communication may be seriously disrupted. There are apt to be difficulties in securing rapid publica-tion and in distributing the journals; in any event, immediate publication of research results may often be ruled out for security reasons.

Part of this problem was met by the periodical *Bulletin of War Medicine*, prepared for the Council by the staff of the Bureau of Hygiene and Tropical Medicine in collaboration with the Council's own publications officer; this gave information about new work published anywhere in the world, including enemy countries. Other-wise, the answer lay in arrangements for the official exchange of unpublished documents between allied countries, and their dis-semination where desirable. The Council's office played its part in this scheme, in respect of relevant subjects.

These international exchanges on paper were supplemented by personal contact. Medical and scientific liaison officers from the Dominions and from the United States were stationed in London. These kept in close touch with the Council's headquarters and appropriate research establishments; they also regularly attended meetings of some of the Council's scientific committees.

In the reverse direction, the Council was able to work through the British Commonwealth Scientific Office in Washington, for purposes of liaison in the United States and Canada; and for part of the time it had its own representative attached to that office, the position being successively held by Professor J. H. Burn of Oxford and Professor A. D. Macdonald of Manchester. In addition, shorter visits were paid for special purposes by other representatives of the Council, not only to North America but to Commonwealth and allied countries elsewhere. Mr (later Sir) Ernest Rock Carling, a member of the Council, was included in a party of British and American surgeons visiting the USSR in 1943; and in the following year Professor H. W. (later Lord) Florey and Dr A. G. Sanders were sent there on a short visit for the exchange of information on recent developments in medical science, and particularly to give information about the uses of penicillin.

Chapter 16
Second War: Personnel Research and Emergency Services

Service personnel research—Flying personnel—Army personnel—Armoured fighting vehicles—Naval personnel—Warships in tropical climates—Continuation of personnel research after the war—Emergency services—Emergency Register of Pathologists—Immunological supplies—Supply of blood for transfusion—The London blood depots in action—Drying of blood products—Determination of blood groups—Blood transfusion research—Permanent gains

Service personnel research

During the Second World War, physiological and psychological research bearing upon the role of the individual participants in war activities became an important concern of the Council. There had been almost no corresponding function in the First World War, except with regard to physiological problems of aviation; and in only a few instances had the Services sought the Council's aid in time of peace. At the request of the Admiralty, for example, a study of colour vision requirements in the Royal Navy had been arranged by the Council, which published a report in 1933. And, later, work on vocational selection for special duties was undertaken for the Fighting Services by investigators of the Council's Industrial Health Research Board.

A characteristic of this type of work is that it relates to the capacities of healthy individuals. For that reason, the problems were often not regarded by the Fighting Services as being within the scope of their Medical Departments, so that the Council had to deal to some extent directly with the operational branches. Eventually, there were also problems that involved the Ministries responsible for the design and production of equipment, not excluding weapons.

'Personnel research', as it came to be called shortly before the war, was defined in the Report for 1939–45 as follows:

> Briefly, the term connotes, in relation to the Fighting Services, the study, by physiological and psychological methods, of the best means of increasing the operational efficiency, safety and comfort of sailors, soldiers and aviators under different environmental conditions, and conversely, the adaptation of ships, fighting vehicles, aircraft and weapons to the convenience and capabilities of those who have to use them.

This work was developed by the appointment of special committees of Service representatives and civilian scientists to plan and direct it on a vastly expanded scale, and by the setting up of a number of new establishments for its intensive prosecution. Much of the information handled, and of the results obtained, was necessarily secret at the time.

317

The first of these special committees to be set up, a few months before the war, was the Flying Personnel Research Committee. In this case the appointment was made by the Air Ministry, which invited Sir Edward Mellanby, Secretary of the Council, to be chairman and to advise on the choice of civilian members. In the other two cases, arising after the war had begun, appointment was by the Council, in agreement with the War Office and Admiralty respectively.

The first problem referred to the Council by the War Office, after the evacuation from Dunkirk in 1940, was that of ear protection against battle noise. This was followed by a request for advice on the controversial question of body armour, and the Council appointed a Body Protection Committee under the chairmanship of the Viscount Falmouth. In the following year, after consultation with the Army Council, this was reconstituted as the Military Personnel Research Committee, with a larger membership and a much wider remit. Dr E. A. Carmichael of the Council's scientific staff was secretary throughout.

In 1942 the Board of Admiralty asked for the establishment of a similar body in respect of its own requirements. It was the Board's suggestion that appointment should be made by the Council, and that Sir Edward Mellanby should be chairman. The Royal Naval Personnel Research Committee was duly set up, with Dr G. L. (later Sir Lindor) Brown of the Council's scientific staff as its secretary.

In retrospect, the Council said:

> It is certain that the practical recommendations arising from investigations promoted by the Personnel Research Committees contributed in no small measure to military success, and the saving of life, in the recent war: and it is already clear that, just as the methods and results of industrial health research have assisted in the solution of various Service problems, so also many of the research methods adopted to solve urgent problems affecting the Fighting Services under war conditions can be effectively applied in peacetime to the solution of numerous problems of the human factor in industry; these include not only the selection of the right worker for the right job, and securing of the best practical environment for the job, but also the design of machines, instrument panels, working benches and other equipment from the points of view of maximal comfort and efficiency. The principle in each case is that of suiting the job to the man, of suiting the man to the job, and of improving the man's performance.

Of personnel research in general, it may be said that under conditions of war much of it was highly satisfying, both to the Council and to its investigators, because it gave quick results that were visibly of immediate use in increasing the efficiency of the Services, as the latter freely acknowledged. Other parts of it, however, were subject to the frustrating factor of a long time-lag in practical application; the theoretical answer to an operational problem might itself be speedily found, but a radical fault in equipment could not be rectified until an improved design had been fully worked out and brought through the stages of production into actual use, perhaps two years later. This consideration led the Council to say:

> The hope may be expressed that whenever in the future vast new problems involving the design and development of instruments, weapons and machinery, which have to be worked by human beings, arise, it will no longer be thought sufficient to have such matters considered only by engineers and physicists. In many cases the main limiting factor in the efficiency of the machine or weapon is the human being working it. The earlier the stage at which the human factor is considered by physiologists and psychologists in relation to machine or instrument design, the more effective will be the end result. This need for taking into consideration the human factor applies not only to machine design but to all matters where human effort is needed, whether in the military or in the civil field.

Only a very brief review of the more important investigations can be given here.

Flying personnel

As already noted, the Committee in this case was appointed by the Air Ministry, which accordingly provided the secretariat and was responsible for executive action. The link with the Council was nevertheless extremely close throughout the war; and the Council's staff made a substantial contribution to the research programme, otherwise carried out largely by regular or temporary officers of the Royal Air Force and notably at the RAF Physiological Laboratory at Farnborough (later the RAF Institute of Aviation Medicine).

Relevant information about other research work promoted by the Council was regularly supplied to the Committee. Various investigations required by the Committee were made in the Council's research establishments by members of its scientific staff. The subjects included special clothing for aircrews, acoustics, visual adaptation, and airsickness. In other cases, members of the Council's staff were seconded to the Air Ministry for work under its direction at Farnborough and elsewhere. Dr A. (later Sir Austin) Bradford Hill became, in this way, statistical adviser to the Director-General of Medical Services at the Ministry.

A major contribution was to make available the whole of the Council's research team under the direction of Professor F. C. (later Sir Frederic) Bartlett in the Psychological Laboratory at Cambridge; this team developed into the Applied Psychology Research Unit, with Dr K. W. Craik as its first director. Among the problems studied were the selection of aircrews, pilot fatigue, human factors in the causation of flying accidents, the selection and training of control personnel, the equipment of operation rooms, the optimal length of watch for radar operators in aircraft on anti-submarine patrol, and the design and positioning of aircraft controls and instruments.

Army personnel

The general scope of the Military Personnel Research Committee is indicated by the subjects for which subcommittees were appointed at various dates. These are named here in alphabetical order: accidents to army vehicles; air-borne troops; analeptic substances; armoured fighting vehicles (tanks); body armour and helmets; clothing for special tasks and conditions; entomology; motion sickness; rations; weapons (biological assay); and vision. Dr E. A. Carmichael was not only secretary of the main committee but also chairman of four of the subcommittees and secretary of two others.

In 1941, the General Staff sought assistance in problems of flame-throwers, and arrangements were made for Dr R. B. Bourdillion of the Council's staff to cooperate with the Petroleum Warfare Board. By courageous experiments involving substantial personal risk, he was able to obtain accurate information on the relative efficiency of different flame-throwing devices, and also to suggest means of protection against them.

The Committee was also consulted about radar equipment, and it was found possible to make improvements in design that increased operational efficiency and reduced fatigue. There had been disquieting rumours among the service personnel concerned, which at home included women, that permanent bodily damage could result from side-effects of the machines generating the rays. Careful measurements showed these fears to be groundless, and an authoritative statement was issued.

The Committee and its subcommittees frequently had need of more definite information about conditions in the field than was readily available. In 1942, therefore, it proposed that skilled observers be attached to Army Headquarters in various theatres of war for the purpose of quickly obtaining accurate scientific data about battle conditions, and of reporting on relevant physiological problems. This commended itself both to the Council and to the War Office, and scientists selected by the former were soon attached to Army Headquarters in Egypt, India and at home, with Army Council directives giving them facilities for entering battle zones and for reporting on urgent matters directly to the Council and the War Office. These were the earliest arrangements for attaching civilian scientists, with temporary commissions, to headquarters in the field; but the practice was afterwards developed on a wider basis, and from it were evolved the Operational Research Groups of later years.

The first implementation of this scheme was the establishment of a Medical Research Section to collect information on the health and well-being of the Middle East Forces, particularly those then operating in North Africa. This was in charge of Professor (Lieut.-Colonel) W. C. Wilson, who held the chair of surgery at Aberdeen, and he had as his colleagues Dr (Major, later Colonel) A. C. Chute from Canada and Dr (Major) E. T. C. Spooner of Cambridge. A wide range of problems was studied, including physiological and other questions relating to tank warfare in the desert, the practical value of body armour as protection against wounds of the trunk, and the medical aspects of parachute jumping. The work of the Section was specially commended by the Army Council; and the more urgent of the recommendations, relating especially to human efficiency in tank warfare, were immediately implemented by the GOC in Cairo. The reports of the observers were of great value in guiding further research under the auspices of the Committee.

Armoured fighting vehicles
An outstandingly interesting and important development of personnel research was a study of the physiological factors affecting the efficiency of the crews of armoured fighting vehicles. In October 1940 the Council offered to provide a research team on this subject, and the proposal was readily accepted by the Army Council. To guide the project, a subcommittee was set up under the chairmanship of Sir Edward Mellanby and including representatives of the War Office directorates concerned and of the Ministry of Supply, together with scientific members nominated by the Council. A Physiological Research Laboratory was established in the Armoured Fighting Vehicle Training School at Lulworth, Dorset, and was in effect a temporary research unit of the Council's organisation. The Laboratory was directed successively by Dr O. M. Solandt (from Toronto), Dr G. L. (later Sir Lindor) Brown, Professor I. de Burgh Daly (University of Edinburgh) and Dr E. E. (later Sir Edward) Pochin—two of them members of the Council's staff, and the others temporarily seconded to it. Civilian scientists and Army medical officers took part in the investigations at Lulworth; special problems were also referred to other establishments of the Council. In all, a very substantial research effort was brought to bear on the subject.

One problem was that of fume hazards due to ineffective disposal of engine exhaust gases, and also to discharge of the vehicle's armament. This involved the Ministry of Supply with regard to design, and also the Admiralty, as the hazards from exhaust fumes were particularly great when the vehicles were being disembarked from tank landing ships and craft. There was likewise collaboration with the Chemical Defence Research Station at Porton. Further, the question of ordinary ventilation, including the use of special ventilated clothing, was very relevant to the operation of the vehicles in hot climates, both dry and wet.

As the Report says, "It early became clear that modern knowledge of lighting, and of the physiological mechanisms of vision, could be effectively applied to increasing the fighting efficiency of the crews". The interior lighting of tanks was at first too dim by day and too bright by night; improvements in design were recommended and adopted, including red lighting of instruments at the right level. A pamphlet instructing tank crews in the more effective use of night vision was written by the staff of the Laboratory and accepted by the War Office as a training manual. As a result, a member of the staff was requested by the Director of Military Training to report on methods of eye training and visual observation in all branches of the Army. Other visual problems successfully tackled were those of dazzle by gunflash, difficulty in observing the fall of shot, and improvement of the field of vision from the cupola and other positions within the vehicle. Again, some of the solutions had wider application and were of value to the Admiralty and the Royal Air Force. This was true also of recommendations that the staff were able to make about the design of optical instruments, such as periscopes and telescopic sights.

Other questions studied were gun-laying, tank driving, and the safety of crews. The account in the Report concludes with the following paragraph:

So valuable was the work of the Armoured Fighting Vehicles Sub-Committee and the Council's research team at Lulworth found to be, that, when the United States of America entered the war, the authorities there sent representatives to report on the work at Lulworth and immediately set up an organisation with generously equipped laboratories to undertake similar studies. A most happy and useful collaboration between the British and American establishments followed, and much of the early work carried out in the Laboratory at Lulworth was confirmed by the American investigators.

Naval personnel
Although it was not until late in 1942 that the Admiralty requested the Council to set up an analogous Royal Naval Personnel Research Committee, this body was thereafter very active. The Admiralty representatives included officers from the Executive and Medical Branches; two members of the Council's staff also served, Dr B. S. Platt and Dr G. L. Brown. The last named, as Secretary, had from 1943 the help of Surgeon Lieut.-Commander (later Captain) F. P. Ellis, RN, as Naval Medical Secretary.

The Committee's first investigation was into living conditions in Coastal Force craft, and this led to recommendations on clothing and on the reduction of condensation and noise. Arrangements were also made for Surgeon Captain M. Critchley, RNVR, to act as a medical observer of the effect of climatic conditions during convoys to Murmansk and Iceland. Later on, as mentioned below, the Committee's attention became directed to climate at the other extreme. Much of the work on living conditions in ships, and indeed also in shore establishments, was coordinated by a Habitability Subcommittee; and that on special clothing by a Clothing Subcommittee. The latter sent Mr J. C. D. Hutchinson as an observer to the cold-weather clothing trials carried out in Canada by the Dominion Armed Forces.

By 1943, developments were taking place in underwater warfare and in extended use of divers for reconnaissance and other purposes. The Admiralty accordingly asked the Committee to undertake further physiological research on diving and cognate matters; a Subcommittee on Underwater Physiology was accordingly set up, and on its recommendation the Admiralty established the Royal Naval Physiological Laboratory, near the submarine base at Fort Block-house and under the direction of Surgeon Commander C. G. L. Pratt, RNVR. The Subcommittee was also able to use the services of Professor J. B. S. Haldane and officers of the Admiralty Experi-mental Diving Unit. Work on some of the problems was undertaken by members of the Council's own staff in the National Institute for Medical Research and in the Neurological Research Unit directed by Dr E. A. Carmichael. In addition, the Subcommittee fostered the development of air-purifying gear for submarines; this work involved sea trials under war conditions.

The Committee was also concerned with some questions of gun-nery and set up a subcommittee on this subject. One problem of major interest, relating primarily to director control towers, was "that of the seated operator working sights and hand-wheels, there being a natural tendency on the part of the designers to assemble components in a manner giving the maximum of constructional simplicity, which too often makes little allowance for the needs of the human operator". Valuable work on this problem was done for the Subcommittee by Professor W. E. (later Sir Wilfrid) Le Gros Clark and Dr A. G. M. Weddell in the Department of Human Anatomy of the University of Oxford. Among other things, they were able "to design seats which provide a secure, stable and comfortable posture for the operator, allow him to use optical instruments or hand-wheels without strain or contortion, and permit of comfortable relaxation during the periods of waiting". The work was later extended to other aspects of gunnery, particularly the design of tracking devices and of sights; in these studies the Psychological Laboratory of the University of Cambridge, and the Council's own Applied Psychology Research Unit there, usefully collaborated.

Other gunnery problems included the conditions inside gun-turrets, and special protective clothing for their crews. In measuring the energy output of turret-crews, Dr J. A. B. (later Sir John) Gray of the Council's staff "found out that certain tasks required of the men in handling-rooms and magazines demanded an energy output equal to or even greater than that of a trained athlete". So that, with the inevitable speeding up of naval warfare, restriction of the rate of fire came to depend on human rather than mechanical limitations. Redesigning of equipment and a reallocation of tasks did much to counteract this difficulty.

Warships in tropical climates
In the spring of 1943, intensive naval operations in tropical waters were clearly imminent, and the attention of the Royal Naval Per-sonnel Research Committee became particularly directed to the problems of life and work in HM ships under such conditions. Arrangements were made to despatch two observers, Surgeon

Captain M. Critchley and Surgeon Lieut.-Commander H. E. Holling, RNVR (of the Council's staff), to the Mediterranean and the Indian Ocean; their subsequent reports showed that the atmospheric conditions in the ships were not conducive to maintaining a high level of efficiency in their complement. The Admiralty asked for more research work, and its Habitability Sub-Committee was set up to coordinate this. A mission consisting of Surgeon Lieut.-Commander Ellis, Surgeon Lieut.-Commander Holling, and Constructor Lieut.-Commander Brokensha, RCNC, with technical assistants and the necessary apparatus, was sent to the Eastern Fleet. As the Report says: "The collaboration of a naval constructor with medical men proved exceptionally valuable, and the mission, in addition to producing unique data on conditions in the Fleet, were able to recommend material improvements in the living conditions in most of the ships which they visited."

At the same time, laboratory investigations were undertaken in the United Kingdom, the Admiralty equipping two climatic chambers at the National Hospital for Nervous Diseases in London, and one in the University Psychological Laboratory at Cambridge, for use by the Council's Research Units at these centres. Experiments soon confirmed that efficiency would suffer at levels of temperature, humidity and air movement which were below those frequently found in ships of the Eastern Fleet. The Admiralty took immediate steps to improve matters by temporary expedients in the first instance, and by alterations in the design of ships under construction or planned. Dr T. Bedford, of the Council's staff, prepared a handbook on environmental warmth and its measurement, which was adopted by the Admiralty for use in HM ships (MRC War Memorandum No. 17).

It was clearly important, however, that research work should be extended to the tropics, instead of being dependent on volunteer subjects living in a temperate climate and temporarily subjected to artificial conditions. In the quest for a suitable location overseas, the Council had the help of Professor H. C. Bazett, a British subject holding a chair in the United States, who had great experience of climatic physiology. The first choice was Bombay, but this idea was dropped when the strategic situation necessitated the formation of a British Pacific Fleet, with a consequent great reduction in the number of ships using Indian ports. Eventually, the cessation of hostilities with Japan made it feasible to place the proposed Tropical Research Unit at Singapore, the Admiralty being anxious that the investigations should be continued in time of peace. Arrangements were made with the King Edward VII Medical College there, and with the Colonial Office, for placing the Unit in the College building; and investigators were appointed by the Council and by the Medical Department of the Navy.

An integral part of this Unit, as originally planned, was a sea-going component that would extend the observations to ships under active service conditions in tropical waters. Surgeon Lieut. J. A. B. (later Sir John) Gray, RNVR, with two technicians, was accordingly attached to the British Pacific Fleet. The favourable course of the war limited the opportunities, but some valuable observations were made.

Continuation of personnel research after the war

Among the Service Departments, the Admiralty in particular was anxious that personnel research should be maintained after the war, and that the Council should continue to advise and the Royal Naval Personnel Research Committee to direct. Lines of investigation for which subcommittees had been set up during the war were extended into the postwar period, even to the present time. Further sub-committees were in fact appointed after the war to deal with the physiological problems related to prolonging survival after shipwreck and to the effects of underwater explosions on men immersed or submerged in the vicinity.

The whole programme was directed entirely towards increasing the comfort, health, safety and efficiency of naval personnel; but the results had important bearings on questions of warship ventilation and the design of diving, gunnery and communication equipment. The actual research work, at this stage, was done mainly by naval scientsts and medical officers, but civilian scientists who had become familiiar with the problems during the war still collaborated.

One of the main continuing interests was in the effects of high temperatures on the mental and physical efficiency of naval personnel serving afloat in the tropics. The Admiralty and the Council accordingly decided to proceed with the plan, already mentioned, for a research unit at Singapore. In 1947, too, the Admiralty sought the help of the Council in examining the effects of cold environments on human efficiency, in relation to shipboard conditions in arctic waters.

Another continuing activity was the examination of human performance in relation to basic principles in the design of weapons and the arrangement of equipment. The complexities of anti-aircraft and anti-submarine defence procedures made this an important study for naval purposes, but many of the new ideas were also capable of wide application in industry. Similarly, the work on methods of escape from sunken submarines, and on the effects of prolonged submergence in submarines fitted with the schnorkel device, had applications to the needs of engineers and industrial workers operating under high pressures during deep tunnelling operations.

Emergency services

During the war, and even in anticipation of it, the Council undertook for the Government the conduct of certain emergency services of a technical nature, with which its staff was particularly fitted to deal. The outstanding example was the Emergency Public Health Laboratory Service; but as this developed into a permanent

organisation of importance it has already been given separate
treatment (Chapter 13).

As the Report says, "a paramount element in the Council's conduct of these technical affairs was scientific control from the centre".
This aspect of the task was at first largely the responsibility of a
member of Council, Professor W. W. C. Topley, who was attached
to the Council's headquarters from the outbreak of war for whole-
time duty as chief adviser in pathology; he had earlier, as the chairman or a member of various *ad hoc* committees, taken a leading part
in planning the emergency services. He was a bacteriologist of high
distinction, holding the University chair in that subject at the London
School of Hygiene and Tropical Medicine. He had an ingenious and
restless mind; and he was a prodigious and persuasive talker. Many
of the ideas were originally his, and later one could assess how far-
seeing they had been. He worked closely with the present writer
and other members of the regular staff in translating these ideas into
administrative action. Topley died suddenly at the beginning of
1944; there is a full obituary notice by Dean and Wilson.

Topley had already left, in 1941, to become Secretary of the
Agricultural Research Council. His former duties were then divided
among a number of experts. Professor G. S. (later Sir Graham)
Wilson, who had been appointed Director of the Emergency Public
Health Laboratory Service on the death of Dr W. M. Scott, became
chief adviser in that respect. Dr A. N. (later Sir Alan) Drury, a
member of the Council's external scientific staff, was brought in to
deal with questions of blood supply and blood transfusion; and when
he in turn left, to become Director of the Lister Institute, his place
was taken by Dr D. P. (later Sir David) Cuthbertson, lent by the
University of Glasgow. Dr (later Sir) Philip Panton of the Ministry
of Health succeeded Topley as chairman of the committee on the
allocation of pathologists and technicians. Dr (later Sir) Percival
Hartley of the National Institute for Medical Research continued to
advise on immunological supplies.

The cost of emergency services was not a charge on the research
funds at the Council's disposal, but was separately provided through
the votes of the appropriate Government Departments. From the outbreak of war, the formula was that the services were conducted on
an agency basis on behalf of the Ministry of Health. There was
nevertheless, as the Report says, "a complete delegation of executive
responsibility, under which both the preliminary planning and the
subsequent administration rested with the Council".

Emergency Register of Pathologists
A purely administrative service was the compilation and maintenance of an Emergency Register of Pathologists and Pathological
Laboratory Technicians. This machinery enabled the Council to
advise the Central Medical War Committee (in respect of medically
qualified personnel) and the Ministry of Labour and National

Service on the allocation of pathologists and technicians to emergency duties, or their reservation in existing employment. Proper use of this category of manpower was especially important, because the wartime demand for its skills was very high in relation to the small total available. Many pathologists and technicians were required to staff the laboratories with the forces and those of the emergency medical services at home; and at the same time the ordinary medical work of the country had to be maintained.

Immunological supplies

While the Therapeutic Requirements Committee was concerned with drugs (Chapter 15), a parallel function was performed—before the war as well as during it—by the Emergency Immunological Supplies Committee, originally appointed by the Council to help it in meeting an assignment from the Committee of Imperial Defence. Sir John Ledingham was chairman, with Dr F. J. C. Herrald of the Council's headquarters staff as secretary.

The original remit to the Council, in 1937, had in view provision against possible bacteriological warfare or sabotage. It soon became apparent, however, that the largest problem was the supply of antitoxins to protect the injured against infections due to the contamination of wounds by soil or other material containing spores of the tetanus bacillus or of organisms of the gas-gangrene group. In peacetime the demand for these antitoxins was small, and the production potential was correspondingly limited. There was thus a need for building up reserve stocks in the first place, and for securing continued large-scale production after the outbreak of war. In making arrangements for this purpose, the Council had the close cooperation of the manufacturers, particularly the Wellcome Foundation Ltd and the Lister Institute of Preventive Medicine. Until 1943, when the responsibility passed to the Ministry of Supply, the Council coordinated and anticipated the demands on the common pool of these products.

The Council was also charged with responsibility for meeting a demand for vaccines and sera that might be required, on an unusually large scale, for the control of possible epidemics of typhoid and paratyphoid fever, bacillary dysentery and cholera in the civilian population. In the event, no serious epidemics occurred; but typhoid–paratyphoid vaccine was required on a large scale for general prophylaxis.

Late in 1940, the Ministry of Health instituted a campaign for the mass immunisation of children against diphtheria, as this protective measure was regarded as having special importance in wartime. The Council was asked at short notice to organise the supply and distribution of the necessary prophylactics. A rapid response from the British manufacturers, helped at the start by a generous gift from the American Red Cross Society, soon enabled supply to overtake demand.

In 1941, the Council undertook to arrange for the supply of typhus vaccine for the protection of Service personnel and of civilians exposed to special risk of infection. The preferred method of manufacture, involving the use of fertile eggs, was impracticable on a large scale in Great Britain under war conditions. The supplies were therefore ordered from the United States and Canada, the Council receiving valuable assistance from the Rockefeller Foundation in making the arrangements. Towards the end of the war, the large-scale production of scrub-typhus vaccine (from the lungs of experimentally infected American cotton-rats) was undertaken in Great Britain with the advice and assistance of members of the Council's scientific staff.

Supply of blood for transfusion

The value of transfusion with blood or blood substitutes, in the treatment of haemorrhage and wound shock, had been indicated by limited experience in the First World War. Methods of blood transfusion had been greatly developed between the wars, and the value of the procedure had been demonstrated during the Civil War in Spain. There was thus every expectation that it would be required on a large scale both by the armed forces and by civil population subjected to air-raids, and the demand for blood, equipment and trained staff was thus likely to be very great.

Early in 1939, Dr J. M. (later Dame Janet) Vaughan raised the question of instituting a broadly based blood transfusion service for air-raid casualties in the Greater London area, believing that the arrangements dependent on individual hospitals were liable to break down under pressure. She initiated discussion among pathologists and others who would be concerned with the problem in the ten sectors into which the area was divided in the Government's plans for an Emergency Medical Service; and this resulted in a project for a supplementary organisation. From this point the Council took over, and an official committee was set up to implement the scheme.

Arrangements were coordinated with those already in hand to meet Army needs. They were also integrated with the arrangements in the separate sectors; equipment and donor enrolment cards were in this way standardised for the whole of the London area. The scheme adopted by the Council to supplement local arrangements within the sectors was based on four blood supply depots on the periphery of the main target area. These depots had to be sited in populous districts from which sufficient volunteer donors could be drawn, and also not too far from the hospitals which they would have to supply.

Eventually, the London Blood Supply Depots, designated N.E., S.E., S.W., and N.W., were respectively located at Luton (Bedfordshire), Maidstone (Kent), Sutton (Surrey), and Slough (Middlesex). Their directors were, in the same order, Dr H. F. Brewer, Dr M. Maizels, Dr J. O. Oliver and Dr Janet Vaughan. (Dr Oliver was later succeeded by Dr O. M. Solandt, and he in turn by Dr. J. F. Loutit.) Coordination was provided by a Blood Depots Committee under the chairmanship of Professor G. Payling Wright, with Dr D. K. M. Chalmers of the Council's staff as secretary. The central administration of the depots by the Council's office was necessarily of a flexible kind, as this entirely new service had to be mobilised before details of organisation could be worked out; this led the directors to develop their depots along individual lines. Moreover, transfusion procedures were continually changing throughout the war, as a result of the experience gained and the progress of research.

A few weeks before the outbreak of war, the scheme was put into operation; before this, premises had been secured and adapted, staff had been recruited and trained, and equipment had been provided—including very large numbers of blood bottles of a special ('MRC') design. The next step was for each depot to enrol a large donor panel and to build up an initial stock of blood.

The call for volunteer donors, both at the depots and in the sectors, involved intensive publicity, and in securing this the Council had the vigorous collaboration of the British Broadcasting Corporation. The Council also had the help, spontaneously offered, of half-a-dozen publicity chiefs of commercial concerns which advertised their wares on a large scale. These were the very kings of their profession, such as had their slogans illuminating the night sky of Piccadilly (but how soon to be switched off for six years). The Council was grateful for this experienced aid; as one medical cynic remarked, "a man who can sell a concept like 'night starvation' can sell anything". This group organised a special office with a distinct telephone number (multiple lines) to which the public announcements could direct volunteers for information about places and times of bleeding; it was obvious that any existing office would have been swamped by calls and put out of ordinary business. There was a slight hitch at the beginning, because these business men were apparently sceptical of the Council's ability to organise the bleeding arrangements by the agreed date and feared that their publicity might end in fiasco; in consequence, the bleeding teams at first stood idle while the excellent publicity arrangements got hastily into gear.

The London blood depots in action

When the war came, the service was favourably placed to cope with whatever situation might arise; but in fact there was little call upon it during the first nine months. Later it was very fully extended at times, and never inactive. Among administrative developments in the course of the war, the depots ceased to be supplementary and took over all responsibility in the Greater London area. The London depots, by request of the Ministry of Health, also extended their fields of operation outwards, so that eventually these covered the whole of south-east England. Further afield the Ministry, as part of a national transfusion service, set up similar depots at several important centres; these were administered regionally.

The depots thus met the needs of hospitals over wide areas; they also drew upon the populations of these areas for supplies of blood, mobile bleeding teams being sent out to temporary clinics at different places on dates that were made known. Transport was a vital necessity for the service, not only for the bleeding teams but even more for supplying the hospitals, especially when there were sudden calls upon these after some bombing incident. The Report describes this latter operation and pays a deserved tribute to the men and women drivers employed by the London Blood Supply Depots:

It was impossible to hold at any hospital a blood bank sufficient to meet the sudden and great demands due to an influx of casualties. The local hospital store could meet only the immediate demand, and the deficiency had to be made good by fresh supplies from a main depot. In theory this arrangement had an aspect of uncertainty, but in practice it proved satisfactory. The depots quickly established close contact with their hospitals and no doubt was left as to what should be done by a hospital in an emergency. Relatively few incidents occurred in which the hospitals did not get an interval between being informed that casualties were to be received and their arrival; in this interval the depot van could be despatched with ample supplies of blood. The deliveries all arrived in time and in many cases before the casualties themselves, a fact which reflected the quality of the drivers employed. Accurate and intimate knowledge of the roads under black-out conditions was essential, but had to be coupled with a willingness to drive while a raid was in actual progress, and a determination to get to the hospital at all costs, however difficult the blocking of roads or other circumstances might make the journey.

One of these depots, for which figures were available for the whole five years to September 1944, enrolled 128 320 donors, made 147 777 bleedings, supplied 38 263 blood-giving sets, issued 49 000 bottles of whole blood, and provided 90 181 bottles for plasma drying. It is estimated that multiplication of these figures by $3\frac{1}{2}$ would give an approximate grand total for the four London depots together.

Drying of blood products

An important development, within the Council's responsibility, was the establishment of a Serum Drying Unit at Cambridge under the direction of Dr R. I. N. Greaves; this passed in 1940 from the experimental stage into production. The method used consisted in freeze-drying blood plasma (blood filtered free of its cellular elements) or serum (the liquid separated after clotting of plasma) in transfusion bottles, where it could be reconstituted with distilled water when required. Thus, blood or blood products were not inevitably wasted through deterioration in store at times of diminished demand, but could be kept indefinitely in cold storage for issue in dry form. From early in 1943 a larger plant presented by the Wellcome Trustees greatly increased the output. This was distributed not only in the London area but throughout the country, to the armed forces, and to Malta and elsewhere. The larger plant alone, in the two and a half years of its operation, dried more than half a million bottles of plasma and serum. A full account of the work of the Unit, by Dr Greaves, was published by the Council in 1946 (MRC Special Report Series No. 258). The enterprise was a pioneer one of its kind and gave guidance to projects elsewhere for the drying of other substances (penicillin for example) as well as blood.

Determination of blood groups

In so far as whole blood was concerned, it was necessary either to restrict its use to group O blood (universal donor) or to determine the blood group of donor and patient to ensure compatibility. This latter procedure involved tests for which high quality grouping sera were required. The task of supplying these sera, on a scale adequate for wartime needs, had been assigned to a Unit that the Council was administering, on behalf of the Rockefeller Foundation, in the Galton Laboratory at University College London. At the beginning of the war, the Galton Laboratory Serum Unit (Dr G. L. Taylor) was moved to Cambridge, where it was able to obtain blood for its special purpose from men passing through an intake depot of the Royal Air Force—and, in the process, close on 200 000 airmen had their blood groups accurately determined and stamped on their identity discs. A guide to the determination of blood groups as then known was published in 1943 (MRC War Memorandum No. 9).

Blood transfusion research

A great deal of research was done during the war on blood groups and on all aspects of blood transfusion. Much of this was done by the staffs of the blood depots, who were constantly seeking to improve their methods. To coordinate this work, a Blood Transfusion Research Committee was appointed by the Council, with Professor Topley and afterwards Dr Drury as chairman; it absorbed the Blood Depots Committee already mentioned, and Dr Chalmers was eventually succeeded by Dr Cuthbertson as secretary.

The questions under review included the collection of blood and the welfare of donors; the substitution of plasma and serum for whole blood; the storage of blood and blood products; the drying of blood products for long-term preservation; and the health of the recipients of transfusion, including the risk of transmitted infections (especially jaundice).

At the end of the war, the Council ceased to have any responsibility for the routine supply of blood for transfusion. Its interest in the subject was maintained, however, by its establishment of a Blood Transfusion Research Unit (Dr P. L. Mollison) at what is now the Royal Postgraduate Medical School. The Galton Laboratory Serum Unit was reconstituted as the Council's Blood Group Research Unit (Dr R. R. Race) at the Lister Institute; and in its more routine aspect it was succeeded by the Blood Group Reference Laboratory

(Dr A. E. Mourant) of the Ministry of Health, administered by the Council as agent and housed likewise at the Lister Institute. The Council also established a Blood Products Research Unit under the supervision of Sir Alan Drury, who had become Director of the Lister Institute; the object was to develop the preparation of various substances that can be fractionated from blood plasma and have been found useful in surgery and immunology. This research unit had a production side, and it eventually became the Blood Products Laboratory (Dr W. d'A. Maycock) of the Ministry of Health, administered for the latter through the Council and situated at the Elstree laboratories of the Institute.

Permanent gains

Of the two principal emergency services directed by the Council during the war, it may be said that their embodiment to some extent reflected an earlier deficiency in normal arrangements as well as a temporary demand for intensive efforts under stress. In the former respect there has been a permanent gain, not only in the acquisition of new knowledge from the associated research, but also in the perpetuation of arrangements that had in war proved their worth for peace-time conditions. The country remains the richer in having a well organised Public Health Laboratory Service (in England and Wales) and greatly improved facilities for the supply of blood and its products for transfusion. The former was the Council's child, and the latter owed much to the part which the Council played in their development.

Appendices

Appendix A
Sources and references

General

Unpublished

Minutes and papers of the Medical Research Committee and Council, and of Boards and Committees of the Council

Correspondence in the files of the Council's office

Annual Reports to Parliament

Reports of the Committee and Council from 1914 onwards, as detailed in Volume One—all published by HMSO, London

Handbooks

Medical Research Council Handbook 1970–71, 1972. MRC, London. Subsequently published annually

NIMR and CRC Scientific Reports

National Institute for Medical Research: scientific report for 1968–69. 1970. MRC, London. Subsequently published annually

Clinical Research Centre: scientific report for 1970–71. 1972. MRC, London. Subsequently published every two years

Chapter 1

Anon. [Fell, H.], n.d. (ca. 1963). *History of the Strangeways Research Laboratory (formerly Cambridge Research Hospital) 1912–1962*. Printed privately, Cambridge

Bardswell, N. D., and Thompson, J. H. R. 1919. *Pulmonary tuberculosis: mortality after sanatorium treatment*. MRC Special Report Series no. 33. HMSO

Brownlee, J. 1918, 1920. *An investigation into the epidemiology of phthisis in Great Britain and Ireland*. MRC Special Report Series nos. 18, 46. HMSO

Burrell, L. S. T., and MacNalty, A. S. 1922. *Report on artificial pneumothorax*. MRC Special Report Series no. 67. HMSO

Greenwood, M., and Tebb, A. E. 1919. *An inquiry into the prevalence and aetiology of tuberculosis among industrial workers, with special reference to female munition workers*. MRC Special Report Series no. 22. HMSO

Griffith, A. S. 1931. *Studies of protection against tuberculosis: results with BCG vaccine in monkeys.* MRC Special Report Series no. 152. HMSO

Hart, P. D'A. 1932. *The value of tuberculin tests in man, with special reference to the intracutaneous test.* MRC Special Report Series no. 164, HMSO

Hartley, P. H-S., Wingfield, R. C., and Thompson, J. H. R. 1924. *An inquiry into the after-histories of patients treated at the Brompton Hospital Sanatorium at Frimley during the years 1905–14.* MRC Special Report Series no. 85. HMSO

Pharmacy and Medicines Act 1941 4 & 5 Geo. 6. Ch. 42

Phthisis in Relation to Occupation, Special Investigation Committee upon the Incidence of. 1915. *First report—the boot and shoe trade.* MRC Special Report Series no. 1. HMSO

Thomson, St. C. 1924. *Tuberculosis of the larynx.* MRC Special Report Series no. 83. HMSO

Vallow, H. 1923. *Tuberculosis in insured persons accepted for treatment by the City o, Bradford Health Committee.* MRC Special Report Series no. 76. HMSO

Chapter 2

Biochemical Research in Psychiatry, MRC Committee on, 1970. *Biochemical research in psychiatry: survey and proposals.* HMSO

Clinical Research Centre: scientific report for 1970–71. 1972. MRC, London.

Department of Health for Scotland. 1957. *Memorandum SHM (57) 60: Scottish Hospital Service—clinical research.* (Official distribution)

Drury, A. N., and Grant, R. T. 1945. Thomas Lewis. *Obituary notices of Fellows of the Royal Society* 5 (1945–48): 179–202

Goodman, N. M. 1970 *Wilson Jameson: architect of national health.* London, George Allen and Unwin

Himsworth, H. P. 1945. Sir Thomas Lewis. *University College Hospital Magazine.* 1945 30: 36–39

Himsworth, H. 1970. Clinical research: its contribution to biological thought. *Lancet* 1970 ii: 835–840

Kuenssberg, E. V. 1971. The James Mackenzie Lecture: General practice through the looking glass. *Practitioner* 206: 129–145

Lancet. 1963. Clinical research in Britain: a survey. *Lancet* 1963 i: 1039–1045

Lewis, T. 1930. Observations on research in medicine: its position and its needs. *British Medical Journal* 1930 i: 479–483. (And editorial article on "Research Physicians", pp. 503–504)

Mair, A. 1962. Mackenzie on records in medical practice. *British Medical Journal.* 1962 i: 1331–1333

Medical Research Council, Ministry of Health, Department of Health for Scotland. 1953. *Clinical research in relation to the National Health Service.* HMSO (White paper)

Ministry of Health. 1957. *Memorandum H.M. (57) 36: National Health Service—clinical research* (official distribution)

Chapter 3

Analgesia in Midwifery, Committee on. 1954. The use of trilene by midwives. MRC Memorandum no. 30

Chain, E. B. 1963. Academic and industrial contributions to drug research. The Trueman Wood Lecture. *Journal of Royal Society of Arts* 1963 iii: 856–882. Abridged version in *Nature* 1963 200: 441–451

Clarke, H. T., Johnson, J. R., and Robinson, R. (eds.) 1949. *The chemistry of penicillin*. Princeton, N.J.

Dale, H. H. 1950. Advances in medicinal therapeutics. *British Medical Journal* 1950 i: 1–7

Foreign Office 1946. Agreement between His Majesty's Government in the United Kingdom and the Government of the United States of America on the Principles applying to the Exchange of Information relating to the Synthesis of Penicillin. *Treaty Series No. 4 (1946)*. HMSO (Cmd. 6757)

Godber, G. 1964. Measurement and mechanisation in medicine. (Address to the Biological Engineering Society.) *Lancet* 1964 ii: 1191–1195

Hadfield, C. F. 1935. The Joint Anaesthetics Committee: a retrospect of eleven years' work. *Proceedings of the Royal Society of Medicine* 28: 1133–1144

Hare, R. 1970. *The birth of penicillin and the disarming of microbes*. London

Pasteur, L. 1854. *Discours prononcé à Douai. Douai*

Platt, Lord. 1967. Medical science: master or servant? (Harveian Oration delivered to the Royal College of Physicians of London.) *British Medical Journal* 1967 4: 439–444

Tennyson, A. 1880. In the children's hospital. *Ballads and other poems*. London

Chapter 4

Air Hygiene Committee (MRC). 1954. *Air disinfection with ultra-violet irradiation: its effect on the health of schoolchildren*. MRC Special Report Series no. 283. HMSO

Colebrook, D. 1929. *Irradiation and health*. MRC Special Report Series no. 131. HMSO

Colebrook, D. 1946. Artificial sunlight treatment in industry. *Industrial Health Research Board Report* no. 89. HMSO

Electro-accoustics, MRC Committee on. 1947. *Hearing aids and audiometers*. MRC Special Report Series no. 261. HMSO

Protection Against Ionizing Radiations, MRC Committee on. 1966. *The assessment of the possible radiation risks to the population from environmental contamination*. HMSO

Radiology Committee (MRC) 1924. *Medical uses of radium: summary of reports from research centres for 1923*. MRC Special Report Series no. 90. (And sixteen further annual summaries in the same series.) HMSO

Russ, S., Lazarus-Barlow, W. S., and others. 1922. *Medical uses of radium: studies of the effects of gamma rays from a large quantity of radium*. MRC Special Report Series no. 62. HMSO

Vonberg, D. D., and Fowler, J. F. 1963. The Cyclotron Unit: Medical Research Council. *Nature* 198: 827–832

Wood, C. A. P., and Boag, J. W., with others. 1950. *Researches on the radiotherapy of oral cancer*. MRC Special Report Series no. 267. HMSO

Chapter 5

Accessory Food Factors Committee (Lister Institute and MRC). 1919. *Report on the present state of knowledge concerning accessory food factors ('vitamins')*. MRC Special Report Series no. 38 (2nd edition 1924). HMSO

Accessory Food Factors Committee (Lister Institute and MRC). 1932. *Vitamins: a survey of present knowledge*. MRC Special Report Series no. 167 (3rd edition of SRS 38). HMSO

Cathcart, E. P., and Murray, A. M. T. 1931. *A study in nutrition: an inquiry into the diets of 154 families of St Andrews*. MRC Special Report Series no. 151. HMSO

Cathcart, E. P., and Murray, A. M. T. 1932. *Studies in nutrition: an inquiry into the diet of families in Cardiff and Reading*. MRC Special Report Series no. 165. HMSO

Chick, H., et al. 1923. *Studies of rickets in Vienna 1919–22*. MRC Special Report Series no. 77. HMSO

Dean, R. F. A. 1953. *Plant proteins in child feeding*. MRC Special Report Series no. 279. HMSO

Dental Disease, Committee for the Investigation of. 1936. *The influence of diet on caries in children's teeth (Final Report)*. MRC Special Report Series no. 211. HMSO

Garry, R. C., Passmore, R., Warnock, G. M., and Durnin, J. V. G. A. 1955. *Studies on expenditure of energy and consumption of food by miners and clerks, Fife, Scotland, 1952*. MRC Special Report Series no. 289. HMSO

Harvey, C. O. 1935. *The determination of iodine in biological substances*. MRC Special Report Series no. 201. HMSO

Iodine Deficiency and Thyroid Disease, MRC Committee on. 1936. *The relationship of the iodine contents of water, milk and pasture to the occurrence of endemic goitre in two districts of England*. MRC Special Report Series no. 217. HMSO

King, J. D. 1940. *Dental disease on the island of Lewis*. MRC Special Report Series no. 241. HMSO

King, J. D., Mellanby, M., Stones, H. H., and Green, H. N. 1955. *The effect of sugar supplements on dental caries in children*. MRC Special Report Series no. 288. HMSO

Korenchevsky, V. 1922. *The aetiology and pathology of rickets from an experimental point of view*. MRC Special Report Series no. 71. HMSO

Mackay, H. M. M., Goodfellow, L., and Hill, A. B. 1931. *Nutritional anaemia in infancy: the influence of iron deficiency on infant health*. MRC Special Report Series no. 157. HMSO

Mann, H. Corry. 1922. *Rickets: the relative importance of environment and diet as factors in causation*. MRC Special Report Series no. 68. HMSO

Mann, H. Corry. 1926. *Diets for boys during the school age*. MRC Special Report Series no. 105. HMSO

McCance, R. A., and Lawrence, R. D. 1929. *The carbohydrate content of foods*. MRC Special Report Series no. 135. HMSO

McCance, R. A., and Shipp, H. L. 1933. *The chemistry of flesh foods and their losses on cooking*. MRC Special Report Series no. 187. HMSO

McCance, R. A., Widdowson, E. M., and Shackleton, L. R. B. 1936. *The nutritive value of fruits, vegetables and nuts*. MRC Special Report Series no. 213. HMSO

McCance, R. A., and Widdowson, E. M. 1940. *The chemical composition of foods*. MRC Special Report Series no. 235. (3rd edition, SRS 297, 1960—omitting "Chemical" from title.) HMSO

McCance, R. A., Widdowson, E. M., and others. 1951. *Studies of undernutrition, Wuppertal 1946–9*. MRC Special Report Series no. 275. HMSO

Mellanby, E. 1921. *Experimental rickets*. MRC Special Report Series no. 61. HMSO

Mellanby, E. 1925. *Experimental rickets: the effect of cereals and their interaction with other factors of diet and environment in producing rickets.* MRC Special Report Series no. 93. HMSO

Mellanby, M. 1929, 1930, 1934, *Diet and the teeth: an experimental study.* Parts I, II and III. MRC Special Report Series nos. 140, 153, 191. HMSO

Murray, M. M., Ryle, J. A., Simpson, B. W., and Wilson, D. C. 1948. *Thyroid enlargement and other changes related to the mineral content of drinking water.* MRC Memorandum no. 18. HMSO

Orr, J. B., and Leitch, I. 1929. *Iodine in nutrition: a review of existing information.* MRC Special Report Series no. 123. HMSO

Orr, J. B. 1931. *Iodine supply and the incidence of endemic goitre.* MRC Special Report Series no. 154. HMSO

Quantitative Problems in Human Nutrition, MRC Committee upon. *Report on the nutrition of miners and their families.* MRC Special Report Series no. 87. HMSO

Widdowson, E. M. 1947. *A study of individual children's diets.* MRC Special Report Series no. 257. HMSO

Widdowson, E. M., and McCance, R. A. 1954. *Studies on the nutritive value of bread and on the effect of variations in the extraction rate of flour on the growth of undernourished children.* MRC Special Report Series no. 287. HMSO

Chapter 6

Begg, T. B., Hill, I. D., and Nicholls, L. C. 1964. Breathalyzer and Kitagawa-Wright methods of measuring breath alcohol. *British Medical Journal* 1964 i: 9–15

Biochemical Research in Psychiatry, MRC Committee on. 1970. *Biochemical research in psychiatry: surveys and proposals.* HMSO

Brown, W. M. Court, Harnden, D. G., Jacobs, P. A., Maclean, N., and Mantle, D. J. 1964. *Abnormalities of the sex chromosome complement in man.* MRC Special Report Series no. 305. HMSO

Clean Air Act 1956. 4 & 5 Eliz. 2. 1956. Ch. 52

Doll, R., and Hill, A. B. 1950. Smoking and carcinoma of the lung: preliminary report. *British Medical Journal* 1950 ii: 739–748

Doll, R., and Hill, A. B. 1952. A study of the aetiology of carcinoma of the lung *British Medical Journal* 1952 ii: 1271–1286

Doll, R., and Hill, A. B. 1956. Lung cancer and other causes of death in relation to smoking: a second report on the mortality of British doctors. *British Medical Journal* 1956 ii: 1071–1081

Durham, F. M., and Woods, H. M. 1932. *Alcohol and inheritance: an experimental study.* MRC Special Report Series no. 168. HMSO

Electro-accoustics, MRC Committee on. 1947. *Hearing aids and audiometers.* MRC Special Report Series no. 261. HMSO

Grüneberg, H., and others. 1966. *A search for genetic effects of high natural radioactivity in South India.* MRC Special Report Series no. 307. HMSO

Hill, L. 1919, 1920. *The science of ventilation and open-air treatment.* Parts I and II. MRC Special Report Series nos. 32, 52. HMSO

House of Commons. 1947. *Third report from the Select Committee on Estimates, Session 1946–47.* Expenditure on Research and Development. HMSO

Medical Research Council. 1958. *Statement on the report of the United Nations Scientific Committee on the Effects of Atomic Radiation.* HMSO (Cmnd. 508)

Medical Research Council. 1960. *The hazards to man of nuclear and allied radiations. A second report.* HMSO (Cmnd. 1225)

Medical Research Council. 1956. *The hazards to man of nuclear and allied radiations.* HMSO (Cmd. 9780)

Medical Research Council Monitoring Report Series, no. 1 *et seq.*, 1960. *Assay of strontium-90 in human bone in the United Kingdom.* HMSO

Medical Research Council. 1966. *The assessment of the possible radiation risks to the population from environmental contamination.* HMSO

Murray, M. B. 1924. *The effect of maternal social conditions and nutrition on birth-weight and birth-length.* MRC Special Report Series no. 81. HMSO

Newman, G. 1939. *The building of the nation's health.* London

Paton, D. Noel, Findlay, L., and others. 1926. *Poverty, nutrition and growth: studies of child life in cities and rural districts of Scotland.* MRC Special Report Series no. 101. HMSO

Physical Training and Recreation Act 1937. 1 Edw. 8 & 1 Geo. 6. c. 46

Physiology of Hearing, MRC Committee upon the. 1932–37. *Reports of the Committee* (various subjects and authors) I–V. MRC Special Report Series nos. 166 207, 219, 221. HMSO

Physiology of Vision, MRC Committee on the. 1929–35. *Reports of the Co mmittee* (various subjects and authors) I–XIV. MRC Special Report Series nos. 104 127, 130, 133, 134, 136, 139, 148, 163, 173, 181, 185, 188, 200. HMSO

Radiological Protection Act 1970. Eliz. 2. 1970. Ch. 46 (see Vol. One, App. B)

Sorsby, A. 1950. *The causes of blindness in England and Wales.* MRC Memorandum no. 24. HMSO

Chapter 7

Air Hygiene Committee. 1954. *Air disinfection with ultra-violet irradiation: its effect on illness among schoolchildren.* MRC Special Report Series no. 283. HMSO

Andrewes, C. 1970. *Viruses and cancer.* London

Andrewes, F. W., and Inman, A. C. 1919. *A study of the serological races of the Flexner group of dysentery bacilli.* MRC Special Report Series no. 42. HMSO

Barnard, J. E. 1925. The microscopical examination of filterable viruses associated with malignant new growths. *Lancet* 1925 ii: 117–123

Bed-bug Committee (MRC). 1942. *Report of the Committee on Bed-bug Infestation, 1935–40.* MRC Special Report Series no. 245. HMSO

Bourdillon, R. B., Lidwell, O. M., and Lovelock, J. E., with others. 1948. *Studies in air hygiene.* MRC Special Report Series no. 262. HMSO

Browning, C. H., with others. 1933. *Chronic enteric carriers and their treatment.* MRC Special Report Series no. 179. HMSO

Burnet, F. M. 1936. *The use of the developing egg in virus research.* MRC Special Report Series no. 220. HMSO

Burnet, F. M. 1968. *Changing patterns—an atypical autobiography.* Melbourne and London, Heinemann

Cummins, S. L., *et al.* 1919. *Studies of influenza in hospitals of the British Armies in France, 1918.* MRC Special Report Series no. 36. HMSO

Department of Health for Scotland. 1933. *Tuberculous infection in milk.* MRC Special Report Series no. 189. HMSO

Dreyer, G. 1923. Some new principles in bacterial immunity; their experimental foundation, and their application to the treatment of refractory infections. *British Journal of Experimental Pathology* 4: 146–176.

Dudley, S. F. 1923. *The Schick test, diphtheria and scarlet fever.* MRC Special Report Series no. 75 (also no. 111, 1926; no. 195, 1934). HMSO

Elton, C. 1931. The study of epidemic diseases among wild animals. *Journal of Hygiene.* 31: 435–452.

Elton, C., Ford, E. B., Baker, J. R., and Gardner, A. D. 1931. The health and parasites of a wild mouse population. *Proceedings of the Zoological Society of London* 1931 ii: 657–721

Erikson, D. 1935. *The pathogenic aerobic organisms of the Actinomyces group.* MRC Special Report Series no. 203. HMSO

Erikson, D. 1940. *Pathogenic anaerobic organisms of the Actinomyces group.* MRC Special Report Series no. 240. HMSO

Gordon, M. H. 1925. *Studies of the viruses of vaccinia and variola.* MRC Special Report Series no. 98. HMSO

Greenwood, M., Hill, A. B., Topley, W. W. C., and Wilson, J. (1936). *Experimental epidemiology.* MRC Special Report Series no. 209. HMSO

Gye, W. E. 1925. The aetiology of malignant new growths. *Lancet* 1925 ii: 109–117 (See also Barnard, above)

Gye, W. E. 1925. Filter-passing viruses and cancer. *British Medical Journal* 1925 ii: 189–191; 290–291

Hoare, C. A., and Mackinnon, D. L. 1950. Clifford Dobell, 1886–1949. *Obituary notices of Fellows of the Royal Society,* 1950–1951, 7 (19): 35–61

Jordon, L. 1933. *The eradication of bovine tuberculosis.* MRC Special Report Series no. 184. HMSO

McIntosh, J. 1922. *Studies in the aetiology of epidemic influenza.* MRC Special Report Series no. 63. HMSO

Medical Mycology Committee (MRC). 1949, 1958, 1967. *Nomenclature of fungi pathogenic to man and animals: Names recommended for use in Great Britain.* MRC Memorandum no. 23. HMSO

Murray, E. G. D. 1929. *The meningococcus.* MRC Special Report Series no. 124. HMSO

Rogers, L. 1926. *Smallpox and climate in India: forecasting of epidemics.* MRC Special Report Series no. 106. HMSO

Savage, W. G., and White, P. Bruce. 1925. *An investigation of the Salmonella group with special reference to food poisoning.* MRC Special Report Series no. 91 (also no. 92, 1925; no. 103, 1926). HMSO

School Epidemics Committee (MRC). 1938. *Epidemics in schools: analysis of the data collected during the first five years of a statistical inquiry.* MRC Special Report Series no. 227 (also no. 271, 1950). HMSO

Stuart-Harris, C. H., Andrewes, C. H., and Smith, W., with others. 1938. *A study of epidemic influenza, with special reference to the 1936–37 epidemic.* MRC Special Report Series no. 228. HMSO

Tuberculin Committee (MRC). 1925. *Tuberculin tests in cattle, with special reference to the intradermal test.* MRC Special Report Series no. 94 (also No. 122, 1928). HMSO

Chapter 8

Bulloch, W. 1925. Emmanuel Klein (1844–1925). *Journal of Pathology and Bacteriology* 28: 684–697. (See also Sanderson, Lady Burdon, *et al.* 1911. *Sir John Burdon Sanderson: a memoir.* Oxford)

Grüneberg, H. 1956. *An annotated catalogue of the mutant genes of the mouse.* MRC Memorandum No. 33. HMSO

Hypogammaglobulinaemia, MRC Working Party on. 1971. *Hypogammaglobulinaemia in the United Kingdom.* MRC Special Report Series no. 310. HMSO

Marrack, J. R. 1934, 1938. *The chemistry of antigens and antibodies.* (First and revised editions.) MRC Special Report Series nos. 194, 230. HMSO

Penrose, L. S. 1938. *A clinical and genetic study of 1280 cases of mental defect.* 1938. MRC Special Report Series no. 229. HMSO

Watson, J. D. 1968. *The double helix: a personal account of the discovery of the structure of DNA.* Atheneum, N.Y.

Chapter 9

Anderson, W. F. 1970. Research on ageing. *Health Trends* 1970, ii: 26–29

Bedford, T. 1936. *The warmth factor in comfort at work. A physiological study of heating and ventilation.* Reports of the Industrial Health Research Board no. 76. HMSO

Browning, E. 1937, 1953. *The toxicity of industrial organic solvents.* Reports of the Industrial Health Research Board no. 80. (Revised edition 1953) HMSO

Carcinogenic Action of Mineral Oils Committee (MRC). 1968. *The carcinogenic action of mineral oils: a chemical and biological study.* MRC Special Report Series no. 306. HMSO

Collis, E. L., and Llewellyn, T. L. 1924. *Report on miners' 'beat knee', 'beat hand', and 'beat elbow'.* MRC Special Report Series no. 89. HMSO

DSIR and MRC, 1954. *First Report of the Joint Committee on Human Relations in Industry. March 1953 to March 1954.* HMSO

DSIR and MRC. 1958. *Report of the Joint Committee on Human Relations in Industry 1954–57* and *Report of the Joint Committee on Individual Efficiency in Industry 1953–57.* HMSO

Fraser, R., and others. 1947. *The incidence of neurosis among factory workers.* Reports of the Industrial Health Research Board no. 90. HMSO

Gilson, J. C., and Hugh-Jones, P. 1955. *Lung function in coal-workers' pneumoconiosis.* MRC Special Report Series no. 290. HMSO

Hill, A. B. 1937. *An investigation of the sickness experience of London transport workers, with special reference to gastric disturbances.* Reports of the Industrial Health Research Board no. 79. HMSO

Industrial Pulmonary Disease, MRC Committee on. 1942, 1943, 1945. *Chronic Pulmonary Disease in South Wales Coalminers. I. Medical studies* (P. D'Arcy Hart *et al.*). *II. Environmental studies* (T. Bedford *et al.*). *III. Experimental studies* (E. J. King *et al.*) MRC Special Report Series nos. 243, 244, 250. HMSO

Miners' Nystagmus Committee (MRC). 1922, 1923. *First and second reports.* MRC Special Report Series nos. 65, 80. HMSO

Prausnitz, C. 1936. *Investigations on respiratory dust disease in operatives in the cotton industry.* MRC Special Report Series no. 212. HMSO

Vernon, H. M. 1919. *The influence of hours of work and of ventilation on output in tinplate manufacture.* Reports of the Industrial Fatigue Research Board no. 1. HMSO

Vernon, H. M., and others. 1926. *Methods of investigating ventilation and its effects* MRC Special Report Series no. 100. HMSO

Vernon, H. M., and Bedford, T. 1927. *The relation of atmospheric conditions to the working capacity and the accident rate of coal-miners.* Reports of the Industrial Fatigue Research Board no. 39. HMSO

Wyatt, S. 1927. *Rest-pauses in industry (a review of the results obtained).* Reports of the Industrial Fatigue Research Board no. 42. HMSO

Wyatt, S., and Langdon, J. N. 1937. *Fatigue and boredom in repetitive work.* Reports of the Industrial Health Research Board no. 77. HMSO

Chapter 10

Burrows, S. M., Matthews, R. J., and Wilcocks, C. (ed. Cummins, S. L.). 1935. Studies of tuberculosis among African natives: reports to the Medical Research Council. *Tubercle, London,* Suppl.

Cinchona Derivatives and Malaria, MRC Committee on. 1925. *Clinical comparisons of quinine and quinidine.* MRC Special Report Series no. 96. HMSO

Colonial Office. 1920. *Report of the Departmental Committee appointed by the Secretary of State for the Colonies to enquire into the Colonial Medical Service.* HMSO (Cmd. 939)

Colonial Office. 1921. *Report of a Committee on Research in the Colonies.* HMSO (Cmd. 1472)

Colonial Office. 1925. *Report of the East Africa Commission.* HMSO (Cmd. 2387)

Colonial Development and Welfare Act 1940 3 & 4 Geo. 6. c. 40; and successors

Hackett, C. 1952. *Bone lesions of yaws in Uganda.* Oxford and Springfield, Ill.

Hunt, J. 1953. *The ascent of Everest.* London

Orr, J. B., and Gilks, J. L. 1931. *Studies in nutrition: the physique and health of two African tribes.* MRC Special Report Series no. 155. HMSO

Rogers, L. 1926. *Smallpox and climate in India: forecasting of epidemics.* MRC Special Report Series no. 106. HMSO

Chapter 11

British Medical Association. 1904. Minute 314 of the Representative Body. (See also Minutes 119, 1909 and 67, 1920 of the Association's Central Ethical Committee)

Cinchona Derivatives and Malaria, MRC Committee on. 1925. *Clinical comparisons of quinine and quinidine.* MRC Special Report Series no. 37. HMSO

Civil Research. 1928. *Report of the Sub-Committee of the Committee of Civil Research on the British Pharmacopoeia.* HMSO (Cmd. 3101)

Development of Inventions Act 1948. 11 & 12 Geo. 6. c. 60

Development of Inventions Act 1954. 2 & 3 Eliz. 2 Ch. 20

Development of Inventions Act 1965. 1965. Ch. 21

General Medical Council. 1968. *British Pharmacopoeia 1968.* London (and earlier editions)

General Medical Council. 1969. *Addendum 1969 to the British Pharmacopoeia 1968.* London

Green, F. H. K. 1944. Clinical evaluation of new remedies in Britain. *British Medical Bulletin* 2: 58–60

Green, F. H. K. 1954. The clinical evaluation of remedies. (Bradshaw Lecture Royal College of Physicians of London.) *Lancet* 1954 ii: 1085–1090

Hill, A. 1952. The clinical trial. *New England Journal of Medicine* 247: 113–119

Hill, A. B. 1962. *Statistical methods in clinical and preventive medicine.* Edinburgh and London

The Medical Act 1858 (21 & 22 Vict. c. 90); and amending or additional measures up to the *Medical Act 1956* (4 & 5 Eliz. 2. Ch. 76)

Medical Research Council, a report to the. 1923. Some clinical results of the use of insulin. *British Medical Journal* 1923 i: 737–740 (and *Lancet* 1923 i: 905–908)

Medical Research Council. 1929. *Memorandum by the Medical Research Council on the patent law in relation to medical research.* (Later published as Appendix A to the Council's Report for 1930–31)

Poliomyelitis Vaccines Committee (MRC). 1957. The assessment of the British, poliomyelitis vaccine. *British Medical Journal* 1957 i: 1271–1277

Poliomyelitis Vaccines Committee (MRC). 1961. Trial of living poliovirus vaccine. *British Medical Journal* 1961 ii: 1037–1044.

Salvarsan and its Substitutes, MRC Committee upon the Manufacture, Biological Testing, and Clinical Administration of. 1919. *First report.* MRC Special Report Series no. 44. HMSO

Tuberculosis Vaccines Clinical Trials Committee (MRC). 1956, 1959, 1963. BCG and vole bacillus vaccine in the prevention of tuberculosis in adolescents ["and in early adult life" on the third occasion]. *British Medical Journal* 1956 i: 413–427; 1959 ii: 379–396; 1963 i: 973–978

Whooping-Cough Immunisation Committee (MRC). 1956, 1959. Vaccination against whooping-cough. *British Medical Journal* 1956 ii: 454–462; 1959, i: 994–1000.

Chapter 12

Biological Standards, Reports on:

I (1922)—*Pituitary extracts* (Burn, J. H., and Dale, H. H.)

II (1929)—*Toxicity tests for novarsenobenzene (neosalvarsan)* (Durham, F. M., Gaddum, J. H., and Marchal, J. E.)

III (1933)—*Methods of biological assay depending on a quantal response* (Gaddum, J. H.)

IV (1935)—*The standardisation and estimation of vitamin A* (Hume, E.M., and Chick, H.)

V (1939)—*Variables affecting the estimation of androgenic and oestrogenic activity* (Emmens, C. W.)

VI (1950)—*The design of toxicity tests.* (Perry, W. L. M.)

MRC Special Report Series nos. 69, 128, 183, 202, 234, and 270. HMSO

Bradstreet, C. M. P. 1965. Fifty years of "Oxford" standards. *Lancet* 1965 i: 1264–1265

Dale, H. H. 1922. Scientific method in medical research. *British Medical Journal* 1950 ii: 1185–1190 (Opening lecture in the series "The scientific basis of medicine", organised by the British Postgraduate Medical Federation)

Dale, H. H. 1957. Percival Hartley 1881–1957. *Biographical memoirs of Fellows of the Royal Society* 3: 81–100

Medical Research Council. 1958. *National collection of type cultures: catalogue of species.* MRC Memorandum no. 35. HMSO

Pathological Methods, Reports of the MRC Committee upon the Standardisation of:

I   (1918)—*The Wassermann test*

II and III (1918)—*The laboratory diagnosis of gonococcal infections. Methods for detection of spirochaetes* (2nd ed. 1923)

IV   (1918)—*The diagnostic value of the Wassermann test*

         (1919)—*The reaction of media.* (2nd ed. 1927)

         (1920)—*The laboratory diagnosis of acute intestinal infections, including the principles and practice of the agglutination tests*

MRC Special Report Series nos. 14 (replaced by No. 129, 1929), 19, 21, 35 and 51 HMSO

Chapter 13

Bradstreet, C. M. P. 1965. See under Chapter 12

Hansard' (House of Commons). 1914. *The parliamentary debates (official report)*, Vol. 62, col. 79, etc.

Howie, J. W. 1965. The Public Health Laboratory Service. *Lancet* 1965 i: 501–505

Howie, J. 1972. A microbiological service for communicable-disease epidemiology. *Lancet* 1972 i: 857–860

Public Health Laboratory Service Act 1960. 8 & 9 Eliz. 2. Ch. 49 (see Vol. One, App. B).

Public Health Laboratory Service Yearbook. 1962 *et seq.* (printed annually for official distribution)

Thomson, A. L. 1943. The organisation of a national Public Health Laboratory Service. *British Medical Bulletin* 1: 38–39

Wilson, G. S. 1948. The Public Health Laboratory Service. *British Medical Journal* 1948 i: 627–631, 677–682. (Milroy Lectures)

Wilson, G. S. 1949. The new organisation of public health laboratory services. In Massey, A. (ed.). *Modern trends in public health.* London

Wilson, G. S. 1951. The Public Health Laboratory Service. *British Medical Bulletin* 7: 147–152. (Followed in the same issue by a symposium of fourteen contributions by members of the Service on particular aspects of its work)

Chapter 14

History of the Great War: Medical Services. 12 vols. 1921 *et seq.* HMSO, London. (The volume on pathology, covering a large part of the research activity, was edited by Macpherson, W. G., Leishman, W. B., and Cummins, S. L., and was published in 1923)

MRC Special Report Series. HMSO. 1915 *et seq.* The following issues relate to the subjects named (in the order in which these appear in the text of the chapter):

Wound infections: nos. 12, 39, 57

Injuries of the nervous system: nos. 54 (282), 88

Surgical shock and allied conditions: nos. 25, 26, 27

Enteric infections: no. 48

Dysentery: nos. 4, 5, 6, 7, 15, 29, 30, 40, 42

Cerebro-spinal fever: nos. 2, 3, 17, 50

Influenza: no. 36

Albuminuria and war nephritis: no. 43

Soldier's heart: no. 8

Air medical investigations: nos. 28, 37, 53

Health of munition workers: nos. 13, 16

T.N.T. poisoning: nos. 11, 58

Alcohol: nos. 31, 34, 56

National Health Insurance: Medical Research Committee. 1915. Interim Report on the work in connection with the war at present undertaken by the Medical Research Committee. HMSO (Cd. 7922)

Chapters 15 and 16

Committee of the Privy Council for Medical Research. *Medical research in war:* Report of the Medical Research Council for the years 1939–45. 1947. HMSO (Cmd. 7335)

History of the Second World War: United Kingdom Medical Series. Medical research. Edited by Green, F. H. K., and Covell, G. 1953. HMSO

Dean, H. R., and Wilson, G. S. 1944. William Whiteman Carlton Topley. *Journal of Pathology and Bacteriology* 56: 451–469

MRC Special Report Series. HMSO. 1939 *et seq.* The following issues relate to the subjects named (in the order in which these appear in the text of the chapters.)

Classification of diseases and injuries: no. 248

Burns: no. 249

Injuries of the nervous system: no. 282

Wound shock: no. 277

Tuberculosis in wartime: nos. 246, 251

Hepatitis: no. 273

Typhus: nos. 255, 256

Nutrition: nos. 235 (297), 252, 254, 264, 269, 280

Hazards to shipwrecked personnel: no. 291

Dust disease in coalminers: nos. 243, 244, 250

Blood transfusion: no. 258

MRC War Memoranda. HMSO. 1940 *et seq.* The following issues relate to the subjects named:

Wounds and wound infections: nos. 2, 4, 5, 6, 7, 10, 12, 13

Wound shock: no. 1 (34)

Economy in use of drugs: no. 3

Nutrition: nos. 14, 16

Survival after shipwreck: no. 8

Blood transfusion: no. 9 (36)

Medical Research Council. Reports of the Industrial Health Research Board HMSO. 1944–47. The following issues relate to the subjects named:

Artificial sunlight: no. 89

Sickness absence: nos. 85, 86

Women on war work: no. 88

Neurosis in factory workers: no. 90

MRC: Emergency Reports of the Industrial Health Research Board. HMSO. 1940–44

The issues relate to the subjects named:

Industrial health in war: no. 1

Hours of work etc.: no. 2

Absenteeism: no. 4

Variations in output: no. 5

Accidents: no. 3

MRC: Industrial Health Research Board Pamphlets. 1943–45. Nos. 1–3 (for titles see text, p. 314). HMSO

Appendix B*
National Institute for Medical Research: senior scientific staff

(Names under highest position attained; titles as at latest date—whether or not after end of service. Unavoidably, it has been necessary to select on a somewhat arbitrary standard of senior status, taking various factors into account.)

Directors

Sir Henry H. Dale, OM, GBE, MD, FRCP, FRS (1928–42; and Director, Department of Biochemistry and Pharmacology, from 1914)

Sir Charles R. Harington, KBE, SCD, FRS (1942–62; later on MRC Headquarters staff as Consultant Adviser and as Acting Second Secretary—see Volume One)

Sir Peter B. Medawar, CH, CBE, DSC, FRS (1962–71; later member of external scientific staff, attached to Clinical Research Centre); now Director Emeritus

A. S. V. Burgen, MD, FRCP, FRS (from 1971; earlier Honorary Director, MRC Molecular Pharmacology Unit)

Deputy Directors

Captain S. R. Douglas, FRS, late IMS (1930–36; and Director of Department of Experimental Pathology and Bacteriology, from 1920; on staff from 1914)

Sir Patrick P. Laidlaw, BCH, FRCP, FRS (1936–40; on staff from 1922)

Sir A. Ashley Miles, CBE, MD, FRCP, FRS (1948–52; and Director, Department of Biological Standards from 1946)

Sir Christopher H. Andrewes, MD, FRCP, FRS (1952–61; on staff from 1927)

J. H. Humphrey, CBE, MD, FRCP, FRS (from 1961; on staff from 1949)

Directors of main departments 1914–30 (see also under Directors and Deputy Directors of the Institute):

Sir Almroth E. Wright, KBE, CB, MD, FRS (Department of Bacteriology, 1914–19)

Sir Leonard E. Hill, MD, FRS (Department of Applied Physiology, 1914–28)

J. Brownlee, MD, DSC (Department of Statistics, 1914–27)

Sir Percival Hartley, DSC, FRS (Department of Biological Standards, 1922–46)

Other senior staff, including Heads of Divisions

A. J. Ewins, DSC, FRS (1914–17; chemistry)

Sir Alexander Fleming, FRCS, FRS (1914–18; bacteriology)

G. Barger, DSC, FRS (1914–19; chemistry)

Martin Flack, CBE, MD (1914–20; applied physiology)

B. Moore, DSC, FRS (1914–20; applied physiology)

* An equivalent list of senior members of staff at MRC Headquarters is given in Appendix J to Volume One. For senior external scientific staff see Appendix C (following)

M. Young, MD (1915–27; statistics and anatomy; later external scientific staff)

L. Colebrook, MB, BSC, FRCS, FRS (1919–22; bacteriology; later external staff—see Appendix C)

Sir Charles A. Lovatt Evans, DSC, FRCP, FRS (1919–22; physiology)

H. W. Dudley, OBE, PHD, FRS (1919–35; biochemistry)

W. E. Gye, MD, DSC, FRS (1919–35; pathology)

C. C. Dobell, MA, FRS (1919–49; protistology)

H. King, DSC, FRS (1919–50; organic chemistry)

J. H. Burn, MB, FRS (1920–25; pharmacology)

J. Argyll Campbell, MD, DSC (1921–44; applied physiology)

J. B. Buxton, FRCVS (1922–23; veterinary superintendent)

W. J. Purdy, MB (1922–42; experimental pathology and bacteriology)

J. Smiles, OBE, ARCS (1922–59; applied optics)

G. W. Dunkin, MRCVS, DVA (1923–37; veterinary superintendent)

W. J. Elford, DSC, FRS (1924–52; biophysics)

J. R. Perdrau, MB (1926–39; pathology)

Sir John H. Gaddum, MRCS, DSC, FRS (1927–34; pharmacology)

P. Bruce White, BSC, FRS (1927–49; bacteriology)

R. B. Bourdillon, CBE, MC, AFC, DM (1928–46; applied physiology; later external scientific staff)

Wilson Smith, MD, FRCP, FRS (1929–39; bacteriology)

R. K. Callow, DPHIL, FRS (1929–66; organic chemistry)

I. W. Rowlands, PHD (1933–45; endocrinology)

Sir G. Lindor Brown, MB, MSC, FRS (1934–49; physiology)

Sir Alan S. Parkes, SCD, FRS (1934–61; endocrinology)

Sir Frank G. Young, DSC, FRS (1936–42; physiology)

C. Rimington, PHD, FRS (1937–45; biochemistry)

D. K. M. Chalmers, MD, DPH (1937–47; medical administrative officer)

C. W. Emmens, PHD (1937–48; endocrinology)

R. E. Glover, BSC, FRCVS (1937–47; veterinary officer; later, see Appendix C)

M. van den Ende, MB, PHD (1938–45; bacteriology)

F. C. MacIntosh, PHD, FRS (1938–49; physiology)

T. S. Work, DSC (1938–present; chemistry)

O. M. Lidwell, DPHIL (1939–46; applied physiology)

J. Walker, DPHIL, DSC (1939–69; chemistry)

D. G. Evans, CBE, DSC, FRS (1940–47, 1955–61; biological standards)

A. T. Fuller, PHD, FRIC (1940–66; chemotherapy)

F. Hawking, DM, DTM (1940–70; parasitology)

J. E. Lovelock, DSC, FRS (1941–61; biochemistry)

J. D. Fulton, MB, PHD (1941–63; chemotherapy)

F. Fulton, DM (1942–49; bacteriology)

Rosalind V. Pitt-Rivers, PHD, FRS (1942–72; biochemistry)

P. G. H. Gell, MB, FRS (1943–48; chemical microbiology)

A. Neuberger, CBE, MD, PHD, FRS (1943–55; biochemistry)

W. D. M. Paton, BM, FRS (1944–52; pharmacology)

A. S. McFarlane, MB, BSC (1944–70; biophysics)

J. N. Davidson, DSC, MD, FRS (1945–46; biochemistry)

G. L. Ada, DSC (1945–48; immunology)

B. Delisle Burns, MRCS, FRS (1946–50 and from 1966; physiology)

Sir John A. B. Gray, MB, SCD, FRCP, FRS (1946–52; physiology; on Council's staff as Second Secretary 1966–68 and as Secretary from 1968)

J. W. Cornforth, MSC, DPHIL, FRS (1946–62; chemistry)

D. F. Elliott, PHD (1946–62; biochemistry)

Audrey U. Smith, BSC, MB (1946–70; experimental biology; on external staff from 1970)

G. J. Popjak, DSC, MD, FRS (1947–53; biochemistry; on external staff 1955–61—see Appendix C)

Sir Walter L. M. Perry, OBE, MD (1947–58; pharmacology, biological standards)

A. W. Gledhill, SCD, MRCVS (1947–67 veterinary officer)

Janet S. F. Niven, MD (1947–67; cytopathology)

A. J. P. Martin, PHD, FRS (1948–56; biochemistry)

D. A. Long, MD (1948–59; biological standards)

H. R. V. Arnstein, PHD (1948–65; biochemistry)

C. E. Dalgleish, PHD (1949–52; biochemistry)

P. N. Campbell, DSC (1949–53; biochemistry)

Major-General G. Brunskill, CB, MC (1949–56; administrative officer)

R. R. Porter, PHD, FRS (1949–60; immunology)

W. S. Feldberg, CBE, MD, FRS (1949–65; physiology)

M. R. Pollock, MB, FRS (1949–65; chemical microbiology)

J. W. Lightbown, DSC (1949–73; biological standards)

O. G. Edholm, BSC, MB (1949–74; applied physiology)

J. S. Porterfield, MB (from 1949; bacteriology)

R. J. W. Rees, BSC, MB (from 1949; bacteriology)

W. W. Douglas, MD (1950–56; physiology and pharmacology)

A. T. James, PHD (1950–62; biochemistry)

A. Isaacs, MB, FRS (1950–67; bacteriology)

A. H. Gordon, PHD (from 1950; biophysics)

L. G. C. E. Pugh, BM (from 1950; field physiology)

G. W. A. Dick, BSC, MD, MRCP (1951–54; bacteriology)

A. T. Roden, MB (1951–56; virology; on external staff from 1948)

W. C. Lister, BSC, MIEE (1951–72; apparatus)

H. G. Pereira, DM, FRS (1951–73; virology)

Marjorie V. Mussett, BSC (1951–74; statistical services)

S. M. Hilton, MB (1952–64; physiology and pharmacology)

J. Mandelstam, PHD, FRS (1952–66; bacterial physiology)

Brigitte A. Askonas, PHD, FRS (from 1952; immunology)

D. R. Bangham, MB, MRCP (from 1952; chemotherapy)

R. K. Macpherson, MSC, MD, MRACP (1953–58; applied physiology)

J. L. Malcolm, BMEDSC, MB (1953–58; pharmacology)

W. E. Brocklehurst, BPHARM, PHD (1953–60; biological standards)

P. H. A. Sneath, MD, DIPBACT (1953–64; bacterial chemistry)

C. R. Austin, DSC, BVSC (1954–61; experimental biology)

H. S. Wolff, BSC (1954–71; biomedical engineering; transferred to Clinical Research Centre)

R. H. Fox, MB, DSC, MRCP (1954–73; physiology)

D. C. Burke, PHD (1955–60; chemistry)

R. C. Valentine, PHD (1955–60; biophysics)

J. A. Armstrong, MB, MSC (from 1955; cytopathology)

G. H. Beaven, PHD (from 1955; physical biochemistry)

F. T. Perkins, PHD (from 1955; biological standards)

C. R. Coid, PHD, MRCVS (1956–61; laboratory animals)

G. P. Lewis, BPHARM, PHD (1956–62; physiology and pharmacology)

H. R. Perkins, PHD (from 1956; bacteriology)

S. Cohen, MD, PHD (1957–60; biophysics)

A. C. Allison, BM, DPHIL (1957–67; virology; transferred to Clinical Research Centre)

R. Goldsmith, PHD, MB (1957–67; applied physiology)

D. A. J. Tyrrell, MD, FRCP, FRC PATH, FRS (1957–67; Common Cold Research Unit; transferred to Clinical Research Centre)

B. M. Wright, MB (1957–69; engineering; transferred to Clinical Research Centre)

S. R. Smithers, DSC (from 1957; parasitology)

E. W. Horton, PHD, MB (1958–60; physiology and pharmacology)

T. Freeman, BM (1958–67; biophysics)

R. H. Gigg, PHD (from 1958; chemistry)

V. C. Abrahams, PHD (1959–63; physiology and pharmacology)

J. L. Turk, DSC, MD (1959–63; immunology)

G. W. Bisset, MB, DPHIL (1960–70; physiology and pharmacology)

R. J. Whitney, PHD (from 1960; human biomechanics)

G. L. Asherson, DM, FRCPE, MRCP, DCH (1961–64; immunology)

O. F. Hutter, PHD (1961–70; physiology and pharmacology)

L. Brent, PHD (1962–65; experimental biology)

N. A. Mitchison, DPHIL, FRS (1962–71; experimental biology; and Director of Studies 1969–70)

D. G. Smyth, PHD (from 1962; chemistry)

J. R. Tata, DES SC, FRS (from 1962; biochemistry)

W. C. Russell, PHD (from 1964; virology)

A. R. Williamson, PHD (1965–74; Director of Studies from 1970)

R. Holliday, PHD (from 1965; genetics)

J. J. Bullen, PHD, MRCVS (from 1968; laboratory animals)

H. J. Rogers, PHD (from 1968; microbiology)

R. M. Gaze, LRCPE, DPHIL, FRS (from 1970; developmental biology)

D. Rothwell, MA, MIEE, CENG (from 1970; engineering)

Librarians:

Katharine M. Baverstock (1918–41)

Ethel G. Wigmore, BSC (1941–49)

Jeannette R. Taylor, BA (1947–59)

L. T. Morton, FLA (1959–72)

R. J. Moore, ALA (from 1972; on staff from 1962)

Appendix C
MRC Research Establishments*

with their directors, and senior members of the external scientific staff

1914   **National Institute for Medical Research**—see Appendix B

1915–46   **Standards Laboratory for Serological Reagents**

School of Pathology, University of Oxford

   (Under the general supervision of Professor G. Dreyer, FRS, 1915–29)

Directors: A. D. Gardner, DM, FRCS (1915–37)

          Lt Col. R. F. Bridges, MB RAMC (retd) (1937–46)

Incorporated in the Public Health Laboratory Service, at Colindale, 1946

1916–74   **(MRC) Department of Clinical Research**

Hampstead Military Hospital, London (1916–17)

University College Hospital Medical School, London (from 1919)

Directors: Sir Thomas Lewis, CBE, MD, FRCP, FRS (1919–45)

          Sir Edward E. Pochin, CBE, MD, FRCP (1945–74)

Disbanded on retirement of Director

1920–49   **National Collection of Type Cultures**

Lister Institute of Preventive Medicine, London (and Elstree, Hertfordshire)

Honorary Director: J. C. G. (later Sir John) Ledingham, DSC, FRCP, FRS (1920–31)

Curators: R. St. John-Brooks, MD (1920–46)

             S. T. Cowan, MD, DSC (1947–49)

Incorporated in the Public Health Laboratory Service, at Colindale, 1949

1926–   **Dunn Nutritional Laboratory** (later **MRC Dunn Nutrition Unit**)

University Field Laboratories, Milton Road, Cambridge (from 1929)

Directors: L. J. Harris, SCD, FRIC (1926–63)

          E. H. Kodicek, CBE, MD, PHD (1963–73)

          R. G. Whitehead, PHD, FIBIOL (from 1973)

---

* In 1968 the titles of research units changed in form: 'MRC' was prefixed and 'Research' dropped before 'Unit'—e.g. 'Rheumatism Research Unit' became 'MRC Rheumatism Unit'; in such cases only the earlier form is usually given.

1927–69   **Statistical Committee Staff,** later (from 1945) **Statistical Research Unit**

National Institute for Medical Research (1927–29)
London School of Hygiene and Tropical Medicine (1929–62)
University College Hospital Medical School, London (1962–69)
Directors: Professor M. Greenwood, DSC, FRCP, FRS (1927–45)
    Professor A. (later Sir Austin) Bradford Hill, CBE, DSC, FRS (1945–61)
    W. R. S. (later Sir Richard) Doll, OBE, MD, DSC, FRCP, FRS (1961–69)
Unit disbanded following appointment of Director to Clinical Research Centre as Deputy Director
See also MRC Statistical Research and Services Unit (p. 368)

1932–39   **Malaria Research Unit**

London School of Hygiene and Tropical Medicine
Director: Brevet Colonel Sir S. Rickard Christophers, CIE, OBE, MB FRS, late IMS (1932–38)
Largely supported by the Leverhulme Trustees
Disbanded after the Director's retirement

1933–61   **Neurological Research Unit**

National Hospital for Nervous Diseases, Queen Square, London
Director: E. A. Carmichael, CBE, FRCP
Disbanded on retirement of Director

1934–49   **Bacterial Chemistry Research Unit**

Middlesex Hospital, London (1934–40); dispersed during much of war period
Lister Institute of Preventive Medicine, London (1946–49)
Director: Sir Paul G. Fildes, OBE, MB, FRS
Absorbed into the National Institute for Medical Research on retirement of Director

1934–57   **Clinical Research Unit**

Guy's Hospital, London
Director: R. T. Grant, OBE, FRCP, FRS
Disbanded on retirement of Director

1938–39   **Unit for Clinical Research in Surgery**

Royal Infirmary and Royal Hospital for Sick Children, Edinburgh
Director: W. C. Wilson, MB, FRCSE
Disbanded on Director's appointment to a chair

1941–46   **Physiological Research Laboratory (AFV)**

Armoured Fighting Vehicles School, Lulworth Camp, Wareham, Dorset
Directors: O. M. Solandt, MD, MRCP (1941–42)
    G. L. (later Sir Lindor) Brown, CBE, MB, MSC, FRS (1942)

Professor I. de Burgh Daly, MD, FRS (1942–45)
E. E. (later Sir Edward) Pochin, MD, FRCP (1945–46)
A wartime project

1941–62   Radiotherapeutic Research Unit

Hammersmith Hospital, London
Director: Constance A. P. Wood, MA, MRCP, FFR
Disbanded on retirement of Director, but part reconstituted as the
Cyclotron Unit (1962)

1942–52   Burns Research Unit

Royal Infirmary, Glasgow (1942–43)
Birmingham Accident Hospital and Rehabilitation Centre (1944–52)
Directors: Leonard Colebrook, MD, FRCOG, FRS (1942–48)
J. R. Squire, MD, FRCP (1948–52)
Combined with Industrial Medicine Research Unit to form the
Industrial Injuries and Burns Research Unit (1952)

1942–45   Wound Infection Research Unit

Birmingham Accident Hospital and Rehabilitation Centre
Director: Professor A. A. (later Sir Ashley) Miles, CBE, MD, FRCP, FRS
A wartime project

1943–63   Department for Research in Industrial Medicine

London Hospital
Director: Donald Hunter, CBE, MD, DSC
Disbanded on retirement of Director

1944–   Applied Psychology Research Unit

Psychological Laboratory, University of Cambridge (1944–52)
15 Chaucer Road, Cambridge (from 1952)
Director: K. W. Craik, PHD (1944–45)
Honorary Director: Professor F. C. (later Sir Frederic) Bartlett, CBE,
MA, FRS (1945–52)
Directors: N. H. Mackworth, MB, PHD (1952–58)
D. E. Broadbent, SCD, FRS (1958–74)
A. D. Baddeley, PHD (from 1974)

1944–62   Chemical Microbiology Research Unit

School of Biochemistry, University of Cambridge
Directors: Marjory Stephenson, SCD, FRS (1944–48)
E. F. Gale, SCD, FRS (1948–62)
Transferred to University of Cambridge in 1962

1944–67   Human Nutrition Research Unit

National Hospital for Nervous Diseases, Queen Square, London
(1944–50)
MRC Laboratories, Hampstead, London (1950–56)

Nutrition Building, National Institute for Medical Research, Mill Hill, London (1956–67)

Director: Professor B. S. Platt, CMG, MB, PHD

(From 1947 to 1953 the Unit had a Field Research Station in the Gambia, which thereafter became an MRC establishment in its own right.)

Responsibility for work of Unit taken over by London School of Hygiene and Tropical Medicine in 1967

1944–67 **Otological Research Unit**

National Hospital for Nervous Diseases, Queen Square, London

Director: C. S. Hallpike, CBE, FRCP, FRCS, FRS (1944–65)

Honorary Director: Sir Terence Cawthorne, FRCS (1965–67)

Disbanded following retirement of the Honorary Director

1945–52 **Blood Products Research Unit**

Lister Institute of Preventive Medicine, London

Honorary Director: Sir Alan Drury, CBE, MD, FRCP, FRS

Disbanded on retirement of Honorary Director

1945–67 **Cell Metabolism Research Unit**

University of Sheffield (1945–54)

Department of Biochemistry, University of Oxford (1954–67)

Director (Honorary from 1954): Professor Sir Hans Krebs, MD, DSC, FRCP, FRS

Disbanded on retirement of Honorary Director

1945–66 **Department of Experimental Medicine**

University of Cambridge and Addenbrooke's Hospital, Cambridge

Director: Professor R. A. McCance, CBE, PHD, FRCP, FRS

Disbanded on retirement of Director

1945– **Pneumoconiosis Research Unit**

Llandough Hospital, Penarth, Glamorgan

Directors: C. M. Fletcher, CBE, MD, FRCP (1945–52)

J. C. Gilson, CBE, MB, FRCP (from 1952)

1946– **Blood Group Research Unit**

Lister Institute of Preventive Medicine, London

Directors: R. R. Race, CBE, PHD, FRCP, FRS (1946–73)

Ruth Sanger, PHD, FRS (from 1973)

1946– **Blood Transfusion Research Unit** (becoming the **Experimental Haematology Research Unit**)

Postgraduate Medical School of London (1946–60); Wright–Fleming Institute of Microbiology, St Mary's Hospital Medical School, London (from 1960)

Director: Professor P. L. Mollison, MD, FRCP, FRCPATH, FRS

1946–51   **Building Research Unit,** later **Group for Research on the Building Industry**

Birkbeck College, London
Honorary Director: Professor C. A. Mace, MA, DLITT
Disbanded

1946–61   **Clinical Chemotherapeutic Research Unit**

Gardiner Institute of Medicine, University of Glasgow (1946–53)
Western Infirmary, Glasgow (1953–61)
Director: J. Reid, MD, MRCP
Disbanded after the death of the Director

1946–73   **Clinical Endocrinology Research Unit**

University and Royal Infirmary, Edinburgh
Honorary Directing Committee (1946–61)
Director: J. A. Loraine, MB, DSC, FRCPE (from 1961)
Disbanded

1946–53   **Dental Research Unit (1)**

King's College Hospital Medical School, London
Director: J. J. D. King, DSC, FDS (1946–52)
Disbanded following death of Director

1946–54   **Electro-medical Research Unit**

Stoke Mandeville Hospital, Aylesbury, Buckinghamshire
Director: R. B. Bourdillon, CBE, MC, AFC, DM
Disbanded on retirement of Director

1946–52   **Industrial Medicine Research Unit**

Birmingham Accident Hospital
Director: J. R. Squire, MD, FRCP
Combined with Burns Research Unit to form Industrial Injuries and Burns Research Unit (1952)

1947–70   **Biophysics Research Unit**

King's College, London
Honorary Director: Professor Sir John Randall, DSC, FRS
Unit disbanded on resignation of Director
Replaced by MRC Muscle Biophysics Unit (1970) and MRC Neurobiology Unit (1970)

1947–64   **Group for Research in Chemotherapy (1),** later **Chemotherapy Research Unit**

Molteno Institute, University of Cambridge
Director: Ann Bishop, SCD, FRS
Disbanded on retirement of Director

1947–59 **Group for Research in Industrial Physiology (1), later Environmental Hygiene Research Unit**

London School of Hygiene and Tropical Medicine, and latterly in part at the MRC Laboratories, Hampstead
Director: T. Bedford, OBE, DSC
Disbanded on retirement of Director; part absorbed by Division of Applied Physiology, National Institute for Medical Research

1947–59 **Group for Research in Industrial Physiology (2), later Group for Research in Occupational Optics**

London School of Hygiene and Tropical Medicine (1947–49)
Institute of Ophthalmology, University of London (1949–59)
Director: H. C. Weston, OBE, FIES
Disbanded on retirement of Director

1947–67 **Group for Research in Industrial Psychology, later Industrial Psychology Research Unit**

Manchester (University), London, and elsewhere (1947–52)
University College London (from 1953–65)
National Institute of Industrial Psychology, London (from 1965)
Director: S. Wyatt, MED, DSC (1947–52)
Honorary Directors: Professor R. W. Russell, DSC (1952–57)
Professor G. C. Drew, MA (1958–65)
C. B. Frisby, PHD (1965–67)

1947– **Laboratory Animals Bureau, later MRC Laboratory Animals Centre**

MRC Laboratories, Hampstead (1947–58)
MRC Laboratories, Carshalton (from 1958)
Directors: R. E. Glover, BSC, MA, FRCVS (1947–49; at NIMR 1937–1947, see Appendix B)
W. Lane-Petter, MB, MA (1949–65)
J. Bleby, BVETMED, MRCVS (from 1965)

1947– **Unit for Research on the Molecular Structure of Biological Systems, later Molecular Biology Research Unit**
Cavendish Laboratory, University of Cambridge; and from 1968
MRC Laboratory of Molecular Biology
University Postgraduate Medical School, Cambridge
Formerly Director, now Chairman of Governing Board: M. F. Perutz, CH, CBE, PHD, FRS
Heads of Divisions: Sir John C. Kendrew, CBE, SCD, FRS
F. H. C. Crick, PHD, FRS
S. Brenner, MB, DPHIL, FRS
F. Sanger, CBE, MD, FRS

1947– **Radiobiological Research Unit, later MRC Radiobiology Unit**
Harwell, Oxford
Directors: J. F. Loutit, CBE, DM, FRCP, FRS (1947–69)
R. H. Mole, MB, FRCP, FRCPATH (from 1969)

1947–59   **Serum Research Laboratory**

MRC Laboratories, Carshalton, Surrey
Director: L. F. Hewitt, DSC, FRIC
Disbanded on transfer of Director to work elsewhere

1947–   **Toxicology Research Unit**

Chemical Defence Experimental Establishment, Porton, Wiltshire (1947–50)
MRC Laboratories, Carshalton (from 1950)
Director: J. M. Barnes, CBE, MB (1947–75)

1947–51   **Vision Research Unit (1)**

Institute of Ophthalmology, London
Director: H. Hartridge, SCD, MRCP, FRS
Reconstituted, on retirement of Director, as the Group for Research on the Physiology of Vision (1951)

1948–53   **Group for Research in Chemotherapy (2)**

Department of Chemistry, Manchester University
Director: J. C. E. Simpson, DSC (1948–52)
Disbanded following death of Director

1948–   **Climate and Working Efficiency Research Unit**

Department of Human Anatomy, University of Oxford, becoming the **Environmental Physiology Research Unit** (from 1962)
London School of Hygiene and Tropical Medicine
Honorary Directors: Professor Sir Wilfrid Le Gros Clark MD, DSC, FRCS, FRS (1948–62)
Professor J. S. Weiner, DSC, MRCS (from 1962)

1948–   **Occupational Psychiatry Research Unit,** later **Unit for Research in Occupational Adaptation,** and still later **MRC Social Psychiatry Unit**

Institute of Psychiatry, Maudsley Hospital, London
Honorary Director: Professor Sir Aubrey Lewis, MD, FRCP (1948–66)
Director: Professor J. K. Wing, MD, PHD, DPM (from 1966)

1948–62   **Ophthalmological Research Unit**

Institute of Ophthalmology, London
Director (part-time): Sir Stewart Duke-Elder, GCVO, FRCS, FRCP, FRS
Transferred to the University of London, except part reconstituted as the Vision Research Unit (2) (1962)

1948–53   **Royal Naval Tropical Research Unit** (jointly with the Admiralty)

University of Malaya, Singapore
Director: Surgeon Commander F. P. Ellis, OBE, MRCP, RN
Disbanded

1948– **Social Medicine Research Unit**

Central Middlesex Hospital, London (1948–56)
London Hospital (1956–66)
London School of Hygiene and Tropical Medicine (from 1966)
Director: J. N. Morris, DSC, FRCP, DPH, DCH (becoming Honorary
Director in 1966 on appointment to chair at School of
Hygiene)

1948– **Tuberculosis Research Unit,** later **MRC Tuberculosis and
Chest Diseases Unit**

MRC Laboratories, Hampstead (1948–65)
Lynton House, Tavistock Square (1965–68)
Brompton Hospital, London (from 1968)
Directors: P. M. D'Arcy Hart, CBE, MD, FRCP (1948–65)
Wallace Fox, MD, FRCP (from 1965)

1949–61 **Antibiotics Research Station**

Clevedon, Somerset
Director: B. K. Kelly, BA
Disbanded on transfer of responsibilities to Microbiological Research
Establishment, Porton

1949–55 **Spectrographic Research Unit**

London Hospital
Director: E. R. Holiday, BM
Disbanded on resignation of Director

1949–65 **Wernher Research Unit on Deafness**

Royal National Throat and Ear Hospital, London (1949–53)
King's College Hospital Medical School, London (1953–65)
Director: T. S. Littler, PHD, FINSTP
Disbanded on retirement of Director

1950–62 **Group for Research in Bilharzia Disease,** later **Bilharzia
Research Unit**

Winches Farm, St Albans, Hertfordshire (London School of Hygiene
and Tropical Medicine)
Director: J. Newsome, MD, DTM & H
Disbanded

1950– **Blood Group Reference Laboratory**

Lister Institute of Preventive Medicine, London
Directors: A. E. Mourant, DM, DPHIL, FRCP, FCPATH (1950–65)
K. L. G. Goldsmith, MB, PHD, MRCPATH, MRCP (from 1965)
Administered by the Council for the Department of Health and Social
Security

1951–55   **Group for Research on the Physiology of Vision**

Institute of Ophthalmology, London
Director: L. C. Thompson, MB, DSC
Attached to the Ophthalmological Research Unit (1948) after death of Director

1952–   **Unit for Research on the Experimental Pathology of the Skin**

Medical School, University of Birmingham
Directors: Professor J. R. Squire, MD, FRCP (1952–62)
C. N. D. Cruickshank, MD, MRCP, FRCPATH, DIH (from 1962)

1952–   **Industrial Injuries and Burns Research Unit**

Birmingham Accident Hospital
(Formed by amalgamating the Industrial Medicine Research Unit (1946–52) and the Burns Research Unit (1942–52))
Director: J. P. Bull, MD, FRCP

1953–62   **Betatron Research Group** (later **Unit**)

Christie Hospital and Holt Radium Institute, Manchester
Honorary Director: Professor Ralston Paterson, CBE, MC, MD, FRCS, FFR
Transferred to Manchester Regional Hospital Board in 1962 on retirement of Director

1953–74   **Experimental Radiopathology Research Unit**

Hammersmith Hospital, London
Directors: G. J. Popjak, MD, FRIC, FRS (1953–62)
Miss T. Alper, MA, MS (ED), DSC, FINSTP (from 1962)
Amalgamated with Cyclotron Unit on retirement of Director

1953–   **Group for Research in Infantile Malnutrition,** later **Infantile Malnutrition Research Unit,** later **MRC Child Nutrition Unit**

Mulago Hospital, Kampala, Uganda
Director: R. F. A. Dean, PHD, FRCP (1953–64)
Honorary Director: Professor R. A. McCance, CBE, MD, DSC, FRCP, FRCOG, FRS (1964–68)
Director: R. G. Whitehead, PHD (from 1968)
Withdrawn in 1973

1953–   **Medical Research Council Laboratories, Gambia**

Fajara, near Bathurst, The Gambia
Directors: J. Newsome, MD, DTM&H (1953–54)
I. A. McGregor, CBE, FRCP, DTM&H (1954–74)
R. S. Bray, DSC (from 1974)
Earlier the Field Research Station of the Council's Human Nutrition Research Unit in London (1944)

1953–71   **Radiological Protection Service** (jointly with Ministry of Health)

Onslow Gardens, London (1955–56)
Downs Nursery Hospital, Sutton, Surrey (1955–56)
Clifton Avenue, Sutton, Surrey (from 1956)
Director: W. Binks, CBE, MSC, FINSTP
Taken over by the new National Radiological Protection Board

1954–69 **Group for Research on Body Temperature Regulation,** later **Body Temperature Research Unit**

St. Mary's Hospital, London (1954–56)
Radcliffe Infirmary, Oxford (1956–69)
Honorary Director: Professor Sir George Pickering, MD, FRCP, FRS
Disbanded on retirement of Honorary Director

1954– **Group** (later **Unit**) **for Research on Drug Sensitivity in Tuberculosis,** later **MRC Unit for Laboratory Studies of Tuberculosis**

Royal Postgraduate Medical School, London
Honorary Director: Professor D. A. Mitchison, MB, FRCP, MRC PATH

1954–66 **Wernher Group** (later **Unit**) **for Research in Ophthalmological Genetics**

Royal College of Surgeons of England, London
Honorary Director: Professor Arnold Sorsby, CBE, MD, FRCS
Disbanded on retirement of Honorary Director

1955– **Group for Research on Atmospheric Pollution,** later **Air Pollution Research Unit**

St Bartholomew's Hospital, London (1955–62)
St Bartholomew's Hospital Medical College (from 1962)
Director: Professor P. J. Lawther, MB, DSC, FRCP

1955–72 **Group for Experimental Research in Inherited Diseases,** late **Experimental Genetics Research Unit**

University College London
Honorary Director: Professor H. Grüneberg, MD, DSC, FRS
Disbanded on retirement of Honorary Director

1955– **Group** (later **Unit**) **for the Experimental Investigation of Behaviour,** later **MRC Unit on Neural Mechanisms of Behaviour**

University College London
Honorary Directors: Professor R. W. Russell, DSC (1955–57)
Professor G. C. Drew, MA (1958–71)
Director: I. S. Russell, PHD (from 1971)

1955–70 **Group** (later **Unit**) **for Research on Occupational Aspects of Ageing**

Department of Psychology, University of Liverpool
Honorary Director: Professor L. S. Hearnshaw, MA (1955–59 and 1963–70)
Director: Alistair Heron, PHD (1959–63)
Disbanded on retirement of Honorary Director

1955–65   **Obstetric Medicine Research Unit**

Department of Midwifery, University of Aberdeen
Honorary Director: Professor Sir Dugald Baird, MD, DSC, FRCOG
On retirement of Director, reconstituted as MRC Medical Sociology
Unit and MRC Reproduction and Growth Unit, q.v.

1955–70   **Tropical Metabolism Research Unit**

University College (later University) of the West Indies, Mona,
Kingston, Jamaica
Director: Professor J. C. Waterlow, CMG, MD, SCD, FRCP
Taken over by the University of the West Indies

1955–67   **Virus Research Group** (later **Unit**)

London School of Hygiene and Tropical Medicine (1955–58)
Medical Research Council Laboratories, Carshalton (from 1959)
Director: F. Kingsley Sanders, DPHIL
Disbanded on resignation of Director

1956–66   **Carcinogenic Substances Research Group** (later **Unit**)

Washington Singer Laboratories, University of Exeter
Honorary Director: Sir James Cook, DSC, FRS
Disbanded on retirement of Honorary Director

1956–   **Group for Research on the General Effects of Radiation,**
later **Clinical Effects of Radiation Research Unit,** later **MRC**
Clinical and Population Cytogenetics Unit

Western General Hospital, Edinburgh
Directors: Professor W. M. Court Brown, OBE, MB, BSC, FRCPE, FFR
(1956–68)
Professor H. J. Evans, PHD (from 1969)

1956–   **Research Unit on Metabolic Disturbances in Surgery,** later
Mineral Metabolism Research Unit

Leeds General Infirmary
Honorary Director: Professor L. N. Pyrah, CHM, MSC, FRCS (1956–64)
Director: Professor B. E. C. Nordin, MD, PHD, FRCP (from 1964)

1956–59   **Group for Epidemiological Research on Respiratory Diseases**
(Air Pollution)

Department of Social and Industrial Medicine, University of Sheffield
Director: J. Pemberton, MD, MRCP (1956–58)
Honorary Director: Professor C. H. Stuart-Harris, MD, FRCP (1958–59)
Disbanded

1956–73   **Trachoma Research Group** (later **Unit**)

Institute of Ophthalmology, London (1956–57)
Lister Institute of Preventive Medicine, London (from 1957)
Honorary Directors: Sir Stewart Duke-Elder, GCVO, DSC, MD, FRCS,
FRCP, FRS (1956–57)

Professor L. H. Collier, MD, DSC, MRCP (from 1957)

Much of the work, although based in London, has been done overseas—at first in Jordan; then at the MRC Laboratories, Gambia (from 1953); and temporarily in Iran

1957– **Clinical Genetics Research Unit**

Institute of Child Health, London
Directors: J. A. Fraser Roberts, MD, DSC, FRCP, FRS (1957–64)
C. O. Carter, DM, FRCP (from 1964)

1957– **Clinical Psychiatry Research Group** (later **Unit**)

Graylingwell Hospital, Chichester, Sussex
Director: P. Sainsbury, MD, MRCP, DPM

1957–74 **Microbial Genetics Research Unit,** later **MRC Molecular Genetics Unit**

Hammersmith Hospital, London (1957–68)
Department of Molecular Biology, Edinburgh (from 1968)
Director: W. Hayes, MB, DSC, FRCPI, FRS (becoming Honorary Director in 1968 on appointment to chair in University of Edinburgh)
Transferred to University of Edinburgh Molecular Genetics Unit on resignation of Director

1957–75 **Neuropsychiatric Research Unit,** later **MRC Neuropsychiatry Unit**

Whitchurch Hospital, Cardiff (1957–61)
Medical Research Council Laboratories, Carshalton (from 1961)
Director: D. Richter, PHD, MRCP, FRCPSYCH (1957–72)
Acting Director: R. Balázs, DMED, DPHIL (from 1972)
In 1975 Dr Balázs became Director of a new Developmental Neurobiology Unit

1957–62 **Virus Culture Laboratory**

Medical Research Council Laboratories, Carshalton
Director: P. D. Cooper, PHD
Disbanded on resignation of Director

1958–63 **Group for Research on the Chemical Pathology of Steroids,** later **Chemical Pathology of Steroids Research Unit**

Jessop Hospital for Women, Sheffield
Director: J. K. Norymberski, DRING
Disbanded

1958–69 **Mutagenesis Research Unit**

Institute of Animal Genetics, University of Edinburgh
Honorary Director: Professor Charlotte Auerbach, DSC, FRS
Disbanded on retirement of Honorary Director

1958– **Neuropharmacology Research Unit**

Department of Experimental Psychiatry, University of Birmingham (1958–62)

Department of Pharmacology (Preclinical), University of Birmingham (from 1962)
Honorary Director: Professor P. B. Bradley, DSC

1958–74   **Population Genetics Research Unit**

Warneford Hospital, Oxford
Director: A. C. Stevenson, MD, BSC, FRCP, DCH
Disbanded on retirement of Director

1958–   **Rheumatism Research Unit (1)**

Canadian Red Cross Memorial Hospital, Taplow
Director: Professor E. G. L. Bywaters, MB, FRCP

1958–63   **Rheumatism Research Unit (2)**

Royal National Hospital for Rheumatic Diseases, Bath
Chairman of directing committee: Professor C. Bruce Perry, MD, FRCP
Disbanded

1959–67   **Blood Coagulation Research Unit**

Churchill Hospital, Oxford
Director (part-time): R. G. Macfarlane, CBE, FRCP, FRS
Disbanded on retirement of Director

1959–67   **Group** (later **Unit**) **for Research on Bone-seeking Isotopes**
Churchill Hospital, Oxford
Honorary Director: Dame Janet Vaughan, DBE, DM, FRCP
Disbanded on retirement of Honorary Director

1959–72   **Environmental Radiation Research Unit**

Department of Medical Physics, University of Leeds
Honorary Director: Professor F. W. Spiers, CBE, DSC
Disbanded

1959–   **Experimental Virus Research Unit,** later **MRC Virology Unit**

Institute of Virology, Glasgow
Honorary Directors: Professor M. G. P. Stoker, MD (1959–68)
                 Professor J. H. Subak-Sharpe, PHD (from 1968)

1959–69   **Psychiatric Genetics Research Unit**

Institute of Psychiatry, London
Director (part-time): E. T. O. Slater, CBE, MD, FRCP, DPM
Disbanded on retirement of Director

1960–   **Unit for Research on the Chemical Pathology of Mental Disorders,** later **MRC Unit for Metabolic Studies in Psychiatry**

Medical School, University of Birmingham (1960–67)
Department of Psychiatry, University of Sheffield (from 1967)
Honorary Directors: Professor I. E. Bush, MB, PHD (1960–64)
                 Professor F. A. Jenner, MB, PHD, MRCP, DPM (from
                 1964)

1960– **Epidemiological Research Unit (South Wales),** formerly part of Pneumoconiosis Research Unit (1945), later **MRC Epidemiology Unit (South Wales)**

Welsh National School of Medicine, Cardiff

Honorary Director: Professor A. L. Cochrane, CBE, FRCP (Director from 1968 on resigning his Chair until 1974)

Director: P. C. Elwood, MD, DPH, DCH (from 1974)

Unit for Research on the Epidemiology of Psychiatric Illness, later **MRC Unit for Epidemiological Studies in Psychiatry**

Department of Psychiatry, University of Edinburgh

Honorary Director: Professor G. M. Carstairs, MD, FRCPE, DPM (1960–70)

Director: N. B. Kreitman, MD, DPM (from 1971)

1961– **Dental Research Unit (2)**

Dental School, University of Bristol

Honorary Director: Professor A. I. Darling, CBE, DDSC, MDS, MRCS, FDSRCS, FRCPATH

1961– **Gastroenterology Research Unit**

Central Middlesex Hospital, London

Director: E. N. Rowlands, MD, BSC, FRCP

1961– **Demyelinating Diseases Research Group** (later **Unit**)

13 Framlington Place, Newcastle upon Tyne (1961–69)

Newcastle General Hospital (from 1969)

Honorary Director: Professor E. J. Field, MD, MS, PHD, FRCP (1961–73)

Acting Director: Professor A. M. Thomson, MB, BSC, FRCOG, DPH (1973–74)

Director: H. M. Wiśniewski, MD, PHD (from 1974)

1962–67 **Atheroma Research Unit**

Western Infirmary, Glasgow

Director: B. Bronte-Stewart, MD, MRCP (1962–65)

Following the Director's death in 1965, the Unit's work was supervised by Sir Edward Wayne until its reconstitution as the Blood Pressure Research Unit (1967)

1962– **Cyclotron Unit**

Hammersmith Hospital, London

Director: D. D. Vonberg, BSC

A residual part of the Radiotherapeutic Research Unit (1942)

1962– **Unit for the Study of Environmental Factors in Mental and Physical Illness**

London School of Economics and Political Science

Director: J. W. B. Douglas, BM, BSC

1962– **Epidemiological Research Unit (Jamaica),** later **MRC Epidemiology Unit (Jamaica)**

University of the West Indies, Mona, Jamaica

Directors: W. E. Miall, MD (1962–70)

A. Davis, MD, FRCPE, DTM&H (1971–74)

G. R. Sergeant, MD, MRCP (from 1974)

1962–	**Human Biochemical Genetics Research Unit**

King's College, London (1962–65)

Galton Laboratories, University College London (from 1965)

Honorary Director: Professor H. Harris, MD, FRS

1962–72	**Neuroendocrinology Research Unit**

Department of Human Anatomy, University of Oxford

Honorary Director: Professor G. W. Harris, CBE, MD, SCD, FRS (1962–1972)

Disbanded following death of Honorary Director

1962–	**Vision Research Unit (2)**

Institute of Ophthalmology, London (1962–69)

School of Biological Sciences, University of Sussex (from 1969)

Director: Professor H. J. A. Dartnall, DSC, FRIC

Formerly part of the Ophthalmological Research Unit (1948)

1963–	**Abnormal Haemoglobin Research Unit**

St Bartholomew's Hospital, London (1963–64)

Department of Biochemistry, University of Cambridge (from 1964)

Honorary Director: Professor H. Lehmann, MB, SCD, FRCP, FRIC, FRCPATH, FRS

1963–74	**Psycholinguistics Research Unit,** later **MRC Speech and Communication Unit**

Institute of Experimental Psychology, Oxford (1963–66)

University of Edinburgh (from 1966)

Director: Professor R. C. Oldfield, MA (1963–72)

Honorary Director: Professor H. J. Walton, MD, PHD, FRCPE, FRCPSYCH (from 1972)

Disbanded

1963–	**Cellular Immunology Research Unit**

Sir William Dunn School of Pathology, University of Oxford

Honorary Director: Professor J. L. Gowans, CBE, MB, DPHIL, FRS

1964–71	**Metabolic Reactions Research Unit**

Biochemistry Department, Imperial College, London

Honorary Director: Professor Sir Ernst Chain, DPHIL, FRS

Disbanded on retirement of Honorary Director

1964–67	**Clinical Pulmonary Physiology Research Unit**

King's College Hospital Medical School, London

Director (part-time): P. Hugh-Jones, MD, FRCP

Taken over by University

1964–68	**Cell Genetics Research Unit**

Department of Genetics, University of Glasgow

Honorary Director: Professor G. Pontecorvo, PHD, FRS

Disbanded on resignation of Honorary Director

1964– **Brain Metabolism Research Unit**

University Department of Pharmacology, Edinburgh
Honorary Director: Professor W. L. M. (later Sir Walter) Perry, OBE,
MD, DSC, MRCPE (1964–68)
Director: G. W. Ashcroft, MB, DSC, FRCPE, DPM (from 1969)

1964– **Microbial Systematics Research Unit**

University of Leicester
Director: Professor P. H. A. Sneath, MD

1965– **Reproduction and Growth Research Unit**

Princess Mary Maternity Hospital, Newcastle upon Tyne
Director: Professor A. M. Thomson, MB, BSC, FRCOG, DPH
The Unit was formed from a section of the former Obstetric Medicine
Research Unit, Aberdeen (1955)

1965– **Medical Sociology Research Unit**

Department of Sociology, University of Aberdeen (1965–68)
Centre for Social Studies, University of Aberdeen (from 1968)
Honorary Director: Professor R. Illsley, PHD
The Unit was set up to carry on work initiated in the former
Obstetric Medicine Research Unit (1955)

1965–74 **Cardiovascular Research Unit**

Royal Postgraduate Medical School of London
Director (part-time): Professor J. P. Shillingford, MD, FRCP
Disbanded

1966–74 **MRC Computer Unit (London)**

242 Pentonville Road, London N1
Director: C. C. Spicer, MRCS
Transferred to Clinical Research Centre

1967– **Blood Pressure Research Unit**

Western Infirmary, Glasgow
Director: A. F. Lever, MB, BSC, FRCP
Reconstituted from the Atheroma Research Unit (1962)

1967–72 **Powered Limbs Research Unit**

West Hendon Hospital, London
Director: A. B. Kinnier Wilson, MB, MRCP, DPM
Disbanded

1967– **Immunochemistry Research Unit** (formerly **Group**)

University Department of Biochemistry, Oxford
Honorary Director: Professor R. R. Porter, PHD, FRS

1967–72 **Molecular Pharmacology Research Unit**

Department of Pharmacology, University of Cambridge
Honorary Director: Professor A. S. V. Burgen, MD, FRCP, FRS
Unit transferred to National Institute for Medical Research follow-
ing Professor Burgen's appointment as Director of the Institute in 1971

1967–   **Clinical Research Centre**

Northwick Park Hospital, Harrow, Middlesex (from 1970). Includes MRC Common Cold Unit, Harvard Hospital, Salisbury, Wiltshire
Director-designate (during planning period): Professor J. R. Squire, MD, FRCP (1960–66)
Director: G. M. Bull, MD, FRCP (from 1966)
Deputy Director: D. A. J. Tyrrell, MD, FRCP, FRCPATH, FRS (from 1970)

1968–   **MRC Developmental Psychology Unit**

Drayton House, Gordon Street, London WCI
Director: N. O'Connor, PHD

1968–   **MRC Biochemical Parasitology Unit**

Molteno Institute, University of Cambridge
Director: B. A. Newton, PHD

1968–   **MRC Neurological Prostheses Unit**

Institute of Psychiatry, London
Honorary Director: Professor G. S. Brindley, MD, MRCP, FRS

1968–   **MRC Social and Applied Psychology Unit**

Department of Psychology, University of Sheffield
Honorary Director: Professor H. Kay, PHD (1968–73)
Director: P. B. Warr, PHD (from 1973)

1969–   **MRC Statistical Research and Services Unit**

University College Hospital Medical School, London
Director: I. Sutherland, DPHIL

1969–   **MRC Leukaemia Unit**

Royal Postgraduate Medical School, London
Honorary Director: D. A. G. Galton, MD, FRCP

1969–   **MRC Unit for Physical Aids for the Disabled**

Princess Margaret Rose Orthopaedic Hospital, Edinburgh
Honorary Director: Professor D. C. Simpson, MBE, PHD

1970–   **MRC Lipid Metabolism Unit**

Hammersmith Hospital, London
Director: N. B. Myant, DM, BSC, FRCP

1970–   **MRC Dental Epidemiology Unit**

Dental School, London Hospital Medical College
Honorary Director: Professor G. L. Slack, OBE, DDS, FDSRCS

1970–   **MRC Cell Mutation Unit**

School of Biological Sciences, University of Sussex
Director: Professor B. A. Bridges, PHD

1970–   **MRC Unit on the Development and Integration of Behaviour**

Sub-Department of Animal Behaviour, University of Cambridge
Honorary Director: Professor R. A. Hinde, SCD, DPHIL, FRS

1970–   **Epidemiology and Medical Care Unit** (jointly with Department of Health and Social Security)

Northwick Park Hospital, Harrow, Middlesex
Director: T. W. Meade, BM, MRCP

1970–74   **MRC Muscle Biophysics Unit**

Department of Biophysics, King's College, London
Director: Professor Jean Hanson, PHD, FRS (died August 1973)
One of two successor units to the Biophysics Unit (1947)
Amalgamated with Neurobiology Unit to form Cell Biophysics Unit

1970–74   **MRC Neurobiology Unit**

Department of Biophysics, King's College, London
Director: Professor M. H. F. Wilkins, CBE, PHD, FRS
One of two successor units to the Biophysics Unit (1947)
Amalgamated with Muscle Biophysics Unit to form Cell Biophysics Unit

1971–   **MRC Hearing and Balance Unit**

Institute of Neurology, London
Director: J. D. Hood, DSC, FINSTP

1971–   **MRC Neurochemical Pharmacology Unit**

Department of Pharmacology, University of Cambridge
Director: L. L. Iversen, PHD

1972–   **MRC Clinical Pharmacology Unit**

Radcliffe Infirmary, Oxford
Honorary Director: Professor D. G. Grahame-Smith, MB, PHD, MRCP

1972–   **MRC Unit on Reproductive Biology**

Department of Obstetrics and Gynaecology, University of Edinburgh
Director: R. V. Short, BVSC, MRCVS, SCD

Senior Members of the External Scientific Staff

The following individual workers of high scientific standing who never became directors of MRC research establishments, and are thus not named above, were attached to the external institutions shown; in some instances they held whole-time grants prior to the staff service for which dates are given.

A. Stanley Griffith, CBE, MD, PHD: University Field Laboratories, Cambridge (1920–40)
E. G. D. Murray, OBE, MD, DSC: University Field Laboratories, Cambridge (1920–1930)

M. H. Gordon, CMG, CBE, MD, FRS: St Bartholomew's Hospital, London (1922–36)

Matthew Young, MD, DSC: Institute of Anatomy, University College London (1927–40; on National Institute for Medical Research staff from 1922)

A. N. (later Sir Alan) Drury, CBE, MD, FRCP, FRS: Department of Pathology, University of Cambridge (1930–43, but attached to MRC headquarters 1940–1943; in Department of Clinical Research, University College Hospital, London, from 1921). Honorary Director of the Blood Products Research Unit 1945–52

R. J. Lythgoe, MD: Institute of Physiology, University College London (1925–40)

L. S. Penrose, MD, FRS: Royal Eastern Counties Institution, Colchester (1930–39)

Julia Bell, FRCP: Galton Laboratory, University College London (1933–44)

F. G. Spear, MD: Strangeways Research Laboratory, Cambridge (1933–60)

Dorothy S. Russell, MD: Institute of Pathology, London Hospital (1933–46)

A. Q. Wells, DM: School of Pathology, University of Oxford (1945–56).

H. Davson, DSC: University College London (from 1954).

D. J. Lewis, SCD: British Museum (Natural History), London (from 1956).

B. O. L. Duke, OBE, MD, DTM&H: Centre Médical de Récherches, Kumba, Federated Cameroon Republic (from 1963).

Appendix D
Nobel Prizewinners on MRC Staff

The following recipients of Nobel Prizes were members of the scientific staff of the Medical Research Council at the time of award (titles here brought up to date):

Sir Henry Hallett Dale, OM, GBE, MD, FRS, Director, National Institute for Medical Research:

  Physiology and Medicine, 1936 (*shared with Professor Otto Loewi*).

Archer John Porter Martin, CBE, PHD, FRS, National Institute for Medical Research:

  Chemistry, 1952 (shared with Dr R. L. M. Synge, *in respect of joint work before he joined the staff*).

Professor Sir Hans Krebs, MD, DSC, FRCP, FRS, Director (part-time), Cell Metabolism Research Unit, Sheffield:

  Physiology and Medicine, 1952 (*shared with Dr F. A. Lipmann*).

Frederick Sanger, CBE, PHD, FRS, member of the Council's External Staff, Cambridge:

  Chemistry, 1958.

Francis Harry Compton Crick, PHD, FRS, member of Laboratory of Molecular Biology, Cambridge; and

Maurice Hugh Frederick Wilkins, CBE, PHD, FRS, Deputy Director, Biophysics Research Unit, King's College, London:

  Physiology and Medicine, 1962 (*shared with each other and with Dr J. D. Watson*).

Max Ferdinand Perutz, CH, CBE, PHD, FRS, Director, Laboratory of Molecular Biology, Cambridge; and

Sir John Cowdrey Kendrew, CBE, SCD, FRS, Deputy Director, Laboratory of Molecular Biology, Cambridge:

  Chemistry, 1962 (*shared with each other*).

The following present member of the staff had previously been a prizewinner:
Sir Peter Brian Medawar, CBE, DSC, FRS:

  Physiology and Medicine, 1960 (*shared with Sir F. Macfarlane Burnet*).

The Council entertained the above (except Professor Wilkins, absent owing to illness) at an informal dinner at the Athenaeum Club, London, on 22 February 1963. The Minister for Science (Lord Hailsham) was also a guest. The Chairman of the Council (Lord Shawcross) presided, and several members of Council,

371

assessors, and senior officers made the total number 26. Lord Shawcross and Lord Hailsham spoke, and Dr Perutz replied on behalf of the laureates.

The following former members of the staff have since been prizewinners:

Professor Rodney Robert Porter, PHD, FRS, formerly of the National Institute for Medical Research and now Honorary Director, MRC Immunochemistry Unit, Oxford:

    Physiology and Medicine 1972 (*shared with Professor G. Edelman*).

John Warcup Cornforth, D PHIL, FRS, formerly of the National Institute for Medical Research: Chemistry 1975 (*shared with Professor V. Prelog*).

Index of general subjects

V

Index of personal names*

* Peers who had that rank at date of first mention are entered under titles other peers and all knights are entered under surnames, with title following with in parenthesis. Where title and surname differ, cross-references are given.

Bennett N. (Sir Norman B.) 87

Bensted H. J. 264

Beresford, Lord Charles 256

Best C. H. 38, 39

Biggam A. (Sir Alexander B.) 302

Binks W. 106, 360

Bishop A. 356

Bishop P. M. F. 238

Bisset G. W. 351

Black D. A. K. (Sir Douglas B.) 28, 310

Bleby J. 357

Blowers R. 136

Boag J. W. 62, 337

Bond C. J. 20

Bourdillon R. B. 68, 80, 136, 225, 320, 340, 349, 356

Bourdillon T. 225

Boyd J. S. K. (Sir John B.) 217

Boyd Orr see Orr

Bradley P. B. 36, 160, 364

Bradstreet C. M. P. 344, 345

Bragg L. (Sir Lawrence B.) 154, 155

Bragg W. (Sir William B.) 306

Breinl A. 44

Brend W. A. 92

Brenner S. 357

Brent L. 351

Brewer H. F. 328

Bridges B. A. 368

Bridges R. F. 352

Brindley G. S. 368

Briscoe H. V. A. 181

Broadbent D. E. 172, 177, 354

Broadhurst P. L. 153

Brocklehurst W. E. 350

Brokensha E. A. 324

Bronte-Stewart B. 365

Brown D. S. 222

Brown G. L. (Sir Lindor B.) 140, 318, 321, 322, 349, 353

Brown T. G. 97

Brown W. M. C. 64, 105, 106, 153, 185, 339, 362

Browning C. H. 45, 114, 215, 280, 340

Browning E. 184, 342

Brownlee J. 8, 92, 110, 277, 278, 335, 348

Brunskill G. 350

Buchanan G. 179

Bull G. M. 33, 368

Bull, J. P. 136, 177, 360

Bullen J. J. 351

Bulloch W. 145, 281, 342

Bullock W. E. 128 and see Gye

Bunbury E. 315

Bunyan 8

Burgen A. S. V. 348, 367

Burke D. C. 350

Burkitt D. P. 128, 220

Burn J. H. 247, 316, 344, 349

Burnet F. M. (Sir Macfarlane B.) 116, 125, 340, 371

Burnie R. M. 215

Burns B. D. 350

Burrell L. S. T. 335

Burrows S. M. 215, 343

Burton K. 146

Bush I. E. 364

Buxton J. B. 119, 349

Buxton P. A. 131, 214, 222, 304

Buzzard R. B. 309

Bywaters E. G. L. 300, 364

C

Cairns H. (Sir Hugh C.) 298, 299

Calder J. A. 197

Callow R. K. 43, 349

Calne R. Y. 27

Campbell J. A. 99, 349

Campbell P. N. 350

Cannon W. B. 282

Canti R. G. 60

Carling E. R. (Sir Ernest Rock C.) 63, 295, 296, 316

Carmichael E. A. 19, 318, 320, 323, 353

Carré E. 120

Carstairs G. M. 159, 365

Carter C. O. 152, 363

Cathcart E. P. 83, 88, 338

Cawthorne T. (Sir Terence C.) 98, 355

Chain E. B. (Sir Ernst C.) 52, 56, 227, 337, 366

Chalmers A. K. 92

Chalmers D. K. M. 329, 331, 349

Chalmers, Lord (Sir Robert C.) 196

Chamberlain J. 202

Chamberlain N. 49

Chick H. (Dame Harriette C.) xii, 75, 78, 79, 338, 344, Plate 1

Christie R. V. 238

H

Dd 505211 K11 2/76
Printed in England for Her Majesty's Stationery Office by
Butler & Tanner Ltd, Frome and London